At a Glance

Color Atlas
of Human Anatomy

in 3 volumes

Volume 1:   Locomotor System
            by Werner Platzer † and
            Thomas Shiozawa-Bayer

Volume 2:   Internal Organs
            by Helga Fritsch and Wolfgang Kuehnel†

Volume 3:   Nervous System and Sensory Organs
            by Werner Kahle †, Michael Frotscher †,
            and Frank Schmitz

Volume 2

Internal Organs

7th Edition
Helga Fritsch, MD

Professor
Head of Department of Anatomy, Histology, and Embryology
Division of Clinical and Functional Anatomy
Medical University of Innsbruck
Innsbruck, Austria

Wolfgang Kuehnel †

213 color plates

Thieme
Stuttgart · New York · Delhi · Rio de Janeiro

Library of Congress Cataloging-in-Publication Data is available from the publisher.

This book is an authorized translation of the 12th German edition published and copyrighted 2018 by Georg Thieme Verlag, Stuttgart , Germany. Title of the German edition: Taschenatlas Anatomie, Band 2: Innere Organe

Translator: Geraldine O'Sullivan, Dublin, Ireland

Illustrated by Professor Gerhard Spitzer, Frankfurt, Germany, in cooperation with Stephan Spitzer, Frankfurt, Germany; Karl Wesker, Berlin, Germany; Holger Vanselow, Stuttgart, Germany; Gay & Sender, Bremen, Germany; Karin Baum, Paphos, Cyprus.

12th German edition 2018

6th English edition 2015

1st Bulgarian edition 2006
2nd Chinese edition 2019
3rd Croatian edition 2012
6th Dutch edition 2012
5th French edition 2015
3rd Greek edition 2022
1st Hungarian edition 1996
2nd Indonesian edition 2000
5th Italian edition 2016
6th Japanese edition 2011
1st Polish edition 1998
2nd Portuguese edition 2007
1st Serbo-Croatian edition 1991
4th Spanish edition 2008
1st Turkish edition 1987

Cover design: © Thieme
Cover image source: the cover image was composed by Thieme using following image:
© Sebastian Kaulitzki/Fotolia

Typesetting by: DiTech Publishing Services
Printed in Germany by
AZ Druck und Datentechnik GmbH

5 4 3 2 1

ISBN 978-3-13-242448-7

Also available as an e-book:
eISBN 978-3-13-242449-4

Important note: Medicine is an ever-changing science undergoing continual development. Research and clinical experience are continually expanding our knowledge, in particular our knowledge of proper treatment and drug therapy. Insofar as this book mentions any dosage or application, readers may rest assured that the authors, editors, and publishers have made every effort to ensure that such references are in accordance with **the state of knowledge at the time of production of the book.**

Nevertheless, this does not involve, imply, or express any guarantee or responsibility on the part of the publishers in respect to any dosage instructions and forms of applications stated in the book. **Every user is requested to examine carefully** the manufacturers' leaflets accompanying each drug and to check, if necessary in consultation with a physician or specialist, whether the dosage schedules mentioned therein or the contraindications stated by the manufacturers differ from the statements made in the present book. Such examination is particularly important with drugs that are either rarely used or have been newly released on the market. Every dosage schedule or every form of application used is entirely at the user's own risk and responsibility. The authors and publishers request every user to report to the publishers any discrepancies or inaccuracies noticed. If errors in this work are found after publication, errata will be posted at www.thieme.com on the product description page.

Some of the product names, patents, and registered designs referred to in this book are in fact registered trademarks or proprietary names even though specific reference to this fact is not always made in the text. Therefore, the appearance of a name without designation as proprietary is not to be construed as a representation by the publisher that it is in the public domain.

Contents

3 Respiratory System 93

4 Alimentary System 141

10 Blood and Lymphatic Systems...................... 391

11 The Integument 421

Preface

The 7th German edition of "Internal Organs," volume 2 of the three-volume *Color Atlas of Human Anatomy*, was published in early 2001 under new authorship with fully revised text and illustrations. A revised 8th edition was published just 2 years later. This was followed by the 9th edition in 2005, with the addition of a chapter on "Pregnancy and Human Development." The clinical correlates were expanded in the 10th edition, with the aid of clinical colleagues. The chapter on "Pregnancy and Human Development" was then also expanded to include a description of the development of the organ systems. Mr. Holger Vanselow assumed responsibility for the illustrations, skillfully incorporating the new ones into the work of Professor Gerhard Spitzer, the book's original illustrator.

To provide a further bridge between theoretical knowledge and clinical application, the 11th edition supplemented cross-sectional illustrations with the corresponding MRI and/or CT images. We acknowledge the assistance of Prof. W. Jaschke of the Department of Radiology of Innsbruck Medical University, and we thank Ms. M. Mauch, Georg Thieme Verlag, for her constructive suggestions and collaboration over many years.

From the 7th to the 11th German edition, Professor Wolfgang Kühnel, one of my mentors, assisted me not only by contributing several chapters to the "Internal Organs" volume but also by advising me on the chapters that I wrote. I would like to express my special thanks to him posthumously.

The content of this new edition, which is based on the 12th German edition, again incorporates suggestions from our readers. The introduction to the "Glands and Secretion" chapter has been updated to reflect the latest scientific understanding. Professor Harald Klein, Director, Medical Department 1, University Hospital Bergmannsheil, Bochum, Germany, provided valuable support in this.

I hope that this new edition will help to ensure the future of the *Color Atlas of Human Anatomy*. Since its first edition, it has been an important companion for students of anatomy, which has always been and must remain an essential and fundamental basis for successful medicine, especially in the era of personalized and molecular medicine.

Innsbruck, 2022
Helga Fritsch

Preface to the 1st edition

While this pocket atlas targets students of medicine, aiming to provide them with a visual overview of the most important findings of human anatomy, it will also give interested laypersons insights into the discipline.

For medical students, exam preparation should primarily entail a repetition of visual experiences. The interplay between text and images helps make anatomical facts easier to visualize.

The three-volume pocket atlas is structured by system: Volume 1 covers the locomotor system, Volume 2 addresses the internal organs, and Volume 3 looks at the nervous system and sensory organs. The topographic relationships of the peripheral conductive pathways, the nerves and blood vessels, are covered in Volume 1, as they are closely connected to the locomotor system. Volume 2 covers only the systematic classification of the vessels. The pelvic floor, which is closely related to the organs of the lesser pelvis, was included in Volume 2, along with the associated topography. The developmental history of the teeth is touched on briefly in Volume 2, because it facilitates understanding of tooth eruption. The common embryonic precursors of the male and female genitals are discussed because they facilitate understanding of their structure and the not uncommon variations and deformities. In the chapter on the female genitals, some questions related to pregnancy and childbirth are touched on. However, the volume in no way covers the knowledge of developmental history required by medical students! The remarks on physiology and biochemistry are certainly rudimentary and serve solely to enhance understanding of distinctive structural features. For more in-depth information, physiology and biochemistry textbooks must be consulted. Finally, we would like to point out that the pocket atlas is obviously no substitute for an in-depth textbook, nor for macroscopic and microscopic courses in medical studies. The list of references includes titles containing references to more in-depth literature, including clinical books, insofar as they have a strong relation to anatomy.

Laypersons interested in learning about the structure of the human body will find easily understandable illustrations of common medical test procedures. In including this information, we responded to the publisher's request to expand the book content to include these aspects.

Frankfurt am Main, Kiel, Innsbruck
The Authors

1 Viscera

Viscera

1.1 Viscera at a Glance

The internal organs contained in the neck and thoracic, abdominal, and pelvic cavities are collectively known as **viscera**. The viscera are responsible for sustaining the life of the human organism.

Arrangement by Function

The book is divided into chapters arranged by organ function.

They are: **Cardiovascular system:** organ system including the *heart, blood vessels,* and *lymphatic vessels*; **Respiratory system:** organ system that is divided into the *gas-exchanging surface of the lungs* and the structures comprising the upper and lower *airways*; **Alimentary system:** organ system that is divided into the part of the gastrointestinal tract contained in the **head** and the **part beginning with the esophagus**, including the *liver* and *pancreas*, which serve as large digestive glands; **Urinary system:** organ system that is divided into the *parts of the kidney responsible for urine formation* and the *urinary passages*; **Male genital system:** system consisting of the *testes, epididymis, ductus deferens, seminal vesicle, penis,* and *accessory sex glands*; **Female genital system:** system consisting of the *female internal genitalia* housed in the lesser pelvis and *female external genitalia* located outside the pelvic floor. **Pregnancy and Human Development:** the organs and processes involved in reproduction, birth, and human development; **Endocrine system:** organ system consisting of numerous specialized *endocrine glands* and *glandular cells* occurring individually or in groups throughout the organism, whose products (*hormones*) are released into the bloodstream or lymph and distributed throughout the body; **Blood and lymphatic systems:** organ system consisting of *blood cells, lymphocytes,* and *lymphatic organs*; **The integument:** As an organ, the skin fulfils a variety of functions, serving to **protect** the body from mechanical, chemical, and thermal trauma, as well as a multitude of pathogens.

Arrangement by Region

Organ systems can also be grouped according to location in various body regions (**A**).

The **head and neck regions** contain the **initial parts of the respiratory and alimentary organs**, mainly found in the *nasal cavity* (**A1**) and *oral cavity* (**A2**). Parts of these organ systems located in the neck also form passageways connecting the head and thoracic cavity. They are situated between the middle and deep layers of cervical fascia (Vol. 1).

In the **trunk** the viscera are divided into **thoracic**, **abdominal**, and **pelvic organs**. The **thoracic cavity** (**A3**) is subdivided into three portions. These are the *right* and *left pleural cavities*, each of which contains one *lung*, and the connective tissue region between them near the midline of the body, known as the *mediastinum*. The mediastinum contains a number of structures, including the *pericardium* which encloses the *heart*. The abdominal cavity is divided into the true **abdominal cavity** (**A4**), which is lined with *peritoneum*, and the connective tissue space behind it known as the **retroperitoneal space**. Below the abdominal cavity, the pelvic organs lie in the lesser pelvis (**A5**) within the **subperitoneal connective tissue space**.

Serous Cavities and Connective Tissue Spaces

There are two ways in which an organ can be embedded in its surroundings. Organs that undergo significant changes in volume affecting adjacent organs are contained in serous cavities. A **serous cavity** is a *completely enclosed space* that contains a small amount of serous fluid and is lined by a smooth, glistening serous membrane. The **serous membrane** has two layers: a *visceral layer* that is in direct contact with the organ and encloses it and a *parietal layer* lining the wall of the serous cavity. The visceral and parietal layers become continuous at sites *or lines of reflection.* The three serous cavities are the **pleural cavities**, which house the lungs; the **pericardial cavity**, which contains the heart; and the **peritoneal cavity** (**C**), which contains most of the abdominal organs.

Organs or parts of organs that are not contained in serous cavities usually lie in **connective tissue spaces**. Smaller connective tissue spaces (**B**) derive their names from adjacent organs; larger ones are the **mediastinum**, **retroperitoneal space**, and **subperitoneal space** (**D**).

Viscera

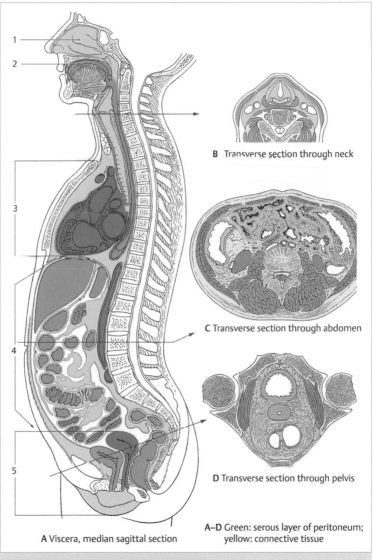

B Transverse section through neck

C Transverse section through abdomen

D Transverse section through pelvis

A Viscera, median sagittal section

A–D Green: serous layer of peritoneum; yellow: connective tissue

Fig. 1.1 Functional and regional organization of the viscera.

2 Cardiovascular System

Cardiovascular System

2.1 Overview

Circulatory System and Lymphatic Vessels

Circulation of blood occurs in a **closed system of tubes consisting of blood vessels**, with the **heart** serving as the **central pump**. The heart can be divided into a *right half* and a *left half*, each consisting of an *atrium* and *ventricle*. Irrespective of blood oxygen level, vessels that carry blood away from the heart are referred to as **arteries** and vessels that carry blood to the heart are referred to as **veins**.

The organization of the human circulatory system demonstrates a high level of differentiation. A distinction is made in postnatal life between **pulmonary circulation** and **systemic circulation**. In systemic circulation, arteries carry oxygen-rich blood away from the heart and veins carry deoxygenated blood toward the heart. In terms of function, pulmonary and systemic circulation are consecutive. Human postnatal circulation can be illustrated schematically as a figure-of-eight, with the heart located at its intersection acting as a suction and pressure pump (**A**). Blood is driven through the circulation by the arterial blood pressure (formula: arterial blood pressure = cardiac output-peripheral resistance).

Pulmonary circulation. Deoxygenated blood from the systemic circulation flows from the **right atrium** (**A1**) into the **right ventricle** (**A2**) of the heart and from there into the pulmonary circulation. Pulmonary circulation begins with the **pulmonary trunk** (**A3**), which bifurcates into **right** (**A4**) and **left pulmonary arteries** (**A5**). These vessels divide in the lungs (**A6**), parallel to the branchings of the airways as far as the **capillaries**, which surround the terminal portions of the airways known as the alveoli. There the blood is enriched with oxygen and carbon dioxide is released into the airways. The oxygenated blood leaves the lungs by the **pulmonary veins** (**A7**) and flows to the **left atrium** (**A8**).

Systemic circulation. Oxygenated blood from the lung flows from the **left atrium** (**A8**) of the heart into the **left ventricle** (**A9**). From there it is pumped through the **aorta** (**A10**) into the systemic circulation, which consists of **numerous separate**

circuits (**A11–A14**) supplying individual organs and regions of the body. Large **arteries** branch off the aorta and pass to the separate circuits, where they divide many times and finally ramify into **arterioles**. These branch into a network of **capillaries**, where exchange of gases and metabolic products occurs. At the capillary plexus, the arterial portion of the systemic circulation passes into the venous portion in which deoxygenated blood is collected in **venules**, which unite closer to the heart, to form **veins**. Venous blood from the legs and lower half of the trunk is conveyed to the **inferior vena cava** (**A15**), and that from the head, arms, and upper half of the trunk to the **superior vena cava** (**A16**). The inferior and superior venae cavae empty into the **right atrium** (**A1**).

Portal circulation is a special part of the systemic circulation. **Venous blood from unpaired abdominal organs** (*stomach, intestine, pancreas,* and *spleen*) does not flow directly into the vena cava. Instead, substances from these organs are absorbed from the intestine, and carried in the blood by the **portal vein** (**A17**), to a capillary bed in the liver. After metabolism in the liver, the blood is collected in the **hepatic veins** (**A18**) and conveyed to the **inferior vena cava**.

Lymphatic system. The lymphatic system (green) (see p. 78) acts within the systemic circulation to shunt lymph to the venous portion of the circulatory system. Unlike the system of blood vessels, the lymph drainage system originates as blind-ended vessels that collect fluid from the extracellular space in the periphery of the body via **lymphatic capillaries** (**A19**) and conveys it via larger **lymphatic vessels** and the main lymphatic trunks, the **thoracic duct** (**A20**), and **right lymphatic duct** to the *superior vena cava*. Biologic filters known as **lymph nodes** (**A21**) are interspersed along the lymph vessels (see p. 94); see also Lymph nodes, thorax, and abdomen (p. 96) and Lymph nodes (p. 424).

Clinical note: Oxygen-rich blood is often referred to in clinical usage as arterial blood and deoxygenated blood is referred to as venous blood.

A22 Chyle (see p. 78)

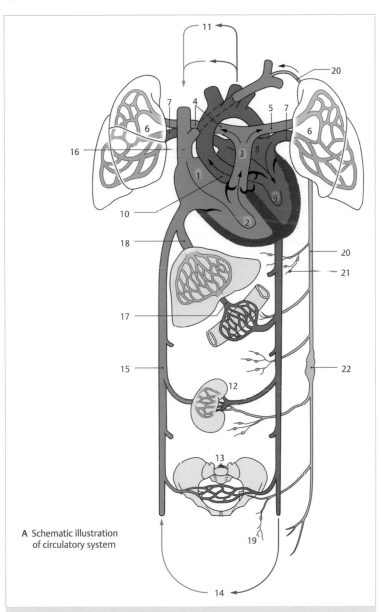

A Schematic illustration
of circulatory system

Fig. 2.1 Blood circulation and lymph vessels.

Fetal Circulation (A)

During prenatal life, the fetus (unborn offspring from the 9th week after fertilization to birth) receives oxygen and nutrients from the mother's blood and releases carbon dioxide and metabolic waste products into it. The **placenta** (**A1**) serves as the connecting organ for exchange between mother and fetus. Oxygen-rich blood carrying abundant nutrients passes from the placenta to the fetus via the **umbilical vein** (**A2**), which initially lies in the umbilical cord. The umbilical vein enters the fetal abdominal cavity at the navel, or umbilicus (**A3**), and passes to the visceral surface of the liver (**A4**), where it connects to the left branch of the *portal vein* (**A5**). Although some of the blood from the umbilical vein thus enters the portal circulation, most bypasses the liver via a shunt called the **ductus venosus** (**A6**) and is carried into the **inferior vena cava** (**A7**). Blood from the ductus venosus thus mixes with deoxygenated blood from the inferior vena cava and *hepatic veins* (**A8**). Owing to the relatively minimal admixture of deoxygenated blood, it remains well oxygenated and passes via the inferior vena cava to the **right atrium** (**A9**). From there, the blood is directed by the *valve of the inferior vena cava* toward the **foramen ovale** (**A10**) that lies in the septum between the right and left atria and connects them. Most of the blood therefore reaches the **left atrium** (**A11**), passes from there into the **left ventricle** (**A12**), and flows via the branches of the **aortic arch** (**A13**) to the heart, head, and upper limbs. Deoxygenated blood from the head and arms of the fetus flows through the **superior vena cava** (**A14**) into the **right atrium** and crosses the bloodstream from the inferior vena cava to reach the **right ventricle** (**A15**), passing from there into the **pulmonary trunk** (**A16**). A minimal amount of blood passes through the *pulmonary arteries* (**A17**) into the lungs, which are not yet aerated, and from there through the *pulmonary veins* (**A18**) to the **left atrium** (**A11**). Most of the blood from the pulmonary trunk flows directly into the **aorta** through the **ductus arteriosus** (**A19**), a shunt connecting the bifurcation of the pulmonary trunk or left pulmonary artery with the aorta. The branches given off by the portion of the aorta after the connection of the ductus arteriosus thus receive blood with a lower oxygen concentration than those before the connection, which supply the head and upper limbs. A considerable amount of blood from the fetal aorta is returned to the placenta through the paired **umbilical arteries** (**A20**).

Circulatory Adjustments at Birth (B)

At birth, the fetal circulation is converted into postnatal circulation. With the first cry of the infant, the *lungs* are *inflated and aerated*, reducing *resistance in the pulmonary circulation*, which in turn increases the volume of blood flowing from the pulmonary trunk into the pulmonary arteries. The blood is oxygenated in the lungs and transported by the pulmonary veins into the left atrium. *Backflow of blood from the lungs increases the pressure in the left atrium*, causing *functional closure of the foramen ovale* as the flaps of the opening overlap. The *foramen ovale* is thus converted into the **oval fossa**, which is normally completely closed. The shunts, the ductus venosus and ductus arteriosus, are closed off by contraction of the muscle within the vessel walls. After obliteration, the *ductus venosus* forms the **ligamentum venosum** (**B21**) and the *ductus arteriosus* forms the **ligamentum arteriosum** (**B22**). Cutting the umbilical cord disrupts the connection between the placenta and umbilical cord vessels, leading to thrombosis and gradual obliteration of the vessels. The *umbilical vein* becomes the **round ligament of the liver** (**B23**) and the *umbilical arteries* become the **cords of the umbilical arteries** (**B24**).

> **Clinical note:** Malformations causing defects in the septum may result in reversed shunts, where venous shunt blood enters the systemic circulation directly, thus reducing arterial oxygen saturation (= cyanosis).

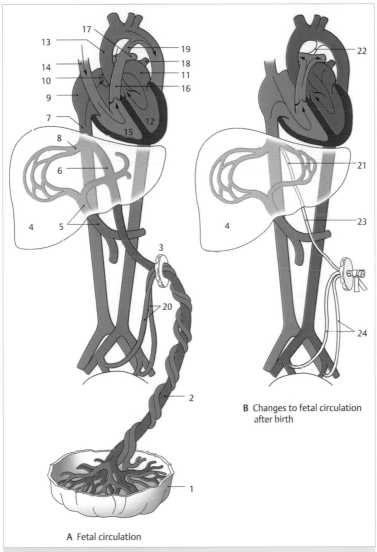

A Fetal circulation

B Changes to fetal circulation after birth

Fig. 2.2 Fetal circulation and perinatal changes.

2.2 Heart

The **heart** (**A1**) is a fibromuscular, hollow organ with a rounded, conical, or three-sided pyramidal shape. It is situated in the thorax (**A**), where it is positioned obliquely to the body's axis so that the **apex of the heart** (**AB2**) is directed to the left, inferiorly and anteriorly, while the **base of the heart** (**A3**) is directed to the right, superiorly and posteriorly. This oblique position means that one-third of the heart is to the right and two-thirds are to the left of the midline. The size of the heart depends upon factors such as the sex, age, and fitness level of an individual.

External Features

Anterior Aspect

Structure. The anterior view of the heart in its natural position with an opened pericardium shows the **sternocostal surface** (**B**), which is mostly formed by the anterior wall of the **right ventricle** (**B4**), the right atrium with its three-cornered auricle, and a narrow strip of the wall of the **left ventricle** (**B5**). The left ventricle extends toward the left to form the **apex of the heart** (**B2**). The boundary between the ventricles is demarcated by a groove known as the **anterior interventricular sulcus** (**B6**). The sulcus contains a branch of the left coronary artery (*anterior interventricular artery*) and the accompanying cardiac vein (*anterior interventricular vein*), embedded in adipose tissue. These vessels fill up the anterior interventricular sulcus, smoothing the anterior surface of the heart. The contour of the right side of the heart is formed by the **right atrium** (**B7**) and superior vena cava (**B8**). The inferior vena cava is not visible in the anterior view. The right atrium has an outpouching known as the **right auricle** (**B9**), which occupies the space between the superior vena cava and the root of the aorta (**B10**). The right atrium and right auricle are separated from the right ventricle by

the **coronary sulcus** (**B11**), which is also filled up by coronary vessels and adipose tissue. The contour of the left side of the heart is formed by a small portion of the **left auricle** (**B12**) and the left ventricle. The left auricle lies adjacent to the pulmonary trunk (**B13**).

Adjacent vessels. Viewing the sternocostal surface of the heart, it can be seen that the **pulmonary trunk** (**B13**), which arises from the right ventricle, lies anterior to the **aorta** (**B10**), which arises from the left ventricle. The aorta and pulmonary trunk wind around each other, with the aorta, which commences posteriorly, passing forward as the **ascending aorta** (**B10 a**) and continuing as the **aortic arch** (**B10 b**), which crosses over the pulmonary trunk, partially covering the pulmonary bifurcation into the *left pulmonary artery* (**B14**) and *right pulmonary artery* (not visible from anterior view). The cut edges of the **left pulmonary veins** (**B15**) are visible below the left pulmonary artery. The vessels supplying the head and arms arise from the aortic arch as the *brachiocephalic trunk* (**B16**), with the *right subclavian artery* (**B17**) and *right common carotid artery* (**B18**), *left common carotid artery* (**B19**), and *left subclavian artery* (**B20**).

The cut edges of the **pericardium** (**B21**) (see p. 30) are visible near the great vessels, the superior vena cava (B8), ascending aorta (**B10 a**), and pulmonary trunk (**B13**). Passing between the inferior aspect of the aortic arch and the superior aspect of the pulmonary bifurcation, there is a short band, the **ligamentum arteriosum** (**B22**), a remnant of the fetal *ductus arteriosus* (see p. 8). The boundary between the sternocostal surface and the diaphragmatic surface is demarcated on the right ventricle by the **right border** (**B23**).

The use of color in the illustrations of internal and external cardiac structures represents as closely as possible the proportions in the living body.

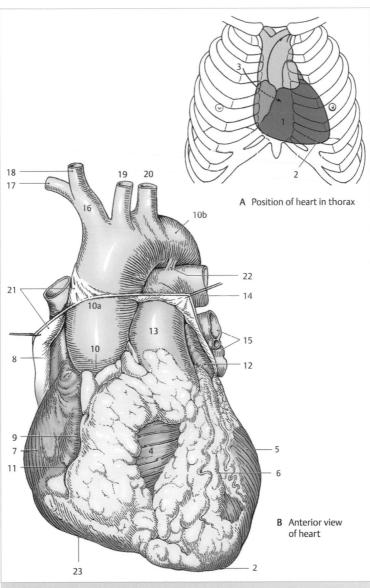

A Position of heart in thorax

B Anterior view of heart

Fig. 2.3 External shape of the heart.

External Features, cont.

Posterior Aspect (A)

Structure and adjacent vessels. In its natural position with the pericardium opened, the **base of the heart** (**I**) and part of the **diaphragmatic surface** (**II**), the inferior surface of the heart, can be seen in the posterior view. This view allows visualization of the openings of the **superior vena cava** (**AB1**) and **inferior vena cava** (**AB2**) into the nearly perpendicular **right atrium** (**AB3**). The long axis of both venae cavae is tilted slightly forward. The venae cavae are separated from the base of the right auricle by a groove known as the **sulcus terminalis cordis** (**A4**). The **right pulmonary veins** (**AB6**) and **left pulmonary veins** (**AB7**) open into the horizontally oriented **left atrium** (**A5**). The cut edge of the **pericardium** (**A8**) is visible on the posterior wall of the left atrium. Above the left atrium, the **pulmonary trunk** bifurcates into the *right pulmonary artery* (**A9**) and *left pulmonary artery* (**A10**). The **aortic arch** (**A11**) crosses over the bifurcation of the pulmonary trunk after giving off the three main branches of the *brachiocephalic trunk* (**A12**), with the *right subclavian artery* (**A13**) and *right common carotid artery* (**A14**) as well as the *left common carotid artery* (**A15**) and *left subclavian artery* (**A16**). After crossing over the pulmonary bifurcation, the aorta continues as the **descending aorta** (**AB17**).

Inferior Aspect (B)

Most of the **diaphragmatic surface of the heart** (**II**) rests on the diaphragm, and it can only be fully visualized when the heart is viewed from the inferior aspect. The view into the **right atrium** (**AB3**) is roughly along the axis of both venae cavae, that is, looking from the opening of the **inferior vena cava** (**AB2**) into the opening of the **superior vena cava** (**AB1**). The diaphragmatic surface of the heart is chiefly formed by the **left ventricle** (**B18**), which is separated from the left atrium by the **coronary sulcus** (**B19**). The coronary sulcus contains the venous *coronary sinus* (**B20**) and a *branch of the left coronary artery*. The left ventricle is separated from the right ventricle (**B21**), which is only visible in the posterior view, by the **posterior interventricular sulcus** (**B22**) (containing the *posterior interventricular branch* and *posterior interventricular vein*).

Clinical note: In clinical practice, especially in **diagnosing** a heart attack, the walls of the left ventricle are referred to as the anterior and posterior walls. The **anterior wall** describes the part of the left ventricular wall that forms the sternocostal surface, while the **posterior wall** is the part that forms the diaphragmatic surface. Myocardial infarctions involving the anterior wall are divided into *anterobasal, anterolateral, anteroseptal,* and *apical infarctions.* In patients with posterior wall involvement, *posterobasal, posterolateral,* and *posteroseptal myocardial infarctions* are distinguished from *posteroinferior* or *diaphragmal myocardial infarctions.*

ECG (electrocardiogram) is used to diagnose a heart attack. Infarcted areas can also be demonstrated by **echocardiography**, as akinetic or dyskinetic regions of myocardium. The effects on the pump function of the left ventricle produced by the heart attack depend on the percentage of contractile substance that has been lost.

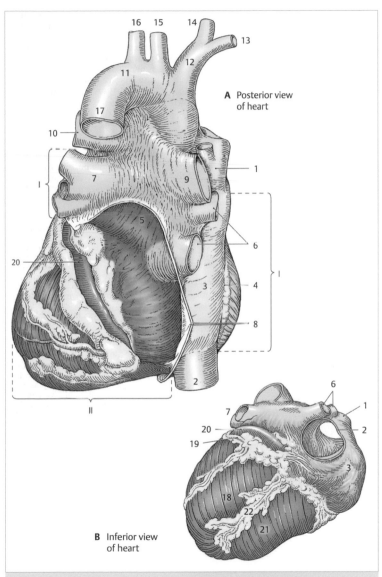

A Posterior view of heart

B Inferior view of heart

Fig. 2.4 External shape of the heart, continued.

Chambers of the Heart

The following sections discuss the chambers of the heart in order of the direction of blood flow.

Right Atrium

The right atrium (**A**) consists of two parts. The two venae cavae, the *superior vena cava* (**A1**) and *inferior vena cava* (**A2**), drain into its posterior portion. The posterior portion of the right atrium has smooth walls arising from its embryological origin and is referred to as the **sinus of the venae cavae** (see p. 320). The **true atrium** lies anterior to this and is derived from the original embryologic atrium. In the true atrium, the cardiac muscle projects into the cavity as trabeculae known as the *pectinate muscles* (**A3**). The true atrium is continuous anteriorly with the **right auricle** (**A4**).

Sinus of the venae cavae. The **opening of the superior vena cava** (**A1 a**) is directed downward and anteriorly and does not have a valve. The inferior vena cava opens at the lowest point of the right atrium. The **opening of the inferior vena cava** (**A2 a**) is shielded by a crescent-shaped valve, the *valve of the inferior vena cava* (**A5**). During fetal life, this valve is large and directs blood from the inferior vena cava directly through the *foramen ovale* (see p. 8) in the **interatrial septum** (**A6**), into the left atrium. After birth, a depression, the **oval fossa** (**A7**), is found at this site. It is bordered by a prominent margin, the *limbus fossae ovalis* (**A7 a**). Medial to the valve of the inferior vena cava, the *coronary sinus*, a venous structure, opens into the right atrium. It returns the greater portion of the backflow of deoxygenated blood from the heart itself. The **opening of the coronary sinus** (**A8**) is also shielded by a valvular fold, the *valve of the coronary sinus*. At various sites, the tiniest cardiac veins empty via minute openings into the right atrium.

True atrium and right auricle. In the interior of the heart, this area is separated from the smooth-walled sinus of the venae cavae by a ridge referred to as the **crista terminalis** (**A9**). On the outer surface of the heart, the crista terminalis, from which the *pectinate muscles* originate, corresponds to a slight depression, the *sulcus terminalis cordis* (see p. 12).

Right Ventricle

The interior of the right ventricle (**B**) is divided by two muscular ridges, the *supraventricular crest* (**B10**) and *septomarginal trabecula* (**B11**), which form the inflow tract located posteroinferiorly (arrows [top left]) and the **outflow tract**, located anterosuperiorly (arrows [top left]). The muscular wall of the right ventricle (**B12**) is thin.

Inflow tract. Muscular ridges, the **trabeculae carneae** (**B13**), project from the wall of the inflow tract in the direction of the lumen. Blood flows through the *atrioventricular orifice*, and the **right atrioventricular valve** (**tricuspid valve**) (**AB14**), out of the right atrium into the inflow tract of the right ventricle. The tricuspid valve has *three cusps, or leaflets* (see p. 22), which are attached by tendinous cords, the *chordae tendineae* (**B15**), to the **papillary muscles** (**B16–17**). The papillary muscles are a special form of trabeculae carneae. The position of the *anterior papillary muscle* (**B16**) and *posterior papillary muscle* is constant, while that of the *septal papillary muscle* varies (**B17**).

Outflow tract. The funnel-shaped **conus arteriosus** (**B18**) (infundibulum) has smooth walls and directs blood flow to the pulmonary valve orifice at the *opening of the pulmonary trunk*. The **pulmonary valve** (**B19**) is located at the origin of the pulmonary trunk (**B20**) and consists of three *semilunar cusps* (see p. 22).

The **interventricular septum**, which bulges into the ventricular cavity, can be seen to consist of a muscular part, which is roughly 1.2-cm thick, and a small membranous part that is only about 1-mm thick, close to the atrium. The septal leaflet of the tricuspid valve arises from this membranous part.

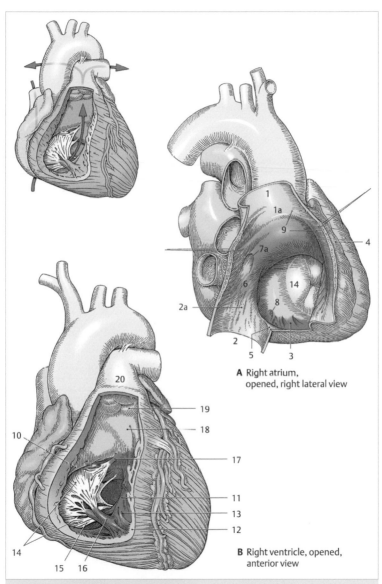

A Right atrium,
opened, right lateral view

B Right ventricle, opened,
anterior view

Fig. 2.5 Internal chambers of the heart.

Chambers of the Heart, cont.

Left Atrium

The predominantly smooth-walled interior of the left atrium (**A**) is smaller than that of the right atrium. Much of the cavity is occupied by the **right and left pulmonary veins (A1–2)**, which are drawn into the left atrium during ontogenetic development. Generally, there are four pulmonary veins, two from each side, which open into the upper portion of the left atrium. There are no valves at the **openings of the pulmonary veins**. The left atrium is continuous anteriorly with the **left auricle**, which contains small *pectinate muscles* that project into its lumen. There is no clear demarcation in the left atrium between the smooth-walled and muscular portions. Near the **interatrial septum** dividing the right and left atria is the **valve of the foramen ovale** (**A3**), which is produced by the *oval fossa* of the right atrium.

Left Ventricle

Like the right ventricle, the inner space of the left ventricle is conical in shape and is divided into an **inflow tract** (arrows [top right]), with jagged *trabeculae carneae* (**B4**), and a smooth-walled **outflow tract** (arrows [top right]). The muscular wall of the left ventricle (**B5**) is about three times thicker than that of the right.

Inflow tract. The **left atrioventricular valve** (**mitral valve**), also called the **bicuspid valve** (**B6**), is located in the *left atrioventricular orifice*. It directs blood from the left atrium into the inflow tract of the left ventricle. The bicuspid valve has two large leaflets, the *anterior* (**AB7**) and *posterior*

cusps (**AB8**). These are attached via the thick and strong *chordae tendineae* (**B9**) to the **papillary muscles**, which have two or more domed projections. The papillary muscles consist of the *anterior papillary muscle* (**B10**) and *posterior papillary muscle* (**B11**). The anterior papillary muscle arises from the sternocostal surface of the left ventricle, and the posterior papillary muscle from the diaphragmatic surface. The anterior cusp of the bicuspid valve is continuous at its origin with the wall of the aorta, dividing the inflow and outflow tracts.

Outflow tract. The smooth-walled outflow tract passes along the interventricular septum (**B12**) to the aorta, at the origin of which lies the **aortic valve** (**B13**). The aortic valve consists of three strong *semilunar cusps*. The largest portion of the **interventricular septum** (**B12**), the *muscular part*, consists of cardiac muscle. A small portion lying just caudal to the right and posterior aortic valve is membranous and is referred to as the *membranous part* (see p. 40). The margins of the interventricular septum correspond to the *anterior interventricular sulcus* (**B14**) and *posterior interventricular sulcus* on the surface of the heart.

Clinical note: Inflammation involving heart valves can be followed by scarring of the valve margins. **Stenosis** refers to narrowing of the valve opening caused by scarring. If scarring shrinks the valve margins, **insufficiency** occurs as they fail to meet completely upon closure of the valve. Valvular heart disease is diagnosed mainly by **echocardiography**, which evaluates the severity of the valvular defect and helps to decide whether surgical treatment is necessary.

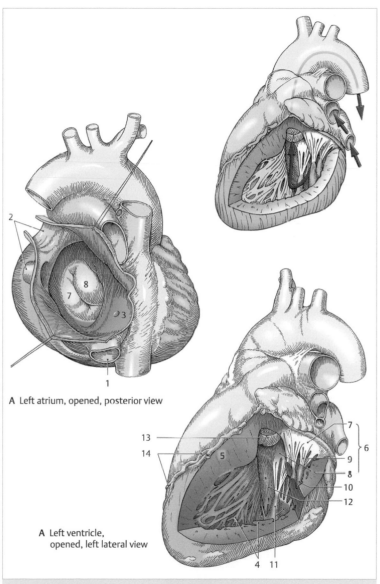

A Left atrium, opened, posterior view

A Left ventricle, opened, left lateral view

Fig. 2.6 Internal chambers of the heart, continued.

Cardiovascular System

Cardiac Skeleton

The heart valves all lie approximately in one plane, the **valvular plane**, which can be visualized when the atria are removed above the level of the coronary sulcus and the base of the heart is viewed from the superior aspect (**A**). In the valvular plane the surrounding connective tissue is thickened to form the fibrous **cardiac skeleton** (**A, B**). The cardiac skeleton separates the muscle of the atria and ventricles completely. The thickest area of condensed connective tissue is found at the site where the *aortic valve* (**AB1**), *tricuspid valve* (**AB2**), and *bicuspid valve* (**AB3**) meet. This area is known as the **right fibrous trigone** (**B4**) or central fibrous body. The site where the *aortic* and *bicuspid valves* meet is referred to as the **left fibrous trigone** (**B5**). The orifices of the *tricuspid valve* and *bicuspid valve* are surrounded by two incomplete fibrous rings, the **right fibrous ring** (**B6**) and **left fibrous ring** (**B7**), which serve for the attachment of the valve flaps. The *pulmonary valve* (**A8**) is not anchored to any considerable extent to the cardiac skeleton. The working muscles of the atria and ventricles have their origin in the right and left fibrous rings.

Layers of the Heart Wall

The wall of the heart is made up of three different layers: the **epicardium**, **myocardium**, and **endocardium**. Its thickness is primarily determined by that of the myocardial layer, which varies in different areas of the heart, depending on functional demands: the walls of the atria contain little muscle while those of the right ventricle are considerably thinner than those of the left ventricle.

Myocardium

Atrial muscle (**C, D**). The atrial myocardium can be divided into superficial and deep layers. The **superficial layer** extends over both atria and is thicker along its anterior aspect (**C**) than its posterior aspect (**D**). The features of the **deep layer** are characteristic for each of the two atria, containing *looped fibers* or *annular fibers* that pass to the respective atrioventricular orifice or surround the openings of the veins.

Ventricular muscle (**C–E**). The walls of the ventricles contain a highly complex arrangement of myocardial fibers, with morphologically distinct subepicardial, middle, and subendocardial layers. In the outer **subepicardial layer** (**C–E**), the fibers of the right ventricle run nearly horizontally around the surface, while those of the left ventricle are directed almost longitudinally toward the diaphragmatic surface. At the apex of the two ventricles, the superficial subepicardial muscle fibers form the *vortex of the heart* (**E9**), where they curve around to form the inner subendocardial layer. The left ventricle and interventricular septum have a thick **middle muscular layer** that is usually circular and is absent in the wall of the right ventricle. The inner, **subendocardial layer** contributes to the formation of the *trabeculae carneae* and *papillary muscles*. The *coronary sulcus* (**CD10**), *anterior interventricular sulcus* (**CE11**), and *posterior interventricular sulcus* (**DE12**) are clearly visible on dissected myocardium.

Endocardium and Epicardium

The inner surface of the myocardium is lined with **endocardium**, a continuation of the inner layer of the vessel walls (see p. 86), consisting of an *endothelial layer* and a thin layer of *connective tissue*. On its outer surface, the myocardium is lined with shiny, smooth **epicardium**, which is formed by *mesothelium*, a thin *layer of connective tissue* and a variably thick subepicardial layer of *fat* that serves to smooth out any unevenness on the surface of the heart.

Clinical note: Inflammation of the inner surface of the heart is called **endocarditis** and is one of the most common diseases of the heart. Endocarditis can be caused directly by disease pathogens (infectious endocarditis) but may also be caused by other mechanisms (thrombotic and rheumatic endocarditis). Infectious endocarditis mainly affects the endocardium of the heart valves.

C13 Left auricle, **CD14** Left ventricle, **CD15** Right ventricle, **CD16** Right atrium, **C17** Right auricle, **CD18** Superior vena cava, **D19** Inferior vena cava, **D20** Pulmonary valves, **D21** Left atrium

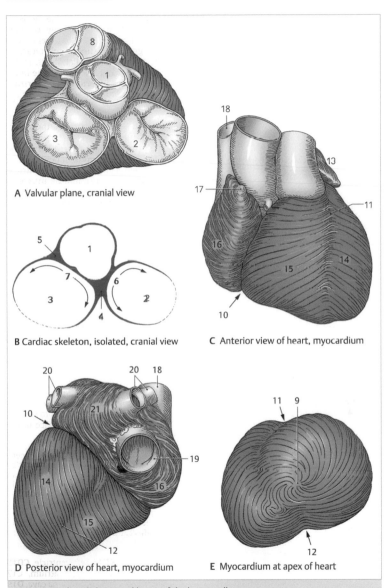

A Valvular plane, cranial view

B Cardiac skeleton, isolated, cranial view

C Anterior view of heart, myocardium

D Posterior view of heart, myocardium

E Myocardium at apex of heart

Fig. 2.7 Cardiac skeleton and layers of the heart wall.

Layers of the Heart Wall, Histology, and Ultrastructure

Working Myocardium

The working myocardium consists of individual muscle cells, which, in a manner similar to skeletal muscle structure, exhibit **transverse striations** produced by the organization of myofibrils. As in skeletal muscle, contractile proteins are arranged in *sarcomeres* (see Vol. 1).

Light Microscopic Appearance (A, B). **Cardiac muscle cells (AB1)** are up to 120 μm long and in the average adult have an average diameter of 20 μm. They are *branched cells* that establish *end-to-end connections* with adjacent cells, and are arranged in *bundles*, thus forming a complex **three-dimensional structure**, with *connective tissue* (**AB2**) containing a *dense capillary network* in its spaces. The pale **nucleus (AB3)** of a cardiac muscle cell is located centrally. Surrounding the nucleus is a **perinuclear zone devoid of myofibrils (A4)**, but with *abundant sarcoplasm and organelles* and containing aggregations of *glycogen granules* and yellow-brown *lipofuscin droplets*. The *transverse cell boundaries*, where cardiac muscle cells abut against each other, are referred to as **intercalated discs (AB5)**.

Electron Microscopic Appearance (C). Hidden behind the intercalated disc is the site where opposing membranes, the **sarcolemma (C6)**, of cardiac muscle cells are intricately interlocked, forming important **cell contacts** consisting of *desmosomes* (**C7**) and *gap junctions* (*nexus*) (**C8**) that act to distribute electrical impulses. At the intercalated disc, the *actin filaments* (**C9**) of a cell end in a condensed **limiting layer** (*zonulae adherens*) (**C10**), although the actin filaments of the adjacent cell continue in the same direction. Cardiac muscle cells contain abundant numbers of large **mitochondria (C11)**, lying between myofibrils, which supply the high amount of energy required for myofibril contraction. Distributed throughout the cardiac muscle cell there are two systems of intracellular canaliculi surrounded by membranes. The system of transverse tubules, or **T-tubules (C12)**, is a special *derivative of the sarcolemma*. The system composed of longitudinal tubules or **L-tubules (C13)** is formed by the *endoplasmic reticulum* of the cardiac muscle cell.

Specialized Conduction Tissue (D)

Cells of the conducting system of the heart (**D14**) (see p. 26) are often *larger in diameter* than those of the working myocardium and usually lie embedded in connective tissue directly beneath the endocardium (**D15**). These cells contain *fewer fibrils*, but have abundant sarcoplasm and *glycogen*, and are capable of producing energy anaerobically. For further information, please refer to textbooks of histology.

Clinical note: Cardiac muscle cells cannot regenerate. Although damage resulting from temporary inadequate blood supply is reversible, prolonged inadequate supply, or **ischemia**, causes irreversible damage involving necrosis and replacement of tissue by connective tissue scarring.

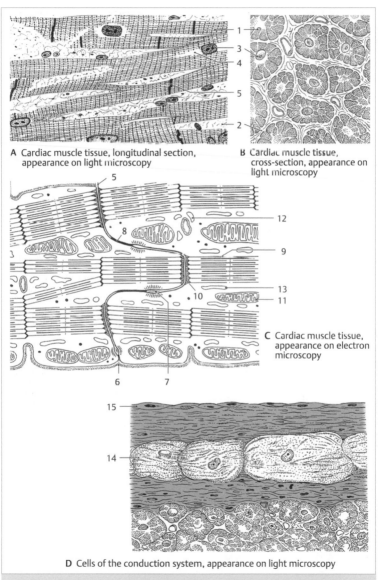

A Cardiac muscle tissue, longitudinal section, appearance on light microscopy

B Cardiac muscle tissue, cross-section, appearance on light microscopy

C Cardiac muscle tissue, appearance on electron microscopy

D Cells of the conduction system, appearance on light microscopy

Fig. 2.8 Layers of the heart wall, microscopic structure and ultrastructure.

Heart Valves

Atrioventricular Valves

The atrioventricular valves close during systole. Each atrioventricular valve consists of a flap of connective tissue that is covered on both sides by endocardium and is devoid of blood vessels. The atrial surface of the flap is smooth; the chordae tendineae arise from its free margins and inferior surface.

Tricuspid valve. The tricuspid valve has three leaflets known as the **anterior cusp** (**A–C1**), **posterior cusp** (**A–C2**), and **septal cusp** (**A–C3**), situated at the interventricular septum. The anterior cusp (**A–C1**) is the largest of the three; its chordae tendineae are attached to the strong *anterior papillary muscle* (**C4**) that is derived from the *septomarginal trabecula*. The attachment site of the septal cusp (**C5**) is at the level of the *membranous part* of the septum, dividing it into an *anterior, interventricular portion* between the two ventricles, and a *posterior, atrioventricular portion* between the right atrium and left ventricle. In between the three large cusps are small **intermediate segments** (**A6–C6**) that do not reach the fibrous ring.

Bicuspid valve. Possessing two leaflets, the bicuspid valve (mitral valve) closes the left atrioventricular opening; it has an anteromedial cusp, the **anterior cusp** (**AB7**), and a posterolateral cusp, the **posterior cusp** (**AB8**). The short and thick chordae tendineae are attached to an anterior and posterior *papillary muscle* in such a manner that each papillary muscle supports adjacent sides of both valve leaflets. The anterior cusp is continuous at its septal origin with the wall of the aorta (**AB9**). In addition to its two large cusps, the mitral valve has two small ones, the **commissural cusps** (**AB10**), which do not extend as far as the fibrous annulus.

Functional anatomy. In the filling phase, **ventricular diastole**, during which blood flows from the atria into the ventricles, the margins of the cusps move apart and the valves open (**A**). In the ejection phase, **ventricular systole**, the ventricular myocardium contracts and the column of blood is forced into the outflow tract (**B**). During this process, the complex attachment of the subvalvular apparatus prevents the cusps from prolapsing into the atrium.

Semilunar Valves

The valves of the pulmonary trunk (**AB11**) and aorta (**AB9**) each consist of three nearly equally sized valves, the **semilunar cusps**, which are formed by **folds of endocardium**. The attachment of the semilunar cusps is curved, and the artery walls near the valves are thin and bulging (**D**). Located in the middle of the free margin of each valve is a *nodule of semilunar cusp* (**D12**). On either side of the nodule, running along the valve margin, there is a thin, crescent-shaped rim called the *lunule of semilunar cusp* (**D13**).

Pulmonary valve. The pulmonary valve is located between the infundibulum and the pulmonary trunk and consists of an **anterior semilunar cusp** (**A14**), **right semilunar cusp** (**A15**), and **left semilunar cusp** (**A16**). The wall of the pulmonary trunk opposite the valve protrudes to form a shallow *sinus* (**A17**).

Aortic valve. The aortic valve is located between the aortic vestibule and the aorta and has a **posterior semilunar cusp** (**A18**), **right semilunar cusp** (**A19**), and **left semilunar cusp** (**A20**). Near the valve, the wall of the aorta bulges outwards, forming the *aortic sinus* (**A21**) and enlarging the luminal diameter of the vessel (*aortic bulb*). The *left coronary artery* (**AD22**) arises from the aortic sinus of the left semilunar cusp (**D**) and the *right coronary artery* (**AD23**) from the aortic sinus of the right semilunar cusp.

Functional anatomy. In **ventricular diastole** (**A**), while the column of blood is exerting pressure on the walls of the pulmonary trunk and aorta, the cusps unfold and the valve closes. The nodules on the margins of the cusps ensure that the valve is fully closed. During **ventricular systole** (**B**), increased pressure in the upstream ventricle causes the margins of the cusps to separate, although turbulent blood flow prevents them from lying directly against the vessel wall.

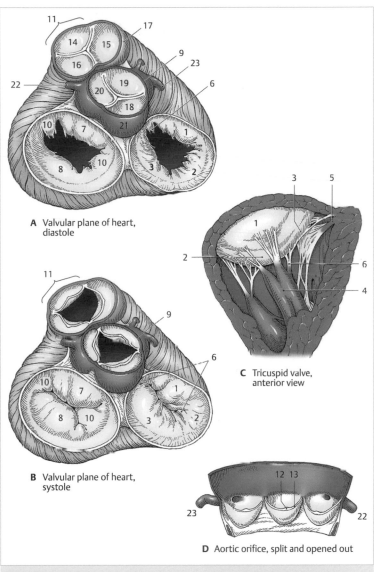

A Valvular plane of heart, diastole

B Valvular plane of heart, systole

C Tricuspid valve, anterior view

D Aortic orifice, split and opened out

Fig. 2.9 Heart valves.

Vasculature of the Heart

The coronary vessels are the blood vessels that **supply the heart itself**, providing nourishment to the cardiac muscle tissue. The vessels responsible for **supplying the body** are the large "functional" vessels, which are situated at the base of the heart. The **coronary vessels** derive their name from the location of their main stems in the coronary sulcus. The short **coronary circulation** comprises the *coronary arteries* (the first branches of the aorta), a *capillary network* lying directly beneath the myocardial surface, and the *coronary veins*, most of which open into the *coronary sinus* and drain into the right atrium.

Coronary Arteries (A–C)

The main stems of the **right coronary artery** (**AC1**) and **left coronary artery** (**AC2**) arise in the *aortic sinuses* of the right and left semilunar valves.

Right coronary artery (**A1**). At the site of its entry into the *coronary sulcus* (**A3**) on the right side, the right coronary artery is initially covered by the right auricle (**A4**). After distributing branches to the right atrium and anterior surface of the right ventricle, and giving off the **right marginal artery** (**A5**), it travels posteriorly in the coronary sulcus to the *posterior interventricular sulcus* (**B6**), where it gives rise to the **posterior interventricular artery** (**B7**). In most people (in **balanced circulation**), the right coronary artery supplies the right atrium, the conducting system of the heart, the greater portion of the right ventricle, the posterior part of the interventricular septum, and the adjacent diaphragmatic surface of the heart.

Left coronary artery (**A2**). The short stem initially passes between the pulmonary trunk (**A8**) and left auricle (**A9**) before dividing into the **anterior interventricular artery** (**A10**), which travels caudally in the *anterior interventricular sulcus* (**A11**), and the **circumflex artery** (**A12**), which runs posteriorly in the *coronary sulcus*. The stems of the coronary arteries, lying superficially in the sulci, are located in the subepicardial fat, but their branches are often surrounded by myocardium or myocardial bridges. In **balanced circulation**, the left coronary artery supplies most of the left ventricle and the anterior portion of the interventricular septum, part of the right ventricle at the sternocostal surface of the heart, and the left atrium.

> **Clinical note:** Although coronary arteries form small anastomoses with one another, these are insufficient for developing collateral circulation if vessels become occluded. Coronary arteries are therefore considered **end arteries** in terms of function. Occluded arteries lead to insufficient blood supply to a portion of myocardium, resulting in a **heart attack**. Over 90% of acute heart attacks arise from fresh coronary thrombosis on a ruptured atherosclerotic plaque.

Coronary Veins (A, B)

Most of the deoxygenated blood leaving the walls of the heart flows through the veins, which accompany the arteries, to the **coronary sinus** (**B13**) lying in the posterior portion of the *coronary sulcus* (**AB3**). The larger tributaries that empty into the coronary sinus are the **anterior interventricular vein** (**A14**), which becomes the **great cardiac vein** (**B15**) in the left coronary sulcus, the **middle cardiac vein** (**B16**) lying in the *posterior interventricular sulcus*, and the **small cardiac vein** (**B17**) from the right side. About two-thirds of deoxygenated blood flows directly into the right atrium via larger veins and the coronary sinus. Smaller veins, the *right ventricular veins*, open directly into the right atrium, and the smallest veins, the *small cardiac veins*, empty directly into the inner spaces of the heart.

Lymphatic Vessels

The dense lymphatic network of the heart can be divided into a **deep endocardial**, **middle myocardial**, and **superficial epicardial network**. Larger collecting vessels travel in the epicardium, accompanying the aorta and pulmonary trunk. The corresponding regional lymph nodes belong to the tracheobronchial and **anterior mediastinal nodes** (see p. 82).

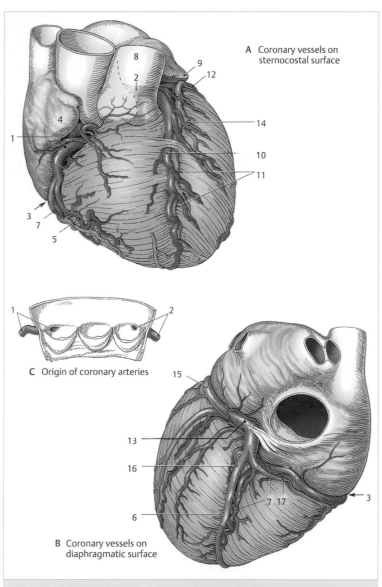

A Coronary vessels on sternocostal surface

C Origin of coronary arteries

B Coronary vessels on diaphragmatic surface

Fig. 2.10 Cardiac blood vessels.

Cardiovascular System

Conducting System of the Heart

Specialized cardiac muscle cells generate and conduct spontaneous rhythmic impulses that stimulate the beating of the heart. These cells are collectively known as the **conducting system of the heart** and they differ in terms of histology and function from the rest of the cardiac muscle, the *working myocardium*. Clusters of cells are found at two sites, where they form **nodular structures** known as the *sinoatrial node* and *atrioventricular node* (*AV node*). Most of these cells, however, are arranged into **bundles**, which can be divided into the *atrioventricular bundle and the right bundle* and *left bundle*, the bundle branches of the ventricular conducting system. The pathway traveled by an impulse, from where it was generated to its functional spread to the working myocardium, is discussed in the following sections on the basis of identifiable morphological structures (**A, B**).

The **sinoatrial node** (**A1**) (Keith-Flack node) lies beneath the epicardium on the posterior surface of the right atrium, near the opening of the superior vena cava (**A2**) in the *sulcus terminalis cordis*. The spindle-shaped node, about 10-mm long, is referred to as the **cardiac pacemaker**, as it generates 60–80 impulses per minute, which travel to the rest of the conducting system. The second component of the specialized cardiac muscle tissue is the **atrioventricular node** (Aschoff-Tawara node) (**A3**), which is about 5-mm long and is located at the atrioventricular septum in the *interatrial septum* (**A4**) between the opening of the coronary sinus (**A5**) and the septal cusp of the tricuspid valve (**A6**). The impulses generated by the sinoatrial node are conducted through the working myocardium of the right atrium to the atrioventricular node, where the bundles belonging to the conducting system begin. These consist of the **atrioventricular bundle** (**A7**) or **bundle of His**, whose trunk, the **trunk of the atrioventricular bundle**, penetrates the cardiac skeleton as it travels toward the ventricles. The atrioventricular bundle reaches the superior margin of the

muscular interventricular septum on the side of the right ventricle and divides into right and left conduction bundle branches.

These travel bilaterally beneath the endocardium in the interventricular septum toward the apex of the heart. The **right bundle** (**A8**) curves downward and enters the *septomarginal trabecula* (**A9**) to reach the *anterior papillary muscle* (**A10**). Its peripheral branches are the **subendocardial branches** (**A11**), which form a subendocardial plexus. The plexus terminates in functional connections with the *papillary muscles* or the *ventricular myocardium near the apex of the heart* and then passes with recurrent bundles in the *trabeculae carneae* to reach the *myocardium of the base of the heart*. A few specialized cardiac muscle cells form pseudo-tendinous cords, **Purkinje fibers**, which pass to the papillary muscles.

The **left bundle** (**B12**) fans out in flat bundles along the interventricular septum. These bundles are usually divided into *two major bundles*, which proceed to the *base of the papillary muscles*, branch off to form *subendocardial networks*, form functional connections with the *ventricular myocardium near the apex of the heart*, and travel as recurrent bundles to reach the *myocardium of the base of the heart*.

Functional anatomy. All components of the conducting system of the heart are theoretically capable of generating impulses. Yet, the impulse frequency of the sinoatrial node, at a rate of about 70 per minute, is faster than that of the AV node, with 50–60 impulses per minute, and that of the ventricles, with 25–45 impulses per minute. Thus, the heartbeat is normally determined and coordinated by the sinoatrial node (**sinoatrial nodal rhythm**), while subsequent components of the conducting system remain silent.

Clinical note: Pathological conditions can disrupt the conducting system of the heart. Diagnosis of abnormalities can be assisted by an **electrocardiogram** (**ECG**). Cardiac arrhythmias can be diagnosed precisely by intracardiac ECG.

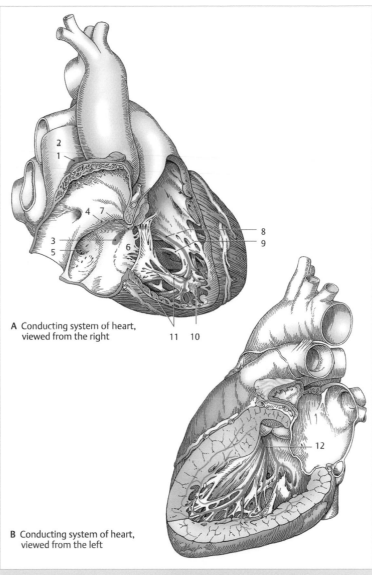

A Conducting system of heart, viewed from the right

B Conducting system of heart, viewed from the left

Fig. 2.11 Impulse generation and conducting system.

Cardiovascular System

Innervation of the Heart

The heartbeat, which is initiated by the sinoatrial node, is influenced by the autonomic nervous system (see Vol. 3). The nerve supply to the heart (**A**) is derived from the sympathetic and parasympathetic parts of the autonomic nervous system. Cardiac nerves carry *autonomic efferent* fibers as well as *viscerosensory afferent* fibers.

Sympathetic innervation. Generally, three cardiac nerves originate from the cervical portion of the sympathetic trunk at the level of the cervical ganglia: the **superior cervical cardiac nerve** (**A1**), **middle cervical cardiac nerve** (**A2**), and **inferior cervical cardiac nerve** (**A3**). Coursing posterior to the neurovascular bundle, they travel caudally to the **cardiac plexus** (**A4**). Additional *thoracic cardiac branches* (**A5**) arise from the upper thoracic ganglia and likewise pass to the cardiac plexus. The cardiac nerves of the sympathetic nervous system carry *postganglionic autonomic fibers*, whose preganglionic segments arise from the upper segments of the thoracic spinal cord. The sympathetic cardiac nerves also contain *viscerosensory fibers*, particularly *pain fibers*, whose perikarya lie in the cervical and thoracic spinal ganglia.

Stimulation of sympathetic cardiac nerves leads to an increased heart rate, greater force of contraction and excitation, and accelerated impulse conduction in the atrioventricular node.

Parasympathetic innervation. The parasympathetic cardiac nerves arise from the **vagus nerve** (**A6**). They branch off at various levels from the cervical portion of the vagus nerve as the *superior* (**A7**) and *inferior* (**A8**) *cervical cardiac branches* and pass to the **cardiac plexus**. The *thoracic cardiac branches* (**A9**) also radiate from the thoracic portion of the vagus nerve and pass to the cardiac plexus. The vagal cardiac nerves contain mostly *preganglionic autonomic fibers* that synapse with postganglionic fibers in subepicardial neurons at the base of the heart. The *viscerosensory fibers* of the parasympathetic cardiac branches mainly conduct impulses from *baroreceptors and stretch receptors*.

Stimulation of parasympathetic cardiac nerves leads to decreased heart rate and force of contraction, and reduced excitation and slower impulse conduction in the atrioventricular node.

Cardiac Plexus

The sympathetic cardiac nerves and parasympathetic cardiac branches ramify and travel along the base of the heart, where they join to form the **cardiac plexus** (**A4**). Based on topographical features, the cardiac plexus can be divided into superficial (**A4 a**) and deep parts (**A4 b**). Embedded within the plexus are smaller and larger collections of nerve cells, including the *cardiac ganglia* (**A10**). The **superficial**, or anterior, portion of the plexus lies below the aortic arch in front of the right pulmonary artery and is supplied mainly by fibers from the *cardiac nerves on the left side*. The **deep**, or posterior, portion of the plexus lies behind the aortic arch and anterior to the tracheal bifurcation (**A11**). It contains fibers from the *cardiac nerves on both sides*. The two portions of the cardiac plexus are interconnected and ultimately give off the *true cardiac branches*, supplying all areas of the heart via *plexuses* lying along the coronary arteries and atria.

Sensory (afferent) innervation. The cardiac plexus also contains viscerosensory fibers, which terminate in the cervical (**C3–C4**) and thoracic spine (mainly T1–T7). This projection to the cervical and thoracic segments of the spine explains why cardiac pain, for example, due to heart attack, is projected to the left shoulder and neck region and to the ulnar side of the left arm (head zone).

A12 Superior cervical ganglion, **A13** Middle cervical ganglion, **A14** Cervicothoracic ganglion (stellate ganglion), **A15** Thoracic ganglia, **A16** Recurrent laryngeal nerve

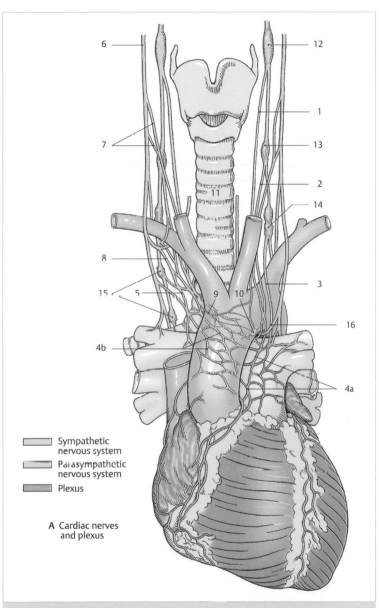

Fig. 2.12 Innervation of the heart.

6

12

7

1

13

11

2

14

8

15   5

9   10

3

16

4b

4a

Sympathetic
nervous system

Parasympathetic
nervous system

Plexus

A Cardiac nerves
and plexus

Pericardium

Like all visceral organs that undergo significant changes in volume and displacement relative to adjacent organs, the heart is contained within a serous cavity, the **pericardial cavity** (**B**).

The **pericardium** (**AB1**) encloses the heart and portions of the great vessels near its base. It consists of two components, an outer fibrous pericardium and an inner serous pericardium. The **fibrous pericardium** is a conical *sac formed by collagenous connective tissue with dense fibers* that surrounds the heart without actually being connected to it. The **serous pericardium** is a dual-layered closed system within the fibrous pericardium. Like all serous membranes, it is composed of a parietal and a visceral layer. The *visceral layer* or *epicardium* lies directly on the surface of the heart and roots of the great vessels. It turns back on itself to become the *parietal layer* (**B2**), which lines the inner surface of the fibrous pericardium (**B3**).

Fibrous pericardium. The fibrous pericardium is fused at various sites with surrounding structures, anchoring the heart in its position in the thorax. Its **caudal** portion is joined to the central tendon of the diaphragm. Its **anterior** portion is attached by the *sternopericardial ligaments*, variable bands, to the posterior surface of the sternum (**B4**). Thicker connective tissue bands also pass **posteriorly** to the trachea and vertebral column. **Laterally**, the fibrous pericardium is separated from the parietal layer of the pleural cavity by loose connective tissue.

Serous pericardium. The **parietal layer** and **visceral layer** can only be visualized when the pericardial cavity is laid open. This also reveals the lines of reflection between these two layers, which form a cranial border around the *superior vena cava* (**A–C5**), *aorta* (**A–C6**), and *pulmonary trunk* (**A–C7**). A segment of the aorta and pulmonary trunk about 3-cm long is contained within the pericardium. Shorter portions of the caudal part of the anterior wall of the *inferior vena cava* (**BC8**) and the posterior walls of the *pulmonary veins* (**BC9**) are also covered by pericardium. The **sites of reflection** are arranged to form two complex tubes (**C**), one enclosing the aorta and pulmonary trunk at the **arterial opening** (red line in **C**) and the other enclosing the pulmonary veins and venae cavae at the **venous opening** (blue line in **C**). Lying between the tubes at the arterial and venous openings there is a groove, the **transverse pericardial sinus** (arrow in **C**). The aorta and pulmonary trunk lie anterior to this passageway and the great veins lie posterior to it. The sites of reflection of the venous opening surround several recesses known as the **pericardial recesses**. Between the inferior pulmonary veins, the inferior vena cava (**BC8**), and the posterior surface of the left atrium, there is the large **oblique pericardial sinus** (**B10**).

The pericardium is covered on its right and left sides by the **pleura** (**A11**). Passing between the pleura and pericardium, the *phrenic nerve* (**A12**) runs bilaterally, accompanying the *pericardiacophrenic artery* (**A13**) and pericardiacophrenic vein.

Blood supply and innervation. The arterial blood supply to the pericardium is mainly provided by the **pericardiacophrenic artery** (**A13**), which arises from the *internal thoracic artery*. Venous drainage runs via the **pericardiacophrenic vein** (**A14**) into the *brachiocephalic vein*. Innervation of the pericardium is provided by the **phrenic nerve** (**A12**), **vagus nerve**, and **sympathetic trunk**.

Clinical note: Under pathological conditions, e.g., pericarditis, larger amounts of fluid can collect in the pericardial recesses (**pericardial effusion**). Following **fibrinous inflammation** adhesions between layers of the serous pericardium can form, potentially severely restricting motion of the heart. These adhesions can ultimately become calcified, causing constrictive pericarditis with severe impairment of cardiac function. A rupture in the wall of the aorta can lead to a rapid outpouring of blood into the pericardial cavity, resulting in **pericardial tamponade**.

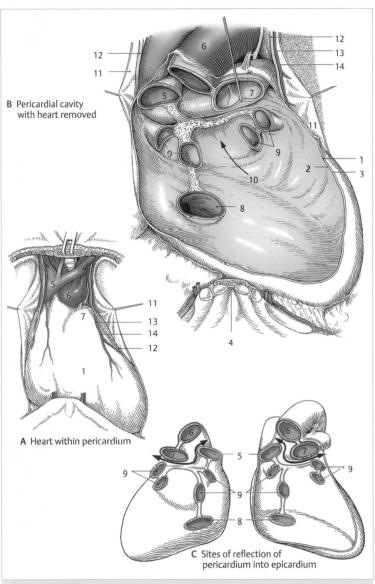

B Pericardial cavity with heart removed

A Heart within pericardium

C Sites of reflection of pericardium into epicardium

Fig. 2.13 Pericardium.

Cardiovascular System

Position of the Heart and Cardiac Borders

Mediastinum (**A**). The heart and pericardium are located in the mediastinum, a *midline region of connective tissue in the thorax*. The mediastinum is bounded **cranially** at the level of the *superior thoracic aperture* (**A1**), where it becomes continuous with the visceral space of the neck, and **caudally** by the *diaphragm* (**A2**). It extends from the *posterior surface of the sternum* (**A3**) to the *anterior surface of the thoracic vertebral column* (**A4**) in the **sagittal plane**. Its **lateral** boundary is formed by the *mediastinal part of parietal pleura*. The mediastinum can be divided into the **superior mediastinum** (**A** red) and **inferior mediastinum** (**A** green/blue). The border between the superior and inferior mediastinum is determined by a *transverse plane* (**A5**) extending from the *sternal angle*. The **superior** mediastinum contains *blood vessel and nerve pathways*, as well as the *thymus* (see p. 406). The **inferior** mediastinum is divided by the anterior and posterior wall of the pericardium into the *anterior mediastinum* (blue-green), *middle mediastinum* (blue), and *posterior mediastinum* (darker blue). The anterior mediastinum is a narrow space filled with *connective tissue*, between the anterior thoracic wall and the anterior surface of the pericardium. The middle mediastinum contains the *heart and pericardium*. It becomes wider and deeper toward the superior mediastinum and contains not only loose connective tissue but also the retrosternal fat body, lymphatic vessels that drain the mammary glands, and branches of the internal thoracic vessels. The posterior mediastinum extends between the posterior wall of the pericardium and the anterior surface of the thoracic vertebral column (T5–12) and contains *large blood vessels and nerve pathways* and the *esophagus* (see p. 176).

Cardiac borders (**B**). In the living body, the heart and pericardium are separated only by a space containing a capillary layer, so that their contours largely conform to each other. For the purposes of describing their location, it is thus sufficient to limit discussion to the heart. Even in healthy individuals, the cardiac borders vary depending on age, sex, and posture. The dimensions described in the following are based on the average adult. In its normal position, two-thirds of the heart lies on the left of the midline. The borders of the heart **projecting toward the anterior thoracic wall** form a trapezoid. The **right border** runs from the sternal attachment of the third rib to the connection to the sixth rib *paralleling the right sternal border*, and about 2 cm away from it. This line corresponds to the *lateral profile of the right atrium*. The continuation of this line cranially marks the *right margin of the superior vena cava*, while its caudal continuation corresponds to the *right margin of the inferior vena cava*. At the connection to the sixth rib, the right border becomes continuous with the contour formed by the *right border* and proceeds to the *apex of the heart*. The **left border** of the heart extends from its apex, located in the fifth intercostal space about 2 cm medial to the *midclavicular line*, curving with a left convexity, to a point located 2 cm lateral to the attachment of the third rib.

A portion of the heart is in direct contact with the anterior thoracic wall, that is, the sternum. Sternal percussion reveals an area of hypophonesis or **absolute cardiac dullness**. The *pleural cavity* (red) extends from either side in front of the heart, covering its lateral portions. Depending on the volume of air in the lung, a variable amount of *lung tissue* (blue) expands into the pleural cavity. Although the percussion sound is clearer at this site than absolute cardiac dullness, it is not as resonant as over adjacent lung tissue. For this reason, the term **relative cardiac dullness** is used. This indicates the true size of the heart, with its area corresponding to the borders of the portion of the heart projecting to the thoracic wall.

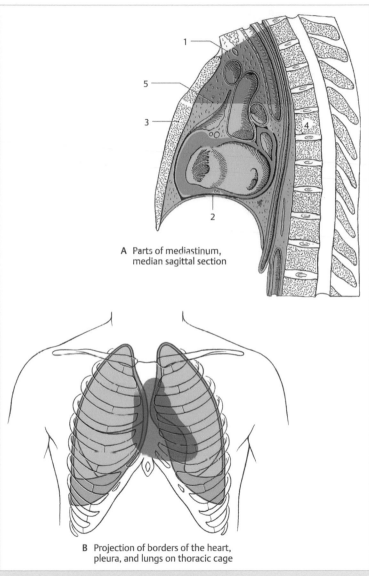

A Parts of mediastinum, median sagittal section

B Projection of borders of the heart, pleura, and lungs on thoracic cage

Fig. 2.14 Position of the heart and cardiac borders.

Cardiovascular System

Radiographic Anatomy

Conventional radiography of the thorax is part of basic diagnostic testing for heart disease. The most common method is to visualize the heart on a **chest radiograph** (**teleradiography**), obtaining a **posteroanterior** view with a **parallel X-ray beam** (**A**). Oblique and lateral views supplement the posteroanterior view.

Posteroanterior View

Most of the heart lies in the **mediastinal shadow**, produced mainly by the *vertebral column, sternum, heart,* and *great vessels*. The mediastinal shadow merges with the neck shadow above and the liver shadow below. Located on either side of the mediastinal shadow are the air-filled, and therefore lucent, **lungs**. The contours of the heart and vessels in the mediastinal shadow normally consist of **two curvatures** on the **right** and **four** on the **left**.

Right side. Comparison of the radiographic image with the orientation of the heart projecting toward the anterior thoracic wall (see p. 33 B) shows that the upper, flattened curvature is produced by the *superior vena cava* (**A1**) and that the lower curvature corresponds to the *right atrium* (**A2**). Deep inspiration can cause the *inferior vena cava* to also appear at the lower right border.

Left side. The uppermost of the four curvatures on the left side of the heart is produced by the distal portion of the *aortic arch* (**A3**). Below the aortic arch, the *pulmonary trunk* (**A4**) produces a variously shaped bulge in the mediastinal shadow. Beneath this is a small and often barely distinguishable curve corresponding to the *left auricle* (**A5**). The lower curvature, which has a left convexity, forms the *margin of the left ventricle* (**A6**). The constriction at the upper margin of the ventricular curvature is also called the "waist" of the heart.

Because the heart shadow is continuous caudally with that of the *diaphragm* (**A7**) and *upper abdominal organs*, it is difficult to precisely discern its inferior margin.

Auscultation

Auscultation, or listening to heart sounds, can provide important information about cardiac function (see p. 42). Heart sounds are vibrations that are caused by the beating of the heart and transmitted to the thoracic wall. The **first heart sound** arises during the **contraction phase of systole**, from vibrations of the ventricular wall. The **second heart sound** arises at the **beginning of diastole**, with closure of the semilunar cusps of the aorta and pulmonary trunk. Pathological **heart sounds** can be produced by *stenosis* or valvular *insufficiency*.

Generally, optimum **auscultation sites** for the heart valves (**B**) do not directly correspond to their surface projection on the anterior thoracic wall. Heart sounds or noises are best heard where the blood flow passing through the respective valve comes closest to the thoracic wall. The following auscultation sites, derived from empirical knowledge, are thus located at some distance from the valves:

- **aortic valve** (**B8**) right second intercostal space near the sternum
- **pulmonary valve** (**B9**) left second intercostal space near the sternum
- **bicuspid valve** (**B10**) midclavicular line in the left fifth intercostal space, near the apex of the heart
- **tricuspid valve** (**B11**) caudal end of the body of the sternum at the level of the right fifth intercostal space.

Clinical note: The **Erb point** is the central auscultation point of the heart in the left third intercostal space beside the sternum; nearly all heart sounds and murmurs can be perceived here, especially the high-frequency sounds of aortic and pulmonary insufficiency.

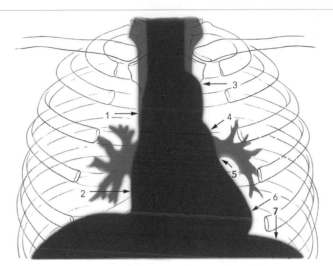

A Schematic illustration of heart radiograph

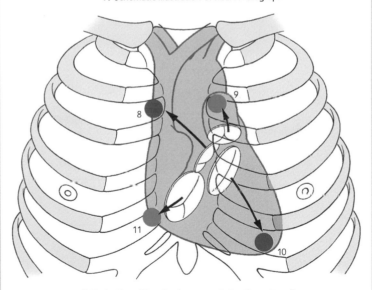

B Projection of heart valves on anterior thoracic wall
and auscultation sites

Fig. 2.15 Radiographic anatomy and auscultation of the heart.

Cross-Sectional Anatomy

Conventional radiography of the heart is supplemented by **cross-sectional** imaging, made possible by modern imaging modalities, such as *computed tomography* (*CT*), *nuclear magnetic resonance imaging* (*MRI*), and *ultrasound*. The most commonly used imaging plane is the **transverse plane**, also referred to in clinical terms as the **axial plane**. Evaluation of sectional images proceeds from caudal with the patient lying in the supine position. On the imaged sections, the *vertebral column*, located posteriorly, is *down* and the thoracic skeleton, located *anteriorly*, is *up*. Also, all *anatomic structures on the right side of the body* are *depicted on the left*. The following section presents examples of three anatomic, nearly transverse imaging planes through the heart and great vessels, from cranial to caudal. Imaging plane levels through the heart and thorax are marked in the illustration showing the position of the heart (**A**).

Transverse Section through the Body at T6 (B)

The image is through the bifurcation of the *pulmonary trunk* (**B1**) into the *right pulmonary artery* (**B2**) and *left pulmonary artery* (**B3**). Anterior to the pulmonary trunk is *subepicardial fat* (**B4**), which extends to the right as far as the section through the *ascending aorta* (**B5**). Anterior to the aorta and subepicardial fat is the *pericardial cavity* (**B6**), which appears somewhat widened in the section, bounded anteriorly by connective tissue and adipose tissue of the *retrosternal fat pad* (**B7**) and the *sternum* (**B8**). On the right side of the ascending aorta, the

superior vena cava (**B9**) is seen. Between the aorta and superior vena cava lies the *transverse pericardial sinus* (**B10**). Posterior to the bifurcation of the pulmonary trunk are sections through the *left* (**B11**) and *right* (**B12**) *main bronchi*. At the site of its ramification in the *right lung* (**B13**), the right main bronchus is accompanied closely by a branch of the *right pulmonary artery* (**B2**), while the root of the *right pulmonary vein* (**B14**) runs at a greater distance from it. Accompanying the branches of the main bronchi are *bronchopulmonary lymph nodes* (**B15**). Posterior to the main bronchi is the section through the *esophagus* (**B16**), which is accompanied on the right side of its posterior aspect by the *azygos vein* (**B17**) and on the left side of its posterior aspect by the *descending aorta* (**B18**). The descending aorta lies directly adjacent to the inferior lobe of the *left lung* (**B19**).

B20 Thoracic duct

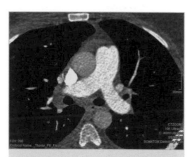

Fig. 2.16C Corresponding plane to Fig. 2.16B on CT.

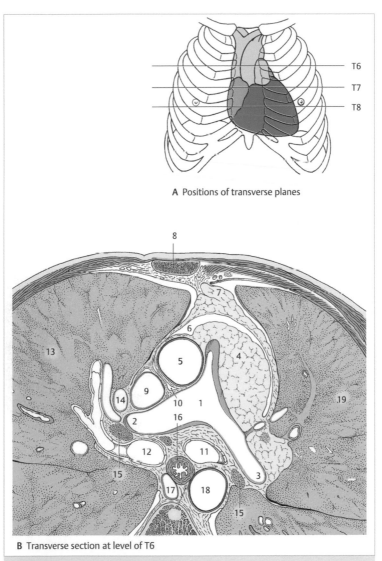

A Positions of transverse planes

B Transverse section at level of T6

Fig. 2.16 Cross-sectional anatomy of the heart.

Cardiovascular System

Cross-Sectional Anatomy, cont.

Transverse Section through the Body at T7 (A)

The image is through the *aorta* at the level of the *semilunar cusps* (**A1**). Anterior to the aorta, the outflow tract of the right ventricle, the *conus arteriosus* (**A2**), can be identified. Curving around the right side of the aorta is the *auricle* (**A3**) of the right atrium. On the left side, in the *subepicardial fat* (**A4**) near the aorta, a section of the *left coronary artery* (**A5**) and *left auricle* (**A6**) is seen. The posterior section of the heart is identified by the *left atrium* (**A7**), which is found in the smooth-walled area of the opening of the inferior *pulmonary veins* (**A8**). Lying posterior and in close proximity to the left atrium, the *esophagus* (**A9**) is shown.

A10 Branch of right pulmonary artery
A11 Branch of left pulmonary artery
A12 Pericardial cavity
A13 Costal cartilage
A14 Right lung
A15 Right inferior pulmonary vein
A16 Azygos vein
A17 Descending aorta
A18 Left lung
A19 Right lobar bronchus
A20 Left lobar bronchus
A31 Thoracic duct

Transverse Section at the Level of T8 (B)

The image is through all four chambers of the heart at the level of the inflow tracts through the atrioventricular valves. The *left ventricle* (**B21**) forms the *apex of the heart* (**B22**), which on the image appears to be directed upward and to the right. The sections through the left and *right ventricle* (**B23**) are easily distinguished by the varying myocardial thickness of the ventricles. On sections through the *subepicardial fat* (**B4**), the *right coronary artery* (**B24**) and *left coronary artery* (**B5**) can be identified. The anterior cusp of the *tricuspid valve* (**B25**) projects into the inflow tract of the right ventricle, and the anterior cusp of the *bicuspid valve* (**B26**) into the inflow tract of the left ventricle. The strong, anterior *papillary muscle group* (**B27**) can also be identified in the left ventricle. The *interatrial septum* (**B28**) can be identified between the two atria, and the *interventricular septum*

(**B29**) between the two ventricles. The close proximity of the left atrium to the *esophagus* (**B9**) is depicted again. The *descending aorta* (**B17**) lies on the left side of the esophagus along its posterior aspect. The *azygos vein* (**B16**) is seen directly anterior to the vertebra.

B10 Branch of right pulmonary artery
B11 Branch of left pulmonary artery
B12 Pericardial cavity (oblique sinus)
B14 Right lung
B15 Right inferior pulmonary vein
B17 Descending aorta
B18 Left lung
B19 Right lobar bronchus
B20 Left lobar bronchus
B30 Right atrium
B31 Thoracic duct

Clinical note: Besides transthoracic echocardiography, the heart can be imaged by transesophageal echocardiography (TEE), because of the proximity of the esophagus and left atrium. This can be enormously helpful in assessing valvular lesions or septal defects and for diagnosing atrial thrombus.

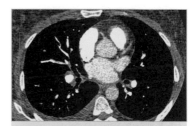

Fig. 2.17C Corresponding plane to Fig. 2.17A on CT.

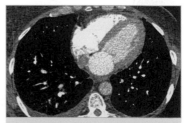

Fig. 2.17D Corresponding plane to Fig. 2.17B on CT.

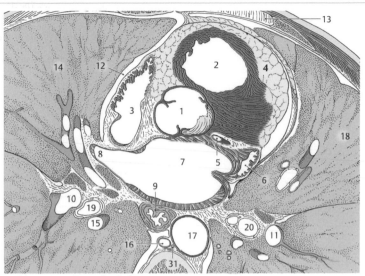

A Transverse section at level of T7

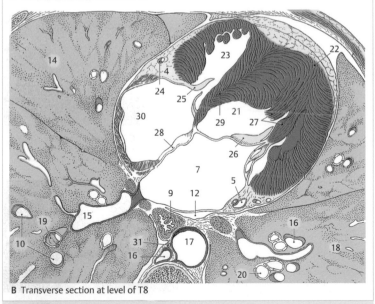

B Transverse section at level of T8

Fig. 2.17 Cross-sectional anatomy of the heart, continued.

Cross-Sectional Echocardiography

Echocardiography, or ultrasound examination of the heart, produces echo signals containing information that can be processed and displayed in various ways. Two-dimensional (2-D) echocardiography obtains pictures from different levels of the patient's heart and vessels, in real-time, instantaneous sectional images. Ultrasound waves travel poorly through bone and are virtually unable to penetrate air, limiting direct access to the heart in the bony thorax to a few acoustic windows for ultrasound examination. Common examinations use parasternal (I), apical (II), subcostal (III), and suprasternal windows (IV). Because the ultrasound transducer can be flexibly manipulated in various positions within a single acoustic window, the planes of 2-D echocardiography can differ considerably from common transverse examination planes applied in other cross-sectional imaging techniques.

Four-chamber view (A). The four-chamber view can be obtained from an apical or subcostal transducer position. This plane runs nearly parallel to the *anterior and posterior wall* of the heart, through the *inflow tract of both ventricles*, so that all four chambers of the heart are imaged simultaneously. The *left atrium* (**A1**) and *left ventricle* (**A2**) are on the right side of the image, the *apex of the heart* (**A3**) at the top, and the *right atrium* (**A4**) and *right ventricle* (**A5**) are on the left side of the image. Additionally, the *interatrial septum* (**A6**) and *interventricular septum* (**A7**), as well as inflow tracts through the *bicuspid* (**A8**) and *tricuspid valves* (**A9**), are visualized. The ventricles can be readily distinguished, as the myocardium of the left ventricle is much thicker than that of the right ventricle. In addition, in the left ventricle, the *anterior* (**A10**) and *posterior* (**A11**) *papillary muscles* are readily visible. The most important feature of this plane is the ability to visualize the *changing position of the bicuspid and tricuspid valves relative to the membranous part of the septum*. In this imaging plane, the tricuspid valve is located higher, that is, originating closer to the apex of the heart, than the bicuspid valve, with part of the membranous septum, the *atrioventricular septum* (**A12**), separating the right atrium and left ventricle.

> **Clinical note:** The four-chamber view is important for **diagnosing congenital heart disease**. It is also useful for evaluating the mitral valve, especially the posterior cusp.

Apical long-axis plane (B). This scan plane is obtained from the **apical window** for imaging the *apical region of the left ventricle* (**B2**), which is directed upward and to the left. The *inflow tract* from the left atrium (**B1**) to the apex of the heart, including the bicuspid valve (**B8**), as well as the *outflow tract* from the apex of the heart to the *aortic valve* (**B13**) are depicted. In front of the aorta (**B15**) is the *outflow tract of the right ventricle* (**B5**). In the left ventricle, the *anterior cusp* (**B14**) of the bicuspid valve can be identified. The *semilunar cusps* (**B13**) of the aorta are also visible when the valve is closed. The section shows how the anterior cusp of the mitral valve separates the inflow and outflow tracts of the left ventricle.

> **Clinical note:** The importance of the apical long-axis view lies in its potential for assessing the **function of the apical region of the heart**, especially following myocardial infarction.

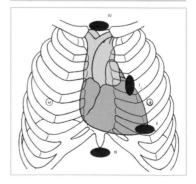

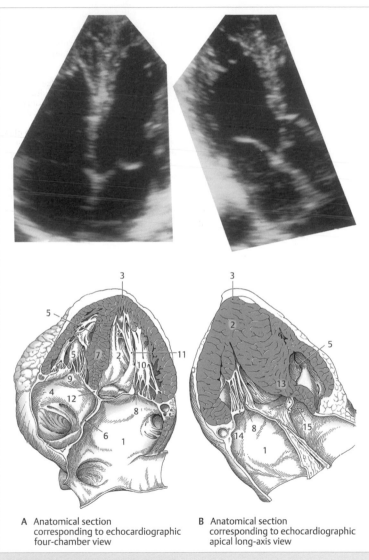

A Anatomical section
corresponding to echocardiographic
four-chamber view

B Anatomical section
corresponding to echocardiographic
apical long-axis view

Fig. 2.18 Cross-sectional echocardiography.

Functions of the Heart

Cardiac Cycle

The heartbeat consists of a **two-phase cardiac cycle**, systole and diastole, continuously repeated throughout life. The ventricles eject blood intermittently into the aorta and pulmonary trunk. In **systole**, the ventricles decrease in width and length, the valvular plane is displaced toward the apex of the heart, and the atria expand (**A**). In **diastole**, the ventricles increase in length and width, the valvular plane is displaced toward the base of the heart, and the atria contract (**B**). The volume of blood ejected during systole from the right or left ventricle (70 mL each) is the **stroke volume**. Proper functioning of the heart's pumping action relies on intact coupling of the conducting system of the heart to the working myocardium. (For further information, please see textbooks of physiology.)

Systole. Contraction of the myocardium at the beginning of systole produces a *rapid increase in pressure* in the ventricles. Both the atrioventricular valves and semilunar cusps of the arteries are initially closed, so that the volume of blood in the ventricles remains unchanged, in what is termed **isovolumetric contraction** (**C**). Once the pressure in the ventricles exceeds that in the aorta and pulmonary trunk, the arterial valves open and the **ejection phase** (**D**) begins. During this phase, a portion of blood, the *stroke volume*, is ejected from the ventricles into the arteries. During the ejection phase, the *valvular plane* (**D1**), along with the atrioventricular valves, is drawn *toward the apex of the heart* (**D2**). This causes the atria to expand, with a suction effect on venous blood from the venae cavae.

Diastole. After blood is ejected during the ejection phase, the ventricular myocardium relaxes and there is a *rapid decrease in pressure*. The pressure in the aorta and pulmonary trunk causes their valves to close, in what is termed the **isovolumetric relaxation phase** (**E**). The *valvular plane* (**E1**) returns to its *original position*. Once the ventricular pressure falls below that of the atria, the atrioventricular valves open, resulting in passive inflow of blood from the atria into the ventricles, in what is known as the **passive ventricular filling phase** (**F**). During ventricular diastole, the atrial musculature is already contracting, actively forcing a small amount of atrial blood into the ventricles at the end of ventricular filling.

During systole, the coronary arteries are strongly compressed by contraction of the ventricular muscle. Nutrient blood supply to the myocardium, especially to the left ventricle, occurs only during diastole. During systole, the coronary veins empty.

Endocrine Function of the Heart

The stretch-sensitive atria, especially the *right auricle*, contain highly differentiated *hormone-producing endocrine myocardial cells* that produce the **atrial natriuretic peptide** (**ANP** or **cardiodilatin**) (see p. 362). This hormone regulates vascular tone, as well as sodium and water excretion from the kidneys. *Atrial distention* is an adequate stimulus for its release.

> **Clinical note:** An elevated BNP level in blood is an early indicator of **heart failure**. BNP stands for B-type natriuretic peptide and is a hormone produced in heart failure by the myoendocrine cells of the left ventricle.

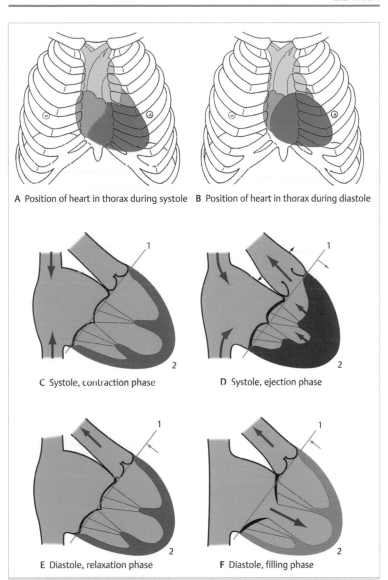

A Position of heart in thorax during systole **B** Position of heart in thorax during diastole

C Systole, contraction phase

D Systole, ejection phase

E Diastole, relaxation phase

F Diastole, filling phase

Fig. 2.19 Functions of the heart.

Cardiovascular System

2.3 Arterial System

Aorta

The aorta arises from the *left ventricle* of the heart and initially ascends behind the pulmonary trunk to the right. The **ascending aorta** (**I**) then curves to form the **aortic arch** (**II**), continues posteriorly over the root of the left lung and, after reaching the level of T4, descends on the left side of the anterior aspect of the vertebral column as the **descending aorta** (**III**).

All arteries of the systemic circulation arise directly or indirectly from the aorta. The following branches arise directly from the aorta:

Ascending aorta. This gives rise to the **right and left coronary arteries** as the first branches of the aorta (see p. 24).

Aortic arch. This gives rise to the great vessels supplying the head, neck, and arms. The first branch arises on the right side as the 2–3-cm long **brachiocephalic trunk** (**A1**). It ascends obliquely to the right over the trachea and divides into the *right subclavian artery* (**A2**), for the right shoulder and arm, and *right common carotid artery* (**A3**), for the right half of the head and neck. Along the left side of the mediastinum, the **left common carotid artery** (**A4**), for the left half of the head and neck, and **left subclavian artery** (**A5**), for the left shoulder and arm, emerge from the aortic arch.

Descending Aorta

Distal to the origin of the left subclavian artery, the aorta tapers slightly to become the **aortic isthmus** (**A6**), forming the junction with the descending aorta. The descending aorta can be divided into the **thoracic aorta** (**III a**), which extends as far as the aortic hiatus of the diaphragm, and the **abdominal aorta** (**III b**), which begins at the aortic hiatus of the diaphragm and extends as far as the aortic bifurcation at the level of L4.

Thoracic aorta. The thoracic aorta gives rise to **parietal branches** segmentally that pass as the **posterior intercostal arteries** (**A7**) to the intercostal spaces 3–11, as well as numerous branches that supply the body wall and spinal cord and its meninges. The **subcostal artery** runs below the 12th rib, hence its name.

Clinical note: The intercostal arteries run along the lower border of the ribs so pleural aspiration should always be sited at the upper border of the ribs.

Smaller, visceral branches include the *bronchial branches*, which branch off at the level of the tracheal bifurcation, and the *esophageal branches*, which arise further distally. The *mediastinal branches* pass to the posterior mediastinum and the *pericardial branches* pass to the posterior aspect of the pericardium. The **superior phrenic arteries** are derived from the inferior portion of the thoracic aorta and are distributed to the diaphragm.

Abdominal aorta. The following **parietal branches** are given off by the abdominal aorta: the **inferior phrenic artery** (**A8**), which arises directly below the diaphragm and gives rise to the *superior suprarenal arteries* (**A9**): the **lumbar arteries** (**A10**), four pairs of segmental arteries which are in a series with the intercostal arteries; and the unpaired **median sacral artery** (**A11**), a small, thin blood vessel that forms the caudal continuation of the aorta.

The **visceral branches** include the **celiac trunk** (**A12**), the common trunk at the level of T12, from which the *left gastric artery* (**A13**), *common hepatic artery* (**A14**), and *splenic artery* (**A15**) arise. Originating about 1-cm distal to the celiac trunk is another unpaired trunk, the **superior mesenteric artery** (**A16**). Arising at some distance is the **inferior mesenteric artery** (**A17**), emerging at the level of L3–4. Arising from the aorta as paired visceral branches, the **middle suprarenal artery**, **renal artery** (**A18**), and **ovarian** or **testicular artery** (**A19**) branch in that order.

At the **aortic bifurcation** (**A20**) at the level of L4, the aorta divides into the *common iliac arteries* (**A21**), which bifurcate at the level of the sacroiliac joint into the *external iliac artery* (**A22**) and *internal iliac artery* (**A23**).

Clinical note: During embryonic development numerous variations involving the aortic arch can arise. The right subclavian artery, for example, can emerge before the end of the aortic arch and pass behind the esophagus to the right side as the arteria **lusoria**. In 10% of cases the **thyroid** ima artery arises from the aortic arch and ascends to the thyroid gland.

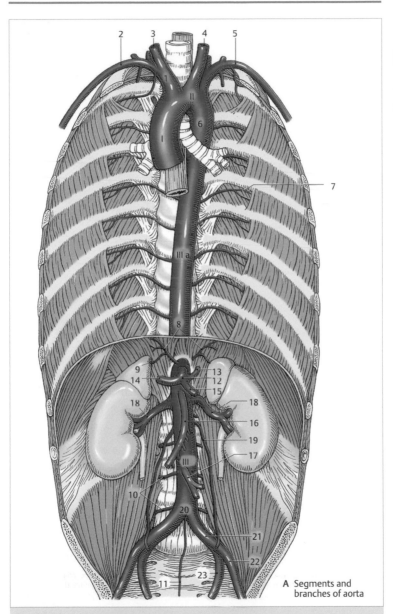

A Segments and branches of aorta

Fig. 2.20 Aorta.

Cardiovascular System

2.4 Arteries of the Head and Neck
Common Carotid Artery

The right common carotid artery (**A1**), originating from the *brachiocephalic trunk* (**A2**), and the left common carotid artery, arising directly from the *aortic arch*, ascend along either side of the trachea and larynx, without giving off any branches.

Together with the *internal jugular vein* and *vagus nerve*, the common carotid artery forms the neurovascular bundle of the neck, which is enclosed in its own connective tissue sheath. Its inferior portion is covered by the sternocleidomastoid. About midway along the neurovascular bundle, the common carotid artery passes to a nonmuscular triangle known as the **carotid triangle** (Vol. 1), where it is covered only by skin, platysma, and superficial cervical fascia. At the level of C6, the common carotid artery can be compressed against the thick anterior tubercle, the **carotid** tubercle (**A3**), and may be compromised.

At the level of C4, the common carotid artery divides into the **external carotid artery** (**A4**) and the **internal carotid artery** (**A5**). The bifurcation of the common carotid artery (**B**) is dilated to form the **carotid sinus** (**B6**), which has *numerous receptors* that monitor changes in blood pressure. Also located at the bifurcation is a chemoreceptor organ, the *carotid body* (**B7**), which responds to the oxygen content of the blood. The internal carotid artery ascends to the interior of the cranium without giving off any branches. The external carotid artery distributes branches to the neck, face, and head.

External Carotid Artery
Anterior Branches

Superior thyroid artery (**AC8**). This arises at the level of the hyoid bone as the first anterior branch of the external carotid artery and curves downward to the anterior surface of the thyroid gland, supplying parts of it. It also gives off a branch, the *superior laryngeal artery* (**AC9**), which pierces the thyrohyoid membrane to supply parts of the inferior of the larynx. Smaller branches, including the sternocleidomastoid and cricothyroid branches, help supply the muscles in the surrounding region.

Lingual artery (**AC10**). This arises near the greater horn of the hyoid bone, as the second anterior branch. It runs under the hyoglossus to the tongue, where it gives rise to the *sublingual artery* (**C11**), which runs anteriorly and inferiorly, sending a terminal branch, the *deep lingual artery* (**C12**), to the tip of the tongue.

Facial artery (**AC13**). This branches off just above the lingual artery and initially lies medial to the mandible and then crosses over the margin of the mandible before the insertion of the masseter. At this site, the pulse of the facial artery can be palpated and the artery can be compromised. The facial artery then follows a tortuous course and ascends to the medial angle of the eye, which it reaches with its terminal branch, the *angular artery* (**A14**). Additional branches include the *ascending palatine artery* (**A15**), *submental artery* (**A16**), *inferior labial branch* (**A17**), and *superior labial branch* (**A18**). The terminal branch of the facial artery anastomoses with the *ophthalmic artery* (see p. 50).

Medial, Posterior, and Terminal Branches

Ascending pharyngeal artery (**A19**). This arises medially from the external carotid artery above the superior thyroid artery and ascends along the lateral wall of the pharynx to the cranial base. Major branches include the *posterior meningeal artery* and *inferior tympanic artery*.

Occipital artery (**A20**). This arises posteriorly and travels in the *occipital groove* medial to the mastoid process (**A21**), to reach the occiput.

Posterior auricular artery (**A22**). The highest posterior branch, this lies between the mastoid process and auricle. Major branches are the *stylomastoid artery* and *posterior tympanic artery*.

Terminal branches. These are the **superficial temporal artery** (**A23**), which divides in the temporal region into the *frontal branch* (**A24**) and *parietal branch* (**A25**) and also gives rise to larger branches, the *transverse facial artery* (**A26**) and *zygomatico-orbital artery* (**A27**), and the largest terminal branch, the **maxillary artery** (**A28**), which supplies the deep facial regions (see p. 48).

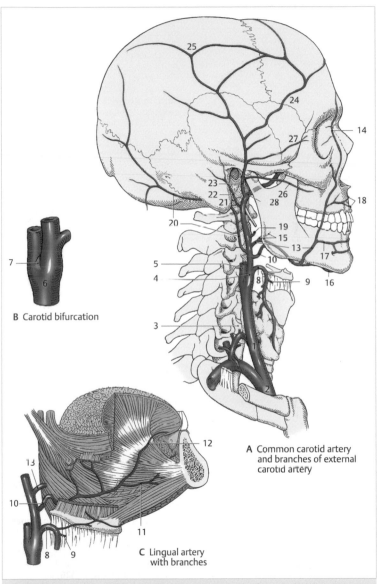

B Carotid bifurcation

A Common carotid artery
and branches of external
carotid artery

C Lingual artery
with branches

Fig. 2.21 Common carotid artery, external carotid artery.

Cardiovascular System

Maxillary Artery

The largest terminal branch of the *external carotid artery* (**A2**), the maxillary artery (**A–C1**), arises below the temporomandibular joint and turns posterior to the *neck of the mandible* (**A3**) to travel to the *deep structures of the face*. There it courses between the *masticatory muscles* and ascends toward the *pterygopalatine fossa* (**A4**).

The course of the maxillary artery can be divided into three parts:

* the first or **mandibular portion** (**I**) passes horizontally behind the neck of the mandible
* the second or **pterygoid portion** (**II**) ascends obliquely at a variable position relative to the masticatory muscles, supplying, in particular, the lateral pterygoid
* the third or **pterygomaxillary portion** (**III**), continues to climb, and passes through the pterygomaxillary fissure to enter the pterygopalatine fossa.

Similarly, the branches of the maxillary artery can be divided into three groups:

Mandibular group. Arising from the first portion of the artery are the **deep auricular artery** (**A5**), which passes to the temporomandibular joint, external acoustic meatus and tympanic membrane, as well as the **anterior tympanic artery** (**A6**), which passes through the petrotympanic fissure to the tympanic cavity. The **inferior alveolar artery** (**A7**) branches off caudally. Before entering the mandibular canal (**A8**), it gives rise to the *mylohyoid branch* (**A9**). The inferior alveolar artery supplies the teeth, bone, and soft tissues of the mandible. It terminates as the *mental branch* (**A10**), which exits through the mental foramen and travels beneath the skin of the chin.

The **middle meningeal artery** (**A11**) is a large, ascending branch that arises from the first part of the maxillary artery. It passes through the foramen spinosum to the middle cranial fossa, where it gives rise to the *frontal branch* (**A11 a**) and *parietal branch* (**A11 b**). The middle meningeal artery is the largest artery supplying the dura mater. It distributes numerous smaller vessels, including the *superior tympanic artery*, which supplies the tympanic cavity.

Pterygoid group. The **arteries supplying the masticatory muscles** arise from the second portion of the maxillary artery. These are the *masseteric artery* (**A12**), *anterior deep temporal artery* (**A13**), *posterior deep temporal artery* (**A14**), and *pterygoid branches*. The **buccal artery** (**A15**) passes to the buccal mucosa and anastomoses with the facial artery.

Pterygomaxillary group. The branches given off by the third portion travel in all directions. The **posterior superior alveolar artery** (**A16**) enters the maxilla and maxillary sinus and terminates as the *dental branches* and *peridental branches*, which supply the back teeth, and fine branches to the nose, lower lid, and lip. The **infraorbital artery** (**A17**) passes forward through the inferior orbital fissure to the orbit, where it travels along the floor of the orbit in the infraorbital canal and passes through the infraorbital foramen (**A18**) to supply the face. In the course of the artery, it distributes the *anterior superior alveolar arteries* (**A19**) to the front teeth, which give off the *dental* and *peridental branches*. The **descending palatine artery** (**A–C20**) arises caudally and passes forward to the hard palate as the *greater palatine artery* (**B22**), through the greater palatine canal (**B21**). The *lesser palatine arteries* are derived directly from the descending palatine artery and supply the soft palate. The *artery of the pterygoid canal* passes backward through the pterygoid canal to the auditory tube and pharynx. The **sphenopalatine artery** (**A–C23**) can be considered the terminal branch of the maxillary artery. It passes through the sphenopalatine foramen to the nasal cavity, where it branches into the *posterior lateral nasal arteries* (**B24**) and *posterior septal branches* (**C25**).

For topography and anatomic variants of the maxillary artery, see Vol. 1.

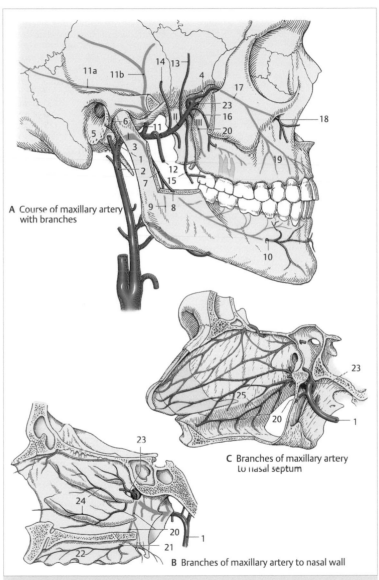

A Course of maxillary artery with branches

C Branches of maxillary artery to nasal septum

B Branches of maxillary artery to nasal wall

Fig. 2.22 Maxillary artery.

Internal Carotid Artery

The internal carotid artery supplies most of the brain, the pituitary, the orbital contents, the forehead, the parts of the face adjacent to the orbits, and also the mucosa of the ethmoid cells, the frontal sinus, and parts of the other paranasal sinuses.

The internal carotid artery can be divided into four portions, based on its course (**A**):

Cervical part (**I**). The cervical part of the internal carotid artery begins at the *carotid bifurcation* (**A1**) and proceeds to the dorsolateral wall of the pharynx, usually without giving off any branches. It accompanies the *vagus nerve* and *internal jugular vein* to the external surface of the cranial base, where it enters the bone through the external opening of the carotid canal.

Petrous part (**II**). The portion of the internal carotid artery that travels in the bony canal is known as the petrous part. This part first ascends in the canal, then curves anteromedially (*carotid knee*) and ascends into the cranial cavity. Important branches of the petrous part of the internal carotid artery include the **caroticotympanic arteries**, which pass to the tympanic cavity.

Cavernous part (**III**). The cavernous part of the internal carotid artery lies in the cavernous sinus and normally has two vascular arches. The vascular arch located near the anterior clinoid process has a pronounced anterior convexity. Together with the initial portion of the cerebral part of the internal carotid artery, it forms the **carotid syphon** (**A2**). The branches of the cavernous part supply the surrounding dura mater, trigeminal ganglion, and, via the **inferior hypophysial artery**, the neurohypophysis.

Cerebral part (**IV**). The cerebral part of the internal carotid artery begins medial to the anterior clinoid process, where the vessel perforates the dura mater. The first branch is the **ophthalmic artery** (**B3**), which travels with the optic nerve into the orbit where it sends branches to the eye, extraocular muscles, and accessory visual structures (see Vol. 3). The cerebral part of the

internal carotid artery typically gives rise to the **posterior communicating artery** (**B4**) posteriorly, which connects to branches of the *vertebral artery* (**B5**) (see below). The next branch is the **anterior choroidal artery**. The internal carotid artery divides into two thick terminal branches, the **anterior cerebral artery** (**B6**) and **middle cerebral artery** (**B7**), each of which supplies large portions of the telencephalon (additional branches and regions supplied by these vessels are described in Vol. 3).

Cerebral Arterial Circle

The **anterior cerebral arteries** are connected with each other via the **anterior communicating artery** (**B8**). The **posterior communicating artery** (**B4**) connects the *internal carotid artery* on either side with *vessels fed by the vertebral arteries* (**B5**), to form the **cerebral arterial circle** (**circle of Willis**), a ring of arteries that form a closed circuit around the sella turcica at the cranial base and supply the brain.

The posterior portion of the arterial circle fed by the vertebral artery is formed as follows: contributing to it from either side is a **vertebral artery** which originates from the *subclavian artery* (see p. 52) and passes through the foramen magnum into the cranial cavity. The two vertebral arteries unite to form the **basilar artery** (**B9**), a large trunk lying on the clivus. The basilar artery gives rise to the *arteries that supply the internal ear* and *cerebellum*, as well as the *posterior cerebral artery* (**B10**). (Additional branches and regions supplied by the arterial circle are described in Vol. 3.)

Branches of the vertebral artery:

B11 Posterior spinal artery

B12 Anterior spinal artery

B13 Posterior inferior cerebellar artery

Branches of the basilar artery:

B14 Anterior inferior cerebellar artery

B15 Labyrinthine artery

B16 Superior cerebellar artery

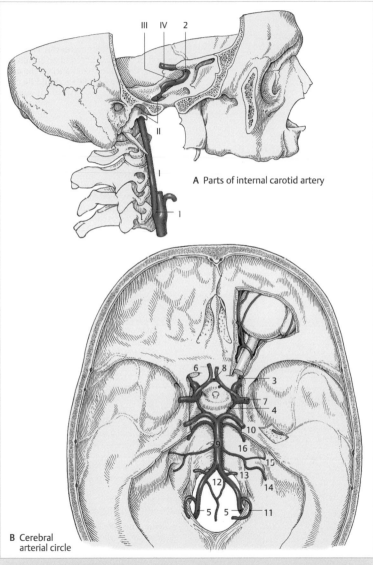

III   IV   2

II

I

I

A Parts of internal carotid artery

6   8

3

7
4

10

9   16

15

13
12   14

5   5   11

B Cerebral
arterial circle

Fig. 2.23 Internal carotid artery.

Subclavian Artery

The subclavian artery conveys blood to part of the neck, the anterior chest wall, the shoulder girdle, and the arm on the same side. It supplies the occipital part of the brain and the cervical spine.

On the **right side**, the subclavian artery (**A1**) arises from the *brachiocephalic trunk* and on the **left**, it arises directly from the *aortic arch*. It can be divided into three parts, based on its relation to the *anterior scalene* (**A2**) muscle: the **first portion** (**I**) extends from the origin of the vessel to the medial margin of the muscle; the **second portion** (**II**) lies posterior to the muscle; and the **third portion** (**III**) extends from the lateral margin of the anterior scalene to the inferior border of the first rib. From that point onward, it is known as the *axillary artery*.

The subclavian artery gives rise to the following large branches:

Vertebral artery (**A3**). The vertebral artery arises from the posterior and superior part of the vessel. From the level of C6 onward, it usually ascends through the foramina in each of the transverse processes. It curves medially on the arch of the atlas and passes through the foramen magnum into the cranial cavity, where it unites with the vertebral artery from the opposite side to form the *basilar artery*. The segments of the vertebral artery are divided with regard to their course, into the *prevertebral part* (**A3 a**), *cervical part* (**A3 b**), *atlantic part* (**A3 c**), and *intracranial part* (**A3 d**) (see p. 50 and Vol. 3).

Internal thoracic artery (**AB4**). The internal thoracic artery arises from the concavity of the origin of the subclavian artery and passes downward and forward to the posterior surface of the first costal cartilage descending parallel to the lateral border of the sternum about 1 cm away from it. It gives rise to the **anterior intercostal branches** (**A5**), which extend toward the diaphragm, and also supplies branches to adjacent structures. Other branches include the **pericardiacophrenic artery**, which supplies the pericardium and diaphragm, as well as the **musculophrenic artery**, which supplies the diaphragm. The terminal branch or prolongation of the internal thoracic artery (**B**) is the **superior epigastric artery**, which, after passing through the diaphragm, enters the rectus sheath. It supplies the abdominal muscles and anastomoses with the *inferior epigastric artery*, which arises from the external iliac artery.

Thyrocervical trunk (**A6**). The thyrocervical trunk usually arises from the anterior and superior part of the vessel and is the common trunk formed by three larger vessels: the **inferior thyroid artery** (**A7**) first ascends, then proceeds medially to reach the posterior side of the thyroid gland, which it supplies along with the pharynx, esophagus, trachea, and parts of the larynx (via the *inferior laryngeal artery*). The *ascending cervical artery* (**A8**), a small ascending branch, is also usually derived from the inferior thyroid artery.

The **suprascapular artery** (**A9**) passes laterally and posteriorly to enter the supraspinous fossa above the superior transverse ligament of the scapula. It continues around the neck of the scapula, where it usually anastomoses with the *circumflex scapular artery* (a branch of the subscapular artery, see p. 54).

The **transverse cervical artery** (**A10**) travels transversely across the neck, passing between the nerves forming the brachial plexus. Its origin, branching pattern, and course are highly variable.

The **posterior scapular artery** (**A11**) arises either as an independent vessel directly from the subclavian artery, or from the *deep branch* of the *transverse cervical artery*. It passes to the levator scapulae.

Costocervical trunk (**A12**). The costocervical trunk arches posteriorly and caudally and gives rise to the **supreme intercostal artery** (**A13**), which runs anteriorly to form the common origin for the two first intercostal arteries, as well as the **deep cervical artery** (**A14**), which passes posteriorly to the muscles of the neck.

Clinical note: The subclavian artery can be constricted in the scalene, particularly in patients with a cervical rib. Certain movements compromise blood flow through the vessel, resulting in symptoms involving the arm and shoulder regions. This is known as scalenus syndrome.

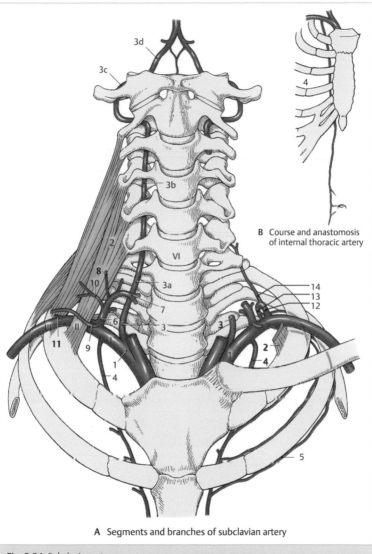

3d

3c

3b

2

VI

8

10

3a

7

6

3

II   II

11   9

1

4

B Course and anastomosis
of internal thoracic artery

4

14
13
12

3

3

2

1

4

5

A Segments and branches of subclavian artery

Fig. 2.24 Subclavian artery.

Cardiovascular System

2.5 Arteries of the Shoulder and Upper Limb

Axillary Artery

The axillary artery (**A1**), the main artery to the arm, passes as the *continuation of the subclavian artery*, from the inferior border of the first rib to the inferior border of the pectoralis major or tendon of the latissimus dorsi (**A2 a**). It is covered on its anterior side by the pectoralis minor (**A2 b**) and pectoralis major.

Arising from the first part of the axillary artery is the variable **superior thoracic artery** (**A3**), which supplies the muscles of the first and second intercostal spaces and the pectoral muscle, subclavius, and upper part of the serratus anterior. Distal to this vessel, a short trunk called the **thoracoacromial artery** (**A4**) arises and divides into numerous branches which pass in all directions, forming the *acromial anastomosis*, a network of arteries near the acromion. The **lateral thoracic artery** (**A5**) runs downward on the serratus anterior, along the lateral thoracic wall. It is thicker in women because it contributes blood to the mammary glands.

The **subscapular artery** (**A6**) arises as a thick vessel at the lateral border of the subscapularis. It divides into the *circumflex scapular artery* (**A7**), which passes through the triangular (medial) space between the teres major and minor muscles, to the infraspinous fossa, and anastomoses with the suprascapular artery (see p. 52 and Vol. 1) and *posterior intercostal artery* (**A8**), which accompanies the thoracoposterior nerve to the latissimus dorsi (**A2 a**). It also supplies the teres major, subscapularis, and serratus anterior. The **anterior circumflex humeral artery** (**A9**) arises from the lateral aspect of the axillary artery and passes anteriorly around the surgical neck of the humerus. The thicker **posterior circumflex humeral artery** (**A10**) passes posteriorly through the quadrangular (lateral) space between the teres major and minor muscles (see Vol. 1) and supplies the shoulder joint and surrounding muscles.

Brachial Artery

The brachial artery (**A11**) is the *continuation of the axillary artery* from the inferior border of the pectoralis major to its division into the arteries of the forearm (**terminal branches:** *ulnar artery* and *common interosseous artery*). Its pulse is palpable in the medial bicipital groove, where it can be compressed against the humerus in an emergency. Its branches mainly supply the humerus, forming part of the **cubital anastomosis**, a vascular plexus around the elbow joint.

The **deep artery of the arm** (**A12**) originates at the lower border of the teres major and passes posteriorly to the humeral shaft. Among the branches given off by the vessel are the *medial collateral artery*, and *radial collateral artery* which pass to the cubital anastomosis.

The **superior ulnar collateral artery** (**A13**) arises distal to the origin of the deep artery of the arm. It runs alongside the ulnar nerve. The **inferior ulnar collateral artery** (**A14**) arises more distally, close to the olecranon fossa above the medial epicondyle. Anatomical variations of the axillary and brachial arteries are common.

Cubital Anastomosis

Encircling the elbow joint is a vascular plexus that is formed by anastomoses between numerous arteries.

The cubital anastomosis is formed by **descending branches** that arise from the *deep artery of the arm* and the *brachial artery* (see above), that is, the *superior ulnar collateral artery* (**A13**), *inferior ulnar collateral artery* (**A14**), *radial collateral artery* (**A15**), and *medial collateral artery* (**A16**). Also contributing to its formation are **ascending branches** (see p. 56) derived from the arteries of the forearm, that is, the *radial artery* (**A17**) and *ulnar artery* (**A18**), which pass as recurrent vessels to the arterial plexus: the *radial recurrent artery* (**A19**), *ulnar recurrent artery* (**A20**), and *recurrent interosseous artery* (**A21**).

Clinical note: The cubital anastomosis permits ligature of the brachial artery distal to the origin of the deep artery of the arm. A patent cubital anastomosis also permits removal of a distal portion of a forearm artery (e.g., radial artery) for use as a graft, as collateral circulation is provided along recurrent vessels via the second large artery of the forearm (ulnar artery).

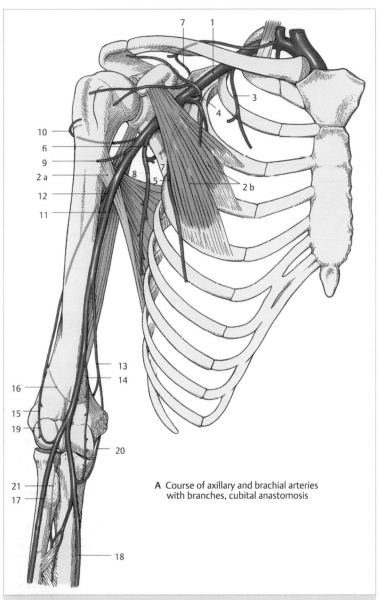

A Course of axillary and brachial arteries with branches, cubital anastomosis

Fig. 2.25 Axillary artery, brachial artery.

Cardiovascular System

Radial Artery

Continuing in the same direction as the *brachial artery* (**A1**) is the *radial artery* (**A2**). The radial artery runs along the radius. Its proximal portion lies between the pronator teres and brachioradialis and its distal portion between the tendons of the brachioradialis and flexor carpi radialis, where its pulse can be palpated. It turns posteriorly and passes between the first two metacarpals, to reach the palm of the hand (see below).

The most important branches of the **radial artery** are:

The **radial recurrent artery** (**A3**) passes as a recurrent vessel to the *cubital anastomosis* (see p. 54).

The **superficial palmar branch** (**A4**) passes to the *superficial palmar arch* (**A5**) (see below).

The **palmar carpal branch** (**A6 a**) passes to the *palmar carpal arch*, a vascular plexus on the palmar side of the wrist.

The **posterior carpal branch** (**B7 a**) passes to the *posterior carpal arch* (**B**), a vascular plexus on the posterior side of the wrist.

The **princeps pollicis artery** (**A8**) arises from the radial artery during its course through the first posterior interosseous and passes to the flexor surface of the thumb.

The **radialis indicis artery** (**A9**) arises either directly from the radial artery or from the princeps pollicis artery and passes to the radial side of the index finger.

The **deep palmar arch** (**A10**) forms the continuation of the radial artery and lies beneath the long flexor tendons (see Vol. 1) on the bases of the metacarpals. It forms anastomoses with the *deep palmar branch of the ulnar artery* (see below).

Ulnar Artery

The ulnar artery (**A11**) is the larger of the two arteries of the forearm. It initially runs deep to the pronator teres in the ulnar direction and then accompanies the flexor carpi ulnaris.

It gives rise to the following branches:

The **ulnar recurrent artery** (**A12**) passes as a recurrent vessel to the *cubital anastomosis*.

The **common interosseous artery** (**A13**) arises embryologically as one of the terminal branches of the brachial artery. It divides into the *posterior interosseous artery* (**A14**), *recurrent interosseous artery* (**A15**), and *anterior interosseous artery* (**A16**).

The **palmar carpal branch** (**A6 b**) arises from the distal portion of the vessel and passes to the *palmar carpal arch*.

The **posterior carpal branch** (**AB7 b**) passes to the *posterior carpal arch*.

The **deep palmar branch** (**A17**) passes to the *deep palmar arch*.

The **superficial palmar arch** (**A5**) is the true terminal branch of the ulnar artery. It lies between the palmar aponeurosis and the long flexor tendons, and anastomoses with the *superficial palmar branch* (**A4**) of the *radial artery*.

Vascular Arches of the Hand

Deep palmar arch. This consists of the **terminal branch of the radial artery** and the **deep palmar branch of the ulnar artery**. It is mainly fed by the radial artery and gives rise to 3–4 thin vessels, the *palmar metacarpal arteries* (**A18**), which pass to the interdigital spaces, as well as the *perforating branches*, which pass to the dorsum of the hand.

Superficial palmar arch. The superficial palmar arch consists of the **terminal branch of the ulnar artery** and the **superficial palmar branch of the radial artery**. It is mainly fed by the ulnar artery and gives rise to three *common palmar digital arteries* (**A19**), each of which sends two *proper palmar digital arteries* (**AC20**) to the radial and ulnar sides of the flexor surfaces of the fingers.

Posterior carpal arch (**B**). The dorsum of the hand is supplied by the **posterior carpal branch of the radial artery** (**B7 a**), which forms a vascular plexus with the **posterior carpal branch of the ulnar artery** (**B7 b**). The plexus gives rise to four *posterior metacarpal arteries* (**B21**), each of which sends two *posterior digital arteries* (**BC22**) to the fingers.

Cardiovascular System

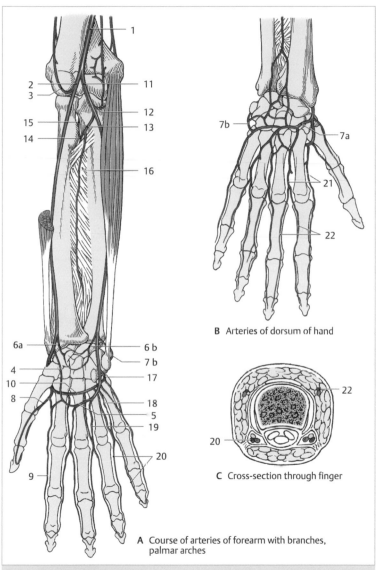

B Arteries of dorsum of hand

C Cross-section through finger

A Course of arteries of forearm with branches, palmar arches

Fig. 2.26 Radial artery, ulnar artery.

Cardiovascular System

2.6 Arteries of the Pelvis and Lower Limb

The abdominal aorta (**A1**) divides in front of L4 into two large trunks known as the **common iliac arteries** (**A2**). They pass on either side toward the plane of the pelvic inlet, without giving off any significant branches, and divide in front of the sacroiliac joint into the **internal iliac artery** (**AC3**) and **external iliac artery** (**AC4**).

Internal Iliac Artery

The internal iliac artery enters the lesser pelvis through the linea terminalis and ramifies at the level of the greater sciatic foramen, usually into two trunks with **parietal branches** to the *wall of the lesser pelvis* and **visceral branches** to the *pelvic viscera*. Its branches are highly variable. Major branches are:

Parietal Branches

The **iliolumbar artery** (**A5**) passes below the psoas major into the iliac fossa and gives rise to an *iliacus branch*, which communicates with the *deep circumflex iliac artery* of the external iliac artery. The **lateral sacral arteries** (**A6**) descend along the lateral portion of the sacrum, sending *spinal branches* to the sacral canal. The **obturator artery** (**A7**) passes anteriorly along the lateral wall of the pelvis, exits the pelvis through the obturator canal, and passes with the *anterior branch* to the adductors of the thigh. It gives rise to a *pubic branch*, which anastomoses with the *inferior epigastric artery* (**AC24**). The *acetabular branch* passes through the ligament of the head of the femur to the head of the femur and a *posterior branch* passes to the deep outer hip muscles.

The **superior gluteal artery** (**AB8**) is the thickest branch. It passes above the piriformis (suprapiriform foramen) to the gluteal muscles, which it supplies via a *superficial branch* and *deep branch*. The **inferior gluteal artery** (**AB9**) passes below the piriformis (infrapiriform foramen) to the surrounding muscles. It gives rise to the *artery to the sciatic nerve* (**B10**), which accompanies the sciatic nerve. In terms of phylogenetic development, it is the principal artery of the leg and in rare situations can serve as such.

Visceral Branches

During fetal life, the **umbilical artery** (**A11**) feeds the placenta (see p. 8). In postnatal life, it is divided into two parts: its proximal, *patent part* (**A11 a**), and an obliterated part, the *occluded part* (**A11 b**), forming the umbilical cord. The patent part of the umbilical artery gives off the *superior vesical arteries* (**A12**), which feed the upper part of the urinary bladder, the *ureteric branches*, and, in the male pelvis, the *artery to the ductus deferens*.

The **uterine artery** (**A13**) corresponds to the *artery to the ductus deferens*, but usually arises directly from the *internal iliac artery*. It supplies the uterus and sends branches to the vagina, ovary, and uterine tube. The **inferior vesical artery** (**A14**) supplies the lower part of the urinary bladder. It sends *vaginal branches* to the vagina and *prostatic branches* to the prostate and seminal vesicle.

The **vaginal artery** (**A15**), often occurring as two or three vessels, supplies the vagina. The variable **middle rectal artery** (**A16**) runs along the pelvic floor to the rectal wall and supplies the muscles of the rectum. The **internal pudendal artery** (**AB17**) usually arises from the internal iliac artery, but occasionally springs from the *inferior gluteal artery*. Its initial portion travels through the infrapiriform foramen, around the ischial spine, and through the lesser sciatic foramen, to reach the lateral wall of the ischioanal fossa. Its branches are: the *inferior rectal artery* (**A18**), *perineal artery* (**A19**), *posterior labial* or *posterior scrotal branches*, *urethral artery* (**A20**), *artery of the bulb of the vestibule* or *bulb of the penis* (**A21**), *deep artery of the clitoris* or *penis* (**A22**) and *posterior artery of the clitoris* or *dorsal artery of the penis* (**A23**).

Clinical note (C): If the vessel connecting the obturator artery (**AC7**) and inferior epigastric artery (**AC24**) is very thick or if the obturator artery arises from the inferior epigastric artery, it can be injured during surgery in the inguinal region, resulting in death from hemorrhage. Hence the name "**aberrant obturator artery**" (**corona mortis**) (**C25**).

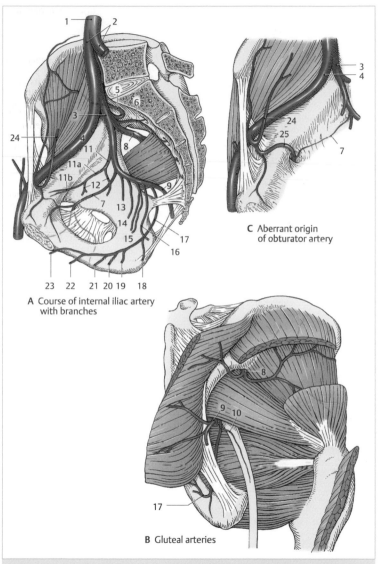

A Course of internal iliac artery with branches

C Aberrant origin of obturator artery

B Gluteal arteries

Fig. 2.27 Internal iliac artery.

External Iliac Artery

The *second branch of the common iliac artery* (**AC1**), the external iliac artery (**AC2**), is wider than the internal iliac artery (**AC3**). It courses parallel to the linea terminalis and medial to the iliopsoas, to the vascular space (see Vol. 1). After traveling through this passage, it continues as the *femoral artery* (**AC4**).

With the exception of smaller muscular branches, the external iliac artery does not give rise to any branches during its course. Arising from the **terminal portion** (**A, B**) of the external iliac artery immediately before it leaves the vascular space is the **inferior epigastric artery** (**AB5**), which originates above the inguinal ligament. It ascends in an arch to the posterior surface of the rectus abdominis, producing the *lateral umbilical fold* on the inner surface of the anterior abdominal wall. It anastomoses with the superior epigastric artery from the internal thoracic artery (see p. 52), at the level of the umbilicus. The inferior epigastric artery gives rise to the *pubic branch*, which gives off an *obturator branch*. The obturator branch anastomoses with the *pubic branch of the obturator artery*. The inferior epigastric artery also gives rise to the *cremasteric artery* or *artery of the round ligament of the uterus*, which passes through the inguinal canal with the round ligament to the labium majus.

The **deep circumflex iliac artery** (**AB6**) arises from the external iliac artery opposite in the inferior epigastric artery and arches laterally behind the inguinal ligament toward the anterior superior iliac spine. One of its branches has anastomoses to the *iliolumbar artery*.

Femoral Artery

The femoral artery (**AC4**) is the *continuation of the external iliac artery* distal to the inguinal ligament where it exits the vascular lacuna. It runs medially and anteriorly past the hip joint to reach the iliopectineal fossa, where it is covered only by skin and the fascia of the thigh. Posterior to the

sartorius, it travels in the adductor canal, which gives it passage to the posterior side of the thigh and popliteal fossa, where it becomes the *popliteal artery*.

The femoral artery gives rise to the following branches:

The **superficial epigastric artery** (**AB7**) arises distal to the inguinal ligament and ascends in the skin of the anterior abdominal wall. The **superficial circumflex iliac artery** (**AB8**), which runs toward the anterior superior iliac spine.

The **external pudendal arteries** (**B9**), which pass medially and give off the *anterior scrotal* or *anterior labial branches*, as well as the *inguinal branches*.

The **descending genicular artery** (**C10**), which divides in the adductor canal into the *saphenous branch*, which passes to the leg, and the *articular branch* which passes to the *genicular anastomosis* (see below). The **deep artery of thigh** (**C11**), which is the thickest branch and arises from the posterolateral part of the vessel about 3–6 cm below the inguinal ligament. Its branches and their twigs are highly variable. In general, they can be divided into: the *medial circumflex femoral artery* (**C12**), which passes medially and posteriorly and distributes branches that supply the surrounding muscles and hip joint. The *lateral circumflex femoral artery* (**C13**) arises laterally. One of its branches usually forms a vascular loop around the neck of the femur with the *medial circumflex femoral artery*. The *perforating arteries* (**C14**) are terminal branches (usually three, but as many as five in number). They pierce the adductors near the femur and pass to the posterior aspect of the thigh, which is supplied by their branches.

Clinical note: Because it lies superficially below the inguinal ligament, the femoral artery can be used for diagnostic and therapeutic purposes. A catheter introduced into the femoral artery can be advanced into the great arteries and left half of the heart. In an emergency, the femoral artery can be compressed against the edge of the pelvis.

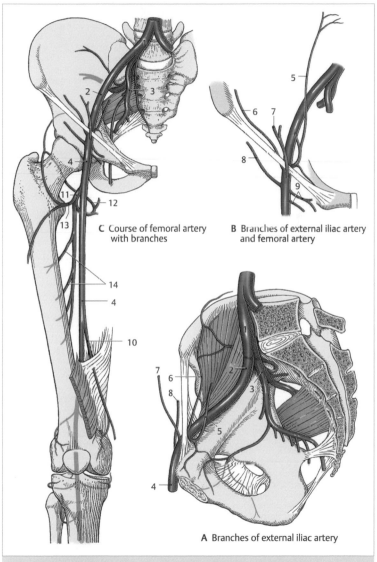

C Course of femoral artery with branches

B Branches of external iliac artery and femoral artery

A Branches of external iliac artery

Fig. 2.28 External iliac artery, femoral artery.

Popliteal Artery

The popliteal artery (**A1**) is the portion of the external iliac artery that courses on the leg from the end of the adductor canal to its division at the inferior border of the popliteus. It lies deep within the popliteal fossa near the capsule of the knee joint and divides into the two arteries that supply the leg, the **anterior tibial artery** (**AB2**), and **posterior tibial artery** (**A3**).

The popliteal artery distributes the following branches to surrounding structures: The **superior lateral genicular artery** (**A4**) and **superior medial genicular artery** (**A5**), which pass laterally and medially forward to the *genicular anastomosis*, an arterial plexus lying on the anterior aspect of the knee joint.

The **middle genicular artery** (**A6**), which passes posteriorly to the joint capsule and cruciate ligaments.

The **sural arteries** (**A7**), which are branches to the calf muscles and the skin and fascia of the lower leg.

The **inferior lateral genicular artery** (**A8**) and **inferior medial genicular artery** (**A9**), which pass anteriorly beneath the lateral and medial heads (origins) of the gastrocnemius, to the *genicular anastomosis*.

Genicular Anastomosis

The genicular anastomosis is an arterial plexus formed by numerous smaller tributaries (see above). Collateral circulation is usually insufficient if the popliteal artery is ligated.

Descending vessels that pass to the genicular anastomosis are the *superior lateral genicular artery* (**A4**), *superior medial genicular artery* (**A5**), and *saphenous branch* of the *descending genicular artery*. **Ascending vessels** are the *inferior lateral genicular artery* (**A8**), *inferior medial genicular artery* (**A9**), *anterior tibial recurrent artery* (**AB10**), and *circumflex fibular branch* of the *posterior tibial artery* (see p. 64).

> **Clinical note:** The popliteal artery must not be ligated, as the collateral circulation through the genicular arteries is insufficient.

Arteries of the Leg and Foot

Anterior tibial artery (**AB2**). The anterior tibial artery pierces the interosseous membrane at the inferior border of the popliteus and passes to the anterior aspect of the leg, where it runs between the extensors to the dorsum of the foot. In addition to *muscular branches*, significant branches include:

The **posterior tibial recurrent artery**, an inconstant vessel that passes to the popliteal fossa.

The **anterior tibial recurrent artery** (**AB10**), which passes as a recurrent vessel to the *genicular anastomosis*. The **anterior lateral malleolar artery** (**B11**) and **anterior medial malleolar artery** (**B12**), which branch to the *lateral malleolar network* and *medial malleolar network* overlying the malleolus.

Posterior artery of the foot (**B13**). The posterior artery of the foot is the *continuation* of the *anterior tibial artery* on the dorsum of the foot (boundary: articular cavity of the talocrural joint). It lies superficially and can be palpated (posterior pedal pulse) between the tendons of the extensor hallucis longus and extensor digitorum longus. It gives rise to the following branches: The **lateral tarsal artery** (**B14**) and **medial tarsal arteries** (**B15**), which supply the area around the posterolateral and posteromedial sides of the tarsus.

The **deep plantar artery** (**B16**), which passes deeply to the sole and contributes to the **deep plantar arch**.

The inconstant **arcuate artery** (**B17**), which runs along the bases of the metatarsals and anastomoses with the *lateral tarsal artery*. Arising from the arcuate artery are the *posterior metatarsal arteries* (**B18**), which pass to the intermetatarsal spaces. These divide distally into the *posterior digital arteries* (**B19**), which pass to the toes.

> **Clinical note:** Compression or bleeding from the anterior tibial artery due to blunt trauma can lead to muscle necrosis (extensor compartment syndrome).

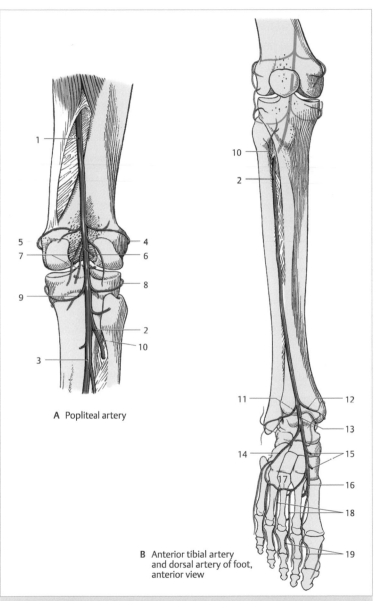

A Popliteal artery

B Anterior tibial artery
and dorsal artery of foot,
anterior view

Fig. 2.29 Popliteal artery, arteries of the leg and foot.

Arteries of the Leg and Foot, cont.

Posterior tibial artery (**A1**). The posterior tibial artery continues in the same direction as the popliteal artery and passes deep to the tendinous arch of the soleus to beneath the superficial flexor group. Its distal portion runs 2 cm in front of the medial border of the Achilles tendon behind the medial malleolus, where its pulse can be palpated. It gives rise to the following branches:

The **circumflex fibular branch** (**A2**), which passes anteriorly through the soleus muscle and around the fibula to the *genicular anastomosis* (see p. 62).

The **fibular artery** (**A3**), which arises in an acute angle from the posterior tibial artery and runs under cover of the flexor hallucis longus near the fibula over the lateral malleolus to the calcaneus. Major branches of the fibular artery are: the *fibular nutrient artery* (**A4**), which passes to the shaft of the fibula; the *perforating branch* (**A5**), which passes to the dorsum of the foot; the *communicating branch* (**A6**), which connects to the posterior tibial artery; and *lateral malleolar branches* (**A7**) to the lateral malleolus. Its branches contribute to the formation of the *lateral malleolar network* (**A8**) and *calcaneal anastomosis* (**A9**). The **tibial nutrient artery** (**A10**), which arises distal and medial to the origin of the fibular artery and passes to the shaft of the tibia.

The medial malleolar branches (**A11**), which pass behind the medial malleolus to the *medial malleolar network* (**A12**). **The calcaneal branches** (**A13**), which pass to the medial surface of the calcaneus and, together with branches from the *fibular artery*, form the *calcaneal anastomosis* on its posterior aspect.

After passing the medial malleolus, the posterior tibial artery divides deep to the abductor hallucis into its two terminal branches, the **medial plantar artery** (**B14**) and **lateral plantar artery** (**B15**).

Medial plantar artery. The medial plantar artery is the medial, and usually thinner, terminal branch that runs along the medial side of the plantar surface of the foot between the abductor hallucis and flexor digitorum brevis. It divides into a **superficial branch** (**B16**), which passes to the great toe, and a **deep branch** (**B17**), which usually connects to the *deep plantar arch* (**B18**).

Lateral plantar artery. The lateral plantar artery is the thicker terminal branch of the posterior tibial artery. It passes in an arch between the flexor digitorum brevis and quadratus plantae, to the lateral side of the plantar surface of the foot, forming the *deep plantar arch* (**B18**) above the metatarsals.

Vascular Arches of the Feet

Deep plantar arch. The deep vascular arch on the plantar surface of the foot corresponds to the deep palmar arch. It gives rise to four **plantar metatarsal arteries** (**B19**), which pass to the intermetatarsal spaces. These send *perforating branches* (**B20**) to the dorsum of the foot. They are continuous with the **common plantar digital arteries** (**B21**), which branch into the *plantar digital arteries proper* (**B22**).

The superficial plantar arch, a superficial arterial arch corresponding to the superficial palmar arch, is usually absent.

> **Clinical note:** Bleeding from the posterior tibial and peroneal arteries can lead to a flexor compartment syndrome, affecting the deep flexor muscles.

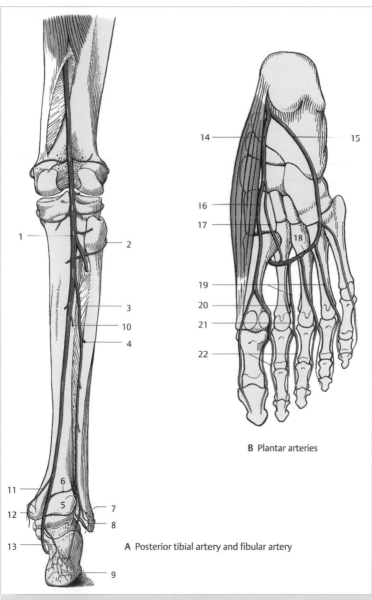

B Plantar arteries

A Posterior tibial artery and fibular artery

Fig. 2.30 Arteries of the leg and foot, continued.

2.7 Venous System

The venous system can be divided into **pulmonary veins** of the pulmonary circulation (see p. 6), the **caval system** of the systemic circulation, and the **portal circulation** to the liver (see p. 216).

The veins of the systemic circulation do not always run parallel to the arteries. A superficial **network of subcutaneous veins**, consisting of vessels lying between the skin and fascia (epifascial veins) without companion arteries, is distinguished from a **network of subfascial veins**, which is usually identical to the pattern of arterial distribution. The deep and superficial systems of veins are usually connected by **perforator veins**.

The **main venous trunks of the systemic circulation** (A) are the *superior vena cava* (**A1**) and *inferior vena cava* (**A2**) (**caval system**). The aorta is accompanied in the thorax by the *azygos vein* (**A3**) and *hemiazygos vein* (**A4**), which are considered remnants of paired longitudinal trunks present during embryonic development (**azygos vein system**). Connections and bypasses between the inferior and superior venae cavae are known as **cavocaval anastomoses**, while connections between the portal vein and venae cavae are referred to as **portal-caval anastomoses**.

Caval System

Superior vena cava. The superior vena cava arises from the union of the **right** (**A5**) and **left brachiocephalic veins** (**A6**), which carry blood to the heart from the head and neck via the *internal jugular vein* (**A7**), as well as from the arms via the *subclavian vein* (**A8**). The main lymphatic trunks open at the union of the subclavian vein and internal jugular vein, the *"venous angle,"* that is, the *right lymphatic duct* (**A9**) on the right side and the *thoracic duct* (**A10**) on the left side.

Inferior vena cava. The inferior vena cava arises from the union of the **common iliac veins** (**A11**), which collect blood from both sides of the body via the *internal iliac vein* (**A12**), which drains blood from the pelvis, and the *external iliac vein* (**A13**), which drains blood from the legs. **Additional tributaries** are the unpaired *median sacral vein* (**A14**), *testicular vein*, or *ovarian vein* on the right side (**A15**), *lumbar veins* (**A16**) and *renal vein* (**A17**) on both sides, and the *right suprarenal vein* (**A18**) on the right side. The *hepatic veins* (**A19**) and *inferior phrenic veins* (**A20**) open just below the diaphragm.

Azygos Vein System

Azygos vein (**A3**). Located on the right side of the body, the azygos vein begins in the abdominal cavity as the **ascending lumbar vein** (**A21**) and empties at the level of L4 or L5, via the *arch of the azygos vein* (**A22**) into the superior vena cava. **Tributaries in the thorax** are: the *right superior intercostal vein* (**A23**) from the second and third intercostal spaces, the *hemiazygos vein* (**A4**) (see below), the variable *accessory hemiazygos vein* (**A24**), which collects blood from the fourth through eighth left intercostal veins (**A25**), and the *esophageal veins, bronchial veins, pericardial veins, mediastinal veins,* and *superior phrenic veins*. The **abdominal portion** of the azygos vein, the ascending lumbar vein (**A21**), receives the *lumbar veins* (**A16**), the *subcostal vein*, and the *right posterior intercostal veins*.

Hemiazygos vein (**A4**). On the left side of the body, the hemiazygos vein also arises from the **left ascending lumbar vein** and receives the corresponding tributaries. It empties at the level of T7 or T8, into the azygos vein.

> **Clinical note:** The azygos system, which drains blood from the chest and abdominal wall through segmental veins, can provide collateral circulation between the superior and inferior vena cava. If the portal vein is occluded, the azygos system forms collateral circulation to the superior vena cava.

Veins of the Vertebral Column

The vertebral column has well-developed venous networks, which may be divided into two groups: **external** and **internal** venous plexuses (**B**).

The **anterior external vertebral venous plexus** (**B26**) forms a network on the anterior aspect of the vertebral bodies. The **posterior external vertebral venous plexus** (**B27**) surrounds the posterior aspect of the vertebral arches and ligament complex. The external vertebral venous plexuses anastomose with the internal plexuses and drain via the *vertebral veins, posterior intercostal veins,* and *lumbar veins*. The **internal vertebral venous plexuses** (**B28** anterior, **B29** posterior) lie epidurally and are better developed than the external vertebral venous plexuses. The internal vertebral venous plexuses are connected to the external vertebral venous plexuses by the **basivertebral veins**.

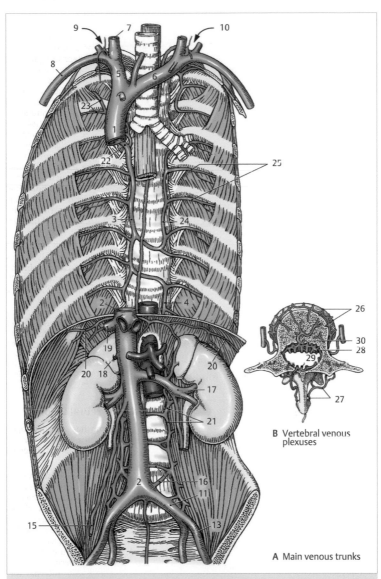

B Vertebral venous plexuses

A Main venous trunks

Fig. 2.31 Caval venous system, azygos system.

2.8 Tributaries of the Superior Vena Cava

The trunk of the **superior vena cava** (**AB1**) is formed by the union of the **right** (**AB2**) and **left** (**A3**) **brachiocephalic veins**. The left brachiocephalic vein is longer than the right one and passes obliquely over the aortic arch (**A4**) and its branches.

Brachiocephalic Veins

The brachiocephalic veins are formed on both sides, by the union of the **internal jugular vein** (**AB5**) and **subclavian vein** (**AB6**). The veins that typically empty into the brachiocephalic veins are:

The **inferior thyroid veins** (**A7**), draining via the **unpaired thyroid plexus** (**A8**) into the left brachiocephalic vein.

Small **veins from surrounding structures**, that is, the thymus, pericardium, bronchi, trachea, and esophagus.

The **vertebral vein** (**AB9**), which communicates with the veins of the cranial cavity and vertebral venous plexuses; the **suboccipital venous plexus**, a venous plexus between the occipital bone and atlas; the **deep cervical vein**.

The **internal thoracic veins** (**A10**), paired companion veins of the internal thoracic artery; the **supreme intercostal vein** and **left superior intercostal vein**.

Jugular Veins

Internal jugular vein. The internal jugular vein is the chief vein draining the neck. Along with the *common carotid artery* and *vagus nerve*, it forms the *neurovascular bundle*, which is enclosed in a common connective tissue sheath. The internal jugular vein commences at the jugular foramen with a dilatation, the **superior bulb of the jugular vein** (**B11**), and extends to the *venous angle*. Immediately before it unites with the subclavian vein, it presents a dilatation known as the **inferior bulb of the jugular vein** (**AB12**). The internal jugular vein drains the cranial cavity, head, and

large portions of the neck. Its extracranial tributaries are:

The **pharyngeal veins** from the *pharyngeal plexus* on the lateral wall of the pharynx; the **meningeal veins**, small veins draining the dura mater.

The **lingual vein** (**B13**), whose course and region of drainage largely corresponds to the distribution area of the lingual artery.

The **superior thyroid vein** (**AB14**), which receives the *superior laryngeal vein*.

The **middle thyroid veins**.

The **sternocleidomastoid vein**.

The **facial vein** (**B15**), which commences at the medial angle of the eye as the *angular vein* (**B16**), which in turn anastomoses with the *ophthalmic* vein. The facial vein receives tributaries from superficial and deep structures of the face. As a large main trunk, it receives the *retromandibular vein* (**B17**), which receives the *superficial temporal veins* (**B18**) from the calvaria and the *pterygoid plexus* (**B19**). The latter lies between the masticatory muscles in the distribution area of the maxillary artery.

External jugular vein (**AB20**). The external jugular vein arises from the union of the **occipital vein** (**B21**) and **posterior auricular vein**. It forms one of the superficial venous trunks of the neck lying on the cervical fascia. It crosses over the sternocleidomastoid and empties near the venous angle, into the *internal jugular vein* or *subclavian vein*.

The second superficial venous trunk of the neck, the **anterior jugular vein** (**AB22**), frequently opens into the external jugular vein. It begins at the level of the hyoid bone and may be connected directly above the sternum by the *jugular venous arch* (**A23**), a transverse vessel connecting it to its counterpart from the opposite side. The **transverse cervical veins** and **suprascapular vein** usually empty into the external jugular vein.

B24 Superior sagittal sinus, **B25** Inferior sagittal sinus, **B26** Straight sinus, **B27** Transverse sinus, **B28** Sigmoid sinus, **B29** Cavernous sinus

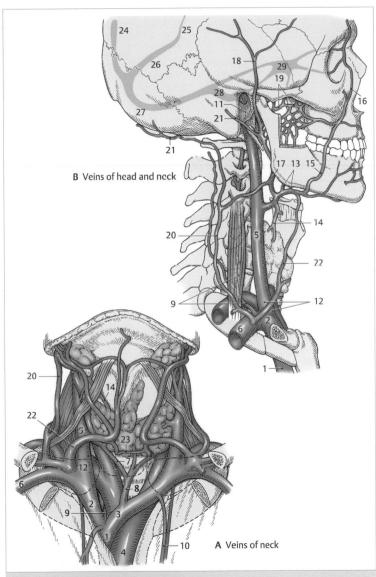

B Veins of head and neck

A Veins of neck

Fig. 2.32 Brachiocephalic veins, jugular veins.

Dural Venous Sinuses

The internal jugular vein receives tributaries from the interior of the cranium via the venous channels of the dura mater known as the dural venous sinuses. The *rigid walls* of these venous channels are formed by the *cranial periosteum* and *dura mater*. The interior of these valveless sinuses is lined with *endothelium*.

At the level of the internal occipital protuberance, several larger dural venous sinuses merge to form the **confluence of sinuses** (**AB1**).

The **transverse sinus** (**AB2**) begins at the confluence of sinuses and continues laterally as the **sigmoid sinus** (**AB3**). The sigmoid sinus travels in an S-shaped course along the posterior inferior border of the petrous part of the temporal bone to the jugular foramen, where the *internal jugular vein* arises.

The **marginal sinus** (**AB4**) encircles the foramen magnum and connects the dural venous sinuses with the *vertebral venous plexuses*.

The unpaired **occipital sinus** (**AB5**) begins at the foramen magnum and travels within the root of the falx cerebelli. It connects the *marginal sinus* with the *confluence of sinuses*.

The **basilar plexus** (**AB6**) refers to the venous plexus lying on the clivus between the *marginal sinus* and *cavernous sinus*.

The **cavernous sinus** (**AB7**) lies on either side of the sella turcica and pituitary gland (**B8**). Passing through the cavernous sinus are the *internal carotid artery* and *abducent nerve*. Lying in its lateral wall are the *oculomotor nerve, trochlear nerve, ophthalmic nerve*, and *maxillary nerve*.

Communicating with the **cavernous sinus** are:

• the *angular vein* (*facial vein*) via the *superior ophthalmic vein* (**B9**)
• the *superior sagittal sinus* via the *sphenoparietal sinus* (**AB10**), which runs on both sides along the margin of the lesser wing of the sphenoid
• the *cavernous sinus* of the opposite side via the *intercavernous sinuses* (**AB11**)
• the *internal jugular vein* via the *inferior petrosal sinus* (**AB12**), which runs on both sides along the inferior border of

the petrous part of the temporal bone and receives the labyrinthine veins from the internal ear
• the *sigmoid sinus* via the *superior petrosal sinus* (**AB13**).

The **superior sagittal sinus** (**A15**), a large venous channel, passes to the *confluence of sinuses* (**AB1**) at the root of the falx cerebri (**AB14**).

The **inferior sagittal sinus** (**A16**) runs within the inferior border of the falx cerebri. It ends above the **straight sinus** (**A17**) in the *confluence of sinuses*. The straight sinus connects the falx cerebri with the tentorium cerebelli (**A18**) and receives the *great cerebral vein* (**A19**).

Additional Intracranial and Extracranial Drainage Pathways

Cerebral veins. Cerebral veins can be divided into **superficial cerebral veins**, superficial vessels, which empty directly into the *dural venous sinuses*, and **deep cerebral veins**, which drain via the *great cerebral vein* into the *dural venous sinuses* (for illustrations and drainage of cerebral veins, see Vol. 3).

Diploic veins. The diploic veins lie in the *diploe* (spongy substance) of the cranial bones and communicate with the *dural venous sinuses*, as well as the *superficial veins of the head*. They receive blood from the dura mater and cranial roof. They can be divided into: *the frontal diploic vein, anterior temporal diploic vein, posterior temporal diploic vein*, and *occipital diploic vein*.

Emissary veins. The emissary veins pass through *preformed cranial openings* and directly connect *cranial venous sinuses* to *extracranial veins*. They are:

• the *parietal emissary vein* (superior sagittal sinus-superficial temporal vein)
• the *mastoid emissary vein* (sigmoid sinus-occipital vein)
• the *condylar emissary vein* (sigmoid sinus-external vertebral venous plexus)
• the *occipital emissary vein* (confluence of sinuses-occipital vein)
• the venous plexus of the hypoglossal canal, venous plexus of the foramen ovale, the internal carotid venous plexus, and portal veins of the hypophysis.

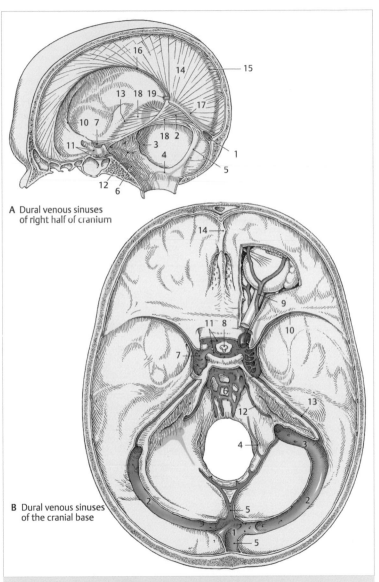

A Dural venous sinuses
of right half of cranium

B Dural venous sinuses
of the cranial base

Fig. 2.33 Dural venous sinuses.

Veins of the Upper Limb

Subclavian vein (A1). The subclavian vein is the *continuation of the axillary vein (A2)*, draining the upper limb to the *venous angle*. It lies between the sternocleidomastoid and anterior scalene muscles and unites behind the sternoclavicular joint with the *internal jugular vein* to form the *brachiocephalic vein*. The **pectoral veins**, **posterior scapular vein** (occasionally), and **thoracoacromial vein** (occasionally) empty into the subclavian vein.

Axillary vein (AC2). The axillary vein runs in the axilla as the companion vein of the axillary artery and collects blood from the area supplied by it via the following **tributaries:** the *subscapular vein, circumflex scapular vein, thoracoposterior vein, posterior circumflex humeral vein, anterior circumflex humeral vein, lateral thoracic vein, thoraco-epigastric veins*, and *areolar venous plexus* around the areola.

> **Clinical note:** Because of their relatively constant position, the deep internal jugular vein and subclavian vein are often used for **central venous** access. The internal jugular vein is more commonly used to obtain access because it can be readily located even by less experienced practitioners, and thus seldom invokes complications. The subclavian vein is the second most commonly used route and is accessed via a supraclavicular or an infraclavicular approach. Subclavian puncture can result in injury to the brachial plexus, subclavian artery, or even pleura, with subsequent pneumothorax.

Deep veins of the upper limb. The deep veins of the arm are *paired* companion veins of arteries. They are divided into: the **brachial veins (A3)**, which accompany the *brachial artery* and unite proximally to form the *axillary vein;* the **ulnar veins (A4)**, lying in the ulnar neurovascular bundle; the **radial veins (A5)**, companion veins of

the *radial artery;* the **anterior interosseous veins (A6)** and **posterior interosseous veins (A7)**, accompanying arteries along the interosseous membrane; the **deep venous palmar arch (A8)**; and **palmar metacarpal veins (A9)** of the palm, of the hand.

Superficial veins of the upper limb. The superficial veins of the arm lie in the subcutaneous tissue above the muscle fascia (epifascial veins). They form an **extensive venous network**, which mainly originates from the **posterior venous network of the hand (B10)**, a well-developed venous plexus on the dorsum of the hand that also receives blood from the less developed *superficial venous palmar arch (C11)* on the palm.

The **cephalic vein (A–C12)** arises from the superficial posterior venous network of the hand (B), passes to the flexor side, ascends proximally on the *radial side* of the forearm and travels along the arm in the *lateral bicipital groove (C)*. It pierces the fascia in the *clavipectoral triangle* and opens into the *axillary vein* (see Vol. 1).

The **basilic vein (AC13)** is a subcutaneous vein that arises above the distal ulna and ascends on the *ulnar side* of the forearm. It pierces the muscle fascia at the middle of the arm, enters the *medial bicipital groove*, and opens into one of the two *brachial veins*.

The cephalic and basilic veins are usually connected at the level of the cubital fossa by the **median cubital vein (C14)**, which passes from inferolateral to superomedial. The subcutaneous veins of the elbow also communicate with deep veins. Subcutaneous veins are highly variable (see Vol. 1).

> **Clinical note:** Subcutaneous veins of the hand and elbow are commonly used for **intravenous injection** or to **draw blood**.

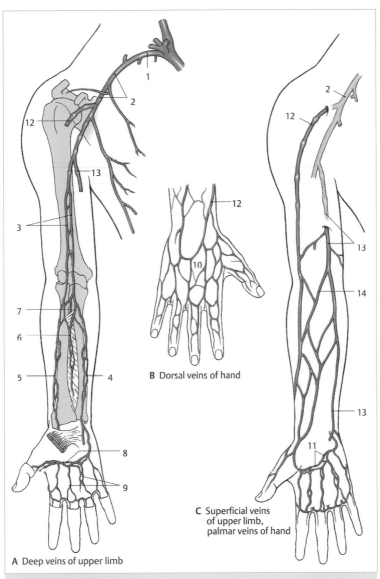

B Dorsal veins of hand

C Superficial veins
of upper limb,
palmar veins of hand

A Deep veins of upper limb

Fig. 2.34 Veins of the upper limb.

2.9 Tributaries of the Inferior Vena Cava

Iliac Veins

Common Iliac Vein

The inferior vena cava (**B1**) arises at the union of the right and left common iliac veins (**AB2**), which extend from the level of L4 to the sacroiliac joint and are derived from the confluence of the **internal** and **external iliac veins**. The **iliolumbar vein** opens into the right and left common iliac veins, and the **median sacral vein** into the left common iliac vein (**AB3**).

Internal Iliac Vein

The valveless **internal iliac vein** (**AB4**) is a short trunk that receives the following veins from the pelvic viscera, pelvic wall, and perineum.

Veins of the Walls of the Trunk

The **superior gluteal veins** (**AB5**) from the buttock region, companion veins of the *superior gluteal artery* that enter the pelvis through the suprapiriform foramen and merge to form a trunk that opens into the internal iliac vein; the **inferior gluteal veins** (**AB6**) from the gluteal region, which accompany the *inferior gluteal artery* and pass through the infrapiriform foramen; the **obturator veins** (**B7**), which drain the adductor muscles of the thigh and emerge from the obturator foramen into the pelvis; and the **lateral sacral veins** (**B8**), which collect blood from the *sacral venous plexus* (**B9**), a venous network lying anterior to the sacrum.

Larger venous plexuses surround the pelvic organs. The **rectal venous plexus** (**AB10**) drains mainly into the *middle rectal veins* (**AB11**) and communicates with the *superior rectal vein*.

Visceral branches. The **vesical venous plexus** (**AB12**) receives the *prostatic venous plexus* or *vaginal venous plexus* (**B13**), as well as the *deep posterior vein of the penis* or *deep posterior vein of the clitoris*. The **uterine venous plexus** (**AB14**) drains into the *uterine veins*. The venous plexuses of the urogenital organs are interconnected.

Venous blood from the pelvic floor and perineum is collected by the **internal pudendal vein** (**B15**). Its tributaries are:

- the *veins of the penis* or *deep veins of the clitoris* (**B16**)
- the *inferior rectal veins*
- the *posterior scrotal veins* or *posterior labial veins*
- the *vein of the bulb of the penis* or *vein of the bulb of the vestibule.*

External Iliac Vein

The external iliac vein (**AB17**) is the proximal *continuation of the femoral vein* (**AB18**) in the vascular lacuna. During its course from below the inguinal ligament to its junction with the *internal iliac vein*, it collects blood from only three tributaries: the **inferior epigastric vein** (**AB19**), which runs on the posterior aspect of the anterior abdominal wall as the companion vein of the *inferior epigastric artery;* the **pubic vein** (**B20**), which *communicates with the obturator vein* and, in rare instances, can replace it (*accessory obturator vein);* the **deep circumflex iliac vein** (**B21**), which arises from companion veins of the deep circumflex iliac artery.

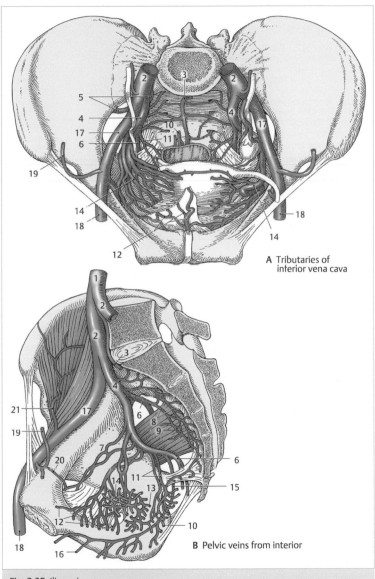

A Tributaries of inferior vena cava

B Pelvic veins from interior

Fig. 2.35 Iliac veins.

Veins of the Lower Limb

Deep Veins of the Lower Limb

Femoral vein (**A1**). The femoral trunk is formed by the deep veins of the lower limb. It accompanies the *femoral artery* and extends from the adductor hiatus of the adductor canal to the inguinal ligament. Near the saphenous opening (see Vol. 1), the femoral vein receives subcutaneous veins from various regions, which drain into it either directly or via the *great saphenous vein* (**ABDE2**):

The **external pudendal veins** (**AB3**), which convey blood from the external genitalia via the *superficial posterior veins of the penis* or *clitoris* and the *anterior scrotal* or *labial veins*. The **superficial circumflex iliac vein** (**AB4**), the companion vein of the superficial circumflex iliac artery in the inguinal region. The **superficial epigastric vein** (**AB5**), which travels along the anterior abdominal wall (**B**) and anastomoses with the *thoraco-epigastric vein* (**B6**) and *paraumbilical veins* (**B7**). The superficial epigastric vein thus forms a connection between the vessels ultimately draining into the inferior vena cava and superior vena cava, that is, it forms a **cavocaval anastomosis**. It is also connected via the *paraumbilical veins* to the portal circulation (see p. 216), forming a **portal-caval anastomosis**.

Another major tributary of the femoral vein is the **deep vein of the thigh** (**A8**), which accompanies the deep femoral artery and receives the following veins:

- the *medial circumflex femoral veins* (**A9**) and *lateral circumflex femoral veins* (**A10**) from the region around the hip joint
- the *perforating veins* from the posterior side of the thigh.

Popliteal vein (**AC11**). The popliteal vein is the companion vein of the *popliteal artery*. It receives the **sural veins** from the leg and the **genicular veins** from the knee. The popliteal vein arises from the union of the paired **anterior tibial veins** (**AC12**) and **posterior tibial veins** (**AC13**), which accompany the anterior and posterior tibial arteries. The *fibular veins* (**AC14**) open into the posterior tibial veins.

The deep veins of the leg communicate via *perforator veins* (**C15**) with the main trunks of the subcutaneous veins. They receive tributaries from the venous plexuses on the posterior and plantar surfaces of the foot.

Superficial Veins of the Lower Limb

Great saphenous vein (**ABDE2**). This is the largest subcutaneous vein of the leg. It begins at the medial border of the foot, ascends medially, and opens at the saphenous opening into the *femoral vein*. It receives the **accessory saphenous vein** (**A16**), which sometimes connects it with the *small saphenous vein* (**ACE17**). It also communicates with the deep veins of the leg, via the **perforating veins** (**C15**), and receives the **external pudendal veins**, **superficial circumflex iliac vein**, and **superficial epigastric vein** at the saphenous opening if they do not open directly into the femoral vein (see above). **Small saphenous vein** (**ACE17**). This arises at the lateral border of the foot and passes over the posterior aspect of the leg to the *popliteal vein*.

Veins that empty into the small saphenous vein (partly also into the great saphenous vein or tibial veins) are: the **posterior venous network of the foot** (**D18**) and **posterior venous arch of the foot** (**D19**) on the dorsum of the foot, which arise from the *posterior digital veins of the foot* (**D20**) and posterior *metatarsal veins;* the **plantar venous network** (**E21**) and **plantar venous arch** (**E22**) on the plantar surface of the foot, which arise from the *plantar digital veins* (**E23**) and *plantar metatarsal veins* (**E24**). The posterior and plantar venous arches of the foot are connected by the *intercapitular veins*.

The **lateral marginal vein** (**E25**) communicates with the *small saphenous vein*, while the **medial marginal vein** (**E26**) communicates with the *great saphenous vein*.

Clinical note: The great and small saphenous veins can become dilated and twisted, forming **varicose veins**. Valves in the vein become insufficient and can no longer move blood toward the heart.

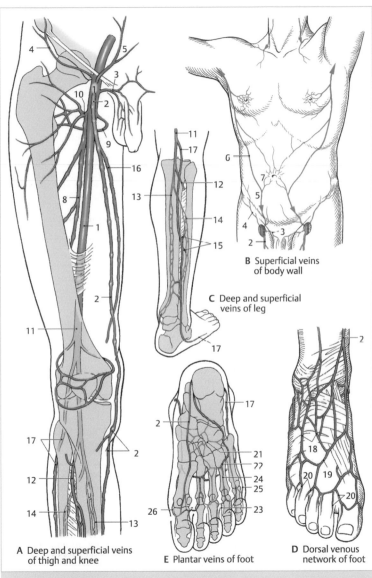

A Deep and superficial veins of thigh and knee

B Superficial veins of body wall

C Deep and superficial veins of leg

E Plantar veins of foot

D Dorsal venous network of foot

Fig. 2.36 Veins of the lower limb.

2.10 Lymphatic System

Lymphatic Vessels

Lymphatic vessels can basically be divided into the following segments:

- lymphatic capillaries
- lymphatic vessels or collectors
- larger lymphatic trunks.

Lymphatic vessel system. The system of lymphatic vessels begins in the periphery of the body, with **lymphatic capillaries**, blind-ended valveless vessels that collect lymph. **Lymph** is a *clear fluid* that arises by *filtration of blood from the arterial part of the capillaries into the interstitial spaces.* It is conveyed through the system of lymphatic vessels to the venous angle and thus returned to the blood circulation. Near their origin, the lymphatic capillaries join to form a network called a **lymphatic rete**, merging to form the thin-walled **lymphatic vessels**, which anastomose freely with each other. Lymphatic vessels possess *valves* and direct the flow of lymph toward the **lymph nodes**, which are interspersed at regular intervals along the course of the lymphatic vessels. Lymphatic vessels can be divided, according to their relation to the general layer of fascia, into *superficial lymph vessels* and *deep lymph vessels.* The lymph collected by lymphatic vessels ultimately flows into two large lymphatic trunks, the **thoracic duct** on the left and the **right lymphatic duct** on the right.

Main Lymphatic Trunks

Thoracic duct (AB1). The thoracic duct is the main trunk of the lymphatic vessel system. It lies below the diaphragm (**A2**) and is derived from a constant, spindle-shaped dilatation, the **chyle cistern** (**AB3**), located on the right side of the aorta (A4). The thoracic duct can be divided into the following portions (**B**): a short **abdominal part** (**I**) in

front of L1, a long **thoracic part** (**II**), a short **cervical part** (**III**) in front of C7, and the **arch of the thoracic duct** (**IV**), the curved portion anterior to the ampulliform dilated opening into the *left venous angle* (**AB5**).

A6 Azygos vein, **A7** Right sympathetic trunk, **A8** Celiac trunk, **A9** Superior mesenteric artery, **A10** Right renal artery

The thoracic duct conveys *lymph from the entire lower half of the body*, as well as *regions on the upper left side of the body.* It receives the following tributaries:

The **right** (**B11**) and **left lumbar trunks** (**B12**), the major tributaries that transport lymph from the *legs, pelvic viscera, pelvic wall*, portions of the *abdominal organs*, and the *abdominal wall* to their union at the *chyle cistern.*

The **intestinal trunks** (**B13**), which convey lymph from the *intestines* and *remaining unpaired abdominal organs* to the thoracic duct. The intestinal trunks unite with the lumbar trunk to form the thoracic duct.

The **left bronchomediastinal trunk** (**B14**), which collects lymph from the *thoracic cavity*. On the left side, it can arise from the union of several lymphatic trunks and open directly into the thoracic duct.

The **left subclavian trunk** (**B15**), which carries lymph from the *left upper limb* and *soft tissues of the left half of the thorax* to the thoracic duct.

The **left jugular trunk** (**B16**), which drains lymph from the *head* and *neck* into the thoracic duct, or directly into one of the two great veins at the venous angle.

Right lymphatic duct (**B17**). The right lymphatic duct drains *regions of the upper right side of the body* and opens into the *right venous angle*. It receives the **right bronchomediastinal trunk** (**B18**), **subclavian trunk** (**B19**), and **right jugular trunk** (**B20**). Tributaries of these vessels correspond to those of the left side of the body.

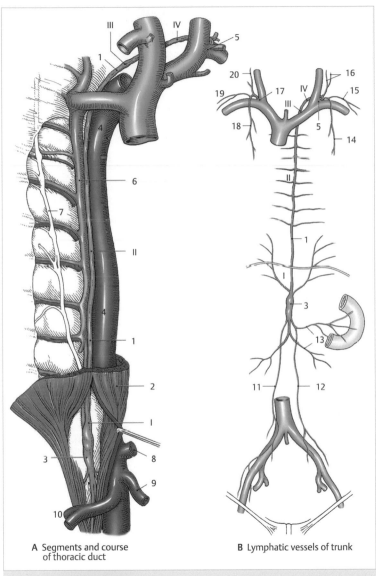

A Segments and course of thoracic duct

B Lymphatic vessels of trunk

Fig. 2.37 Lymphatic vessels.

Regional Lymph Nodes of the Head, Neck, and Arm

Regional lymph nodes are groups of lymph nodes found within a specific region of the body or organ that drain into **central** or **collecting lymph node stations**.

Head. The **occipital nodes** (**A1**) located at the border of the trapezius receive lymph from the *occiput and neck;* the **mastoid nodes** (**A2**), located on the mastoid process, receive lymph from *parts of the ear* and *scalp;* and the **superficial parotid nodes** (**A3**), lying on the parotid fascia, and the **deep parotid nodes** (**A4**), underlying the fascia, receive lymph from the *parotid gland*, parts of the *eyelids, external acoustic meatus*, and *external nose*. These three groups of lymph nodes share a common drainage pathway to the *deep cervical lymph nodes*.

The **facial nodes** (**A5**) are inconstant. They receive lymph from the *eyelids, nose, palate*, and *pharynx*. The **lingual nodes** (**AB6**) mainly drain lymph from the *tongue*, while the **submental nodes** (**AB7**) drain the *floor of the oral cavity, tip of the tongue*, and *lower lip*. All three groups of lymph nodes drain via the **submandibular nodes** (**AB8**), which are located between the mandible and submandibular gland and act as first and second filtering stations. These receive drainage directly from the *medial angle of the eye, cheek, nose, lips, gingiva*, and parts of the *tongue*. They drain into the *deep cervical lymph nodes*.

Neck. The **anterior cervical nodes** can be divided into a **superficial** group of lymph nodes, the *superficial nodes* (**A9**) lying along the anterior jugular vein, and a **deep** group, the *deep nodes* (**B10**), which can be divided into various subgroups by cervical viscera. All anterior lymph nodes ultimately drain into the *deep cervical lymph nodes*.

The **lateral cervical nodes** lie in the lateral part of the neck and can also be divided into

a **superficial** group, the *superficial nodes* (**A11**), situated along the external jugular vein, which collect lymph from the *auricle* and inferior part of the *parotid gland*, and a **deep** group. The latter is usually divided into two groups, the *superior deep nodes* (**B12**), the second lymph node station for nearly all lymph nodes of the head, and *inferior deep nodes* (**B13**), the second lymph node station for nearly all lymph nodes of the neck and the last filtering station for the lymph nodes of the head. The deep cervical lymph nodes drain into the respective *jugular trunk*.

Upper limb. Lymph from the hand and forearm first drains to the elbow, where the superficial and deep **cubital nodes** (**C14**) are located. One or two **supratrochlear nodes** (**C15**) lie medial to the brachial vein, and scattered **brachial nodes** (**C16**) may sometimes be situated further along the course of the brachial vessels.

The **axillary lymph nodes** (**C17**) are major lymph node stations serving the upper limb and anterior thoracic wall. They are interconnected by lymphatic vessels to form a network in the axilla known as the **axillary lymphatic plexus**. Various classifications of axillary lymph nodes into groups are found in the literature. Based on the anatomic nomenclature, they can be divided into *apical nodes* (**C18**) at the superior border of the pectoralis minor, *brachial nodes* (**C16**) along the brachial or axillary artery, *subscapular nodes* (**C19**), *pectoral nodes* (**C20**) at the inferior border of the pectoralis minor, *central nodes* (**C21**), *interpectoral nodes* (**C22**) between the pectoralis major and pectoralis minor, and *deltopectoral nodes* (**C23**) in the deltopectoral triangle. The axillary lymph nodes serve as **regional lymph nodes draining the mammary gland** and *breast* and are extremely important in clinical practice.

C24 Parasternal nodes on the inner aspect of the thoracic wall (see p. 82)

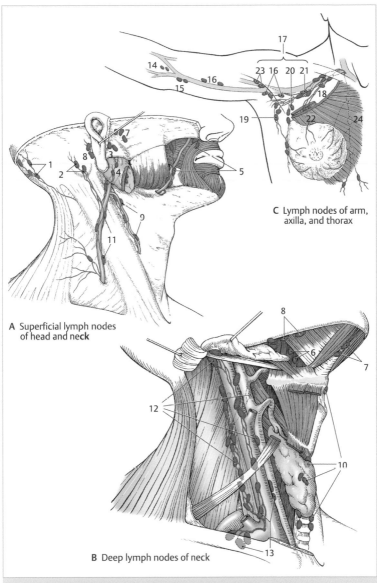

C Lymph nodes of arm, axilla, and thorax

A Superficial lymph nodes of head and neck

B Deep lymph nodes of neck

Fig. 2.38 Regional lymph nodes of the head, neck, and arm.

Regional Lymph Nodes of the Thorax and Abdomen

The lymph node groups of the body cavities can be roughly divided into **parietal lymph nodes**, or **nodes that drain the walls of a body cavity**, and **visceral lymph nodes**, or **nodes lying adjacent to organs**.

Thorax

The **paramammary nodes** lie outside the thorax on the lateral border of the mammary gland.

On the inner aspect of the thoracic wall, lying along the internal thoracic vessels, are the **parasternal nodes** (see p. 80), which receive lymph from the *mammary gland, intercostal spaces, pleura,* and parts of the *liver* and *diaphragm*.

The **intercostal nodes** (**A1**) lie in the posterior portions of the intercostal spaces and receive lymph from the *pleura* and *intercostal spaces;* the **prevertebral nodes** (**AC2**) lie between the esophagus and vertebral column and receive lymph from surrounding regions; the **superior diaphragmatic nodes** (**A3**) are located at the large openings in the diaphragm and receive lymph from the *diaphragm* and *liver;* the **prepericardial nodes** (**B4**), situated between the sternum and pericardium, and the **lateral pericardial nodes** (**B5**) between the mediastinal pleura and pericardium receive lymph from the neighboring areas; the group of nodes comprising the **anterior mediastinal nodes** (**B6**) lies anterior to the aortic arch and receives lymph from the adjacent structures. The **posterior mediastinal nodes** (**C7**) lie in the posterior part of the mediastinum. They are divided into subgroups by the adjacent organs and include the *tracheobronchial nodes* and *paratracheal nodes* along the trachea. The posterior mediastinal nodes receive lymphatic drainage from the *lungs, bronchi, trachea, esophagus, pericardium, diaphragm,* and *liver.*

Abdomen

Parietal lymph nodes. These include the **left lumbar nodes** (**D8**), lying along the abdominal aorta, and **right lumbar nodes**

(**D9**) along the inferior vena cava. Each of these groups of lymph nodes is divided into subgroups of nodes, which receive lymph from the *adrenal glands, kidneys, ureters, testes,* and *ovaries,* as well as the *fundus of the uterus* and *abdominal wall.* Situated between these two groups of lymph nodes are the **intermediate lumbar nodes** (**D10**), which drain the same regions. The **inferior diaphragmatic nodes** (**DE11**) lie on the inferior surface of the diaphragm and drain lymph from this area. The **inferior epigastric nodes** lie on the inner surface of the abdominal wall along the inferior epigastric artery.

Visceral lymph nodes. The **celiac nodes** (**DE12**) lie around the celiac trunk and form the second filtering station for the upper abdominal organs.

The **gastric nodes** (right/left) (**E13**) lie along the lesser curvature of the stomach, and the **gastro-omental nodes** (right/left) (**E14**) lie along the greater curvature of the stomach. The **pyloric nodes** (**E15**) usually lie behind the pylorus.

The **pancreatic nodes** (**DE16**) are arranged along the superior and inferior borders of the pancreas.

The **splenic nodes** (**DE17**) lie at the splenic hilum.

The **pancreaticoduodenal nodes** (**E18**) lie between the pancreas and duodenum. The **hepatic nodes** (**E19**) are located near the porta hepatis.

The 100–150 **mesenteric lymph nodes** (**EF20**) are situated along the root of the mesentery and drain via the *celiac nodes.* The **ileocolic nodes** (**F21**) lie along the ileocolic artery.

The **prececal nodes** (**F22**) and **retrocecal nodes** are located anterior and posterior to the cecum; the **appendicular nodes** (**F23**) lie along the appendicular artery.

The **mesocolic nodes** (**F24**) lie along the mesocolon. Groups of mesocolic nodes receive lymph from the large intestine. The **inferior mesenteric nodes** (**F25**) lie along the inferior mesenteric artery and receive lymph from the descending colon, sigmoid colon, and rectum.

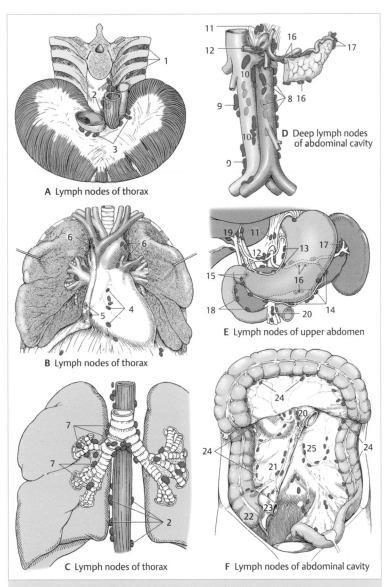

A Lymph nodes of thorax

B Lymph nodes of thorax

C Lymph nodes of thorax

D Deep lymph nodes of abdominal cavity

E Lymph nodes of upper abdomen

F Lymph nodes of abdominal cavity

Fig. 2.39 Regional lymph nodes of the thorax and abdomen.

Regional Lymph Nodes of the Pelvis and Lower Limb

Pelvis

Pelvic lymph nodes can also be divided into **parietal** and **visceral lymph nodes** (**A**).

Parietal groups. The **common iliac nodes** (**A1**) are several groups of parietal lymph nodes lying along either side of the common iliac vessels. They serve as the second filtering station and collect lymph from most of the *pelvic viscera, inner surface of the abdominal wall*, and the *gluteal* and *hip muscles*. They drain into the *lumbar trunk*.

The **external iliac nodes** (**A2**) are numerous groups of lymph nodes that surround the external iliac vessels. They serve as the second filtering station for the *inguinal lymph nodes* and as the first filtering station for parts of the *urinary bladder* and *vagina*.

The parietal **internal iliac nodes** (**B3**) accompany the internal iliac vessels and drain the *pelvic viscera, perineal region*, and *inner* and *outer pelvic walls*.

Visceral groups. These are groups of lymph nodes lying near individual pelvic organs: The **paravesical nodes** (**B4**), arranged in various groups around the *urinary bladder*, draining it as well as the *prostate*. The **parauterine nodes** (**B5**), lying adjacent to the uterus and mostly draining the *cervix of the uterus*.

The **paravaginal nodes** (**B6**), lying adjacent to the *vagina* and draining part of it. The **pararectal nodes** (**B7**), located in the connective tissue lateral and posterior to the rectum. They drain lymph from the *rectum* toward the *inferior mesenteric nodes*. The **anorectal nodes** (**B8**), despite their anatomic nomenclature, should not be considered synonymous with pararectal nodes.

The anorectal nodes receive lymph from the *anal canal* and drain via the *superficial inguinal nodes*.

Lower Limb

The **superficial inguinal nodes** (**C9**) serve as major lymph node stations at the *border between the lower limb* and *trunk*. They are located in the subcutaneous fat of the inguinal region and can be easily palpated if they become enlarged. They receive lymph from the *superficial* vessels of the *leg* as well as the *anus, perineum*, and *external genitalia*. They drain via the parietal *external iliac nodes*.

The **deep inguinal nodes** (**C10**) lie deep to the fascia lata and receive lymph from the *deep* vessels of the *leg*. The uppermost lymph node belonging to this group, the *Rosenmüller node (proximal node)*, can be very large and can be found in the femoral canal.

In the *lower limb*, lymph nodes are often found in the popliteal fossa. The **superficial popliteal nodes** (**D11**) lie at the proximal end of the small saphenous vein, and the **deep popliteal nodes** (**D12**) along the popliteal artery. These serve as the filtering station for lymph from the *foot* and *leg*, on which occasionally an *anterior tibial node, posterior tibial node*, or *fibular node* is found.

Clinical note: Precise knowledge of the regional lymph nodes adjacent to an organ is essential to **removal of cancerous tumors**. Surgery usually removes both the affected organ and its lymph nodes, since the cancerous cells may already have spread to the nodes (metastasis). It should be noted that not all cancers metastasize via the lymphatic system. Because of their clinical importance, regional lymph nodes are also discussed in the sections on individual organs.

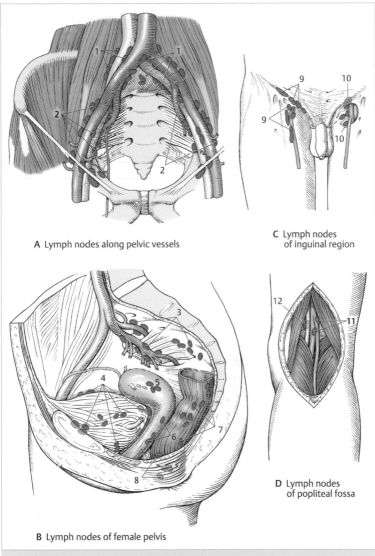

A Lymph nodes along pelvic vessels

C Lymph nodes of inguinal region

B Lymph nodes of female pelvis

D Lymph nodes of popliteal fossa

Fig. 2.40 Regional lymph nodes of the pelvis and lower limb.

Cardiovascular System

2.11 Structure and Function of Blood and Lymphatic Vessels

The walls of blood and lymphatic vessels are very similar in terms of basic structure. The appearance of the vessel wall may vary by location, presenting characteristic modifications to accommodate functional demands and stresses.

Vessel Wall

The vessel wall basically consists of **three layers**, the **tunica interna** (**A1**), or intima; **tunica media** (**A2**), or media; and **tunica externa** (**A3**), or adventitia.

Tunica interna (**intima**). This consists of a layer of longitudinally arranged, flat endothelial cells (**A1 a**) (simple epithelium) that usually rest on a *basement membrane*. Underneath this layer of cells, there is a small amount of connective tissue known as the subendothelial layer (**A1 b**). Arterial walls additionally contain a fenestrated, elastic membrane, the internal elastic membrane (**A1 c**). The tunica intima allows the *exchange of substances, fluids, and gases* through the vessel wall. It is directly affected by the sheer force of blood flowing through the vessel.

In all blood vessels, the endothelial cells are connected by cell-cell contacts (consult a histology textbook for a detailed description). These vary in number and density, according to the vessel segment and organ. Intercellular junctions between arterial endothelial cells tend to be tight, while those in capillaries and postcapillary venules are generally more permeable. The capillaries of some organs, however, have an especially dense barrier (*blood-brain barrier, blood-thymus barrier, blood-testis barrier*, etc.).

Tunica media. The tunica media is the muscular layer and consists of nearly concentric, flat spirals of smooth muscle cells (**A2 a**), as well as interwoven elastic fibers. It forms an especially thick layer in arteries and is usually thinner in veins. The tunica media must counteract the expansion of the vessel wall caused by the pressure of

the blood and, by changing the tension in the smooth muscle, it can adjust the luminal diameter of the vessel.

The media includes the **external elastic membrane** (**A3 a**), which constitutes the border with the tunica externa (adventitia).

Tunica externa (**A3**). The tunica externa consists of connective tissue (**A3 b**) which, in the walls of veins, is accompanied by smooth muscle cells. The cells and interwoven fibers of the tunica externa are arranged longitudinally.

The tunica externa embeds the vessel in the surrounding tissues, and also counteracts external forces such as longitudinal stretching. In most veins, it is therefore especially prominent. In areas where vessels are not subject to longitudinal stretching forces, such as the brain, the tunica externa may be less prominent or even entirely absent.

In large vessels, the vasa vasorum (**A3 c**), blood vessels supplying the vessel walls, penetrate the tunica externa to the outer layers of the vessel wall. The inner layers are supplied by the blood flowing through the vessel. Autonomic nerves, which supply vessel musculature, enter the vessel wall through the tunica externa.

Integration of blood vessels in the musculoskeletal system. Arteries and their companion veins generally pass over the flexor surface of a joint (**B**). When a joint is flexed, the vessels are neither stretched nor compressed. The risk of kinking is avoided by the enclosure of blood vessels and accompanying nerves in a malleable fat body. This allows the vessels to reduce their longitudinal tension and, thus, their absolute length, so that they can accommodate strong flexion.

Special Forms of Arteries

Arteries, mainly small ones, which can close actively to reduce or completely interrupt blood flow to the microcirculation are known as contractile arteries. They have a particularly thick media and obvious internal longitudinal muscle bundles without an internal elastic membrane. Helicine arteries are convoluted, tortuous small arteries. They are found in the penis and uterus.

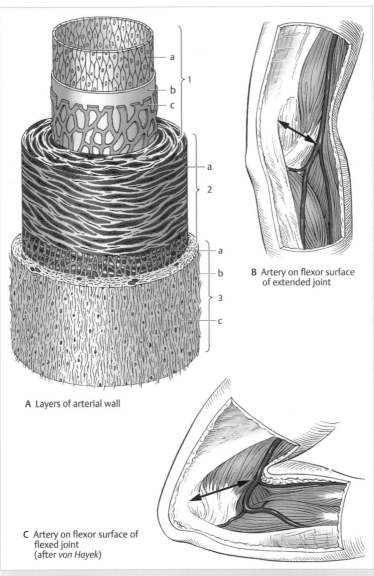

A Layers of arterial wall

B Artery on flexor surface
of extended joint

C Artery on flexor surface of
flexed joint
(after *von Hayek*)

Fig. 2.41 Vessel wall.

Regional Variation in Vessel Wall Structure—Arterial Vessels

The walls of arteries vary in structure depending on their function and proximity to the heart:

The aorta and large arteries near the heart are **elastic arteries**. Their walls have a distinct **three-layered structure**. The *tunica intima* (**A1**) is thick owing to its prominent subendothelial layer. The *tunica media* (**A2**) consists mainly of densely arranged and nearly concentric elastic lamellae, with the appearance of fenestrated membranes on horizontal section. The smooth muscle cells of the tunica media insert directly into these membranes and can adjust and regulate their tension. The *tunica externa* (**A3**) contains vasa vasorum and autonomic nerves within its connective tissue.

Functional anatomy. The aorta and arteries close to the heart are directly exposed to pulsatile cardiac output. During systole (**B**), a portion of the blood ejected with each heartbeat is stored in the vessel wall, the expansion of which is facilitated by the elastic membrane. During diastole (**C**), the elastic membrane acts as a type of "**pressure reservoir**," releasing the stored energy into the blood and propelling it toward the periphery of the body.

Arteries further away from the heart include large peripheral arteries (**D**), as well as all medium-sized and smaller arteries of the systemic circulation (**E**). These are **muscular arteries**. Their *tunica intima* often consists of only endothelium and a small amount of subendothelial connective tissue. The *internal elastic membrane* (**D4**) is a distinct layer composed of elastic fibers and lying between the tunica intima and tunica media. Moving away from the heart, the *tunica media* contains fewer elastic fiber mesh-works, and smooth muscle cells predominate. The *tunica externa* is best developed in medium-sized arteries and is often separated from the tunica media by an *external elastic membrane* (**D5**).

Arterioles (**F**) are precapillary vessels (terminal branches of arteries) with a diameter of only 20–40 μm. Their *tunica intima* consists of endothelium and an *internal elastic membrane*, which may be incomplete. The *tunica media* of arterioles is composed of one or two *concentric* layers of smooth muscle cells, which facilitates their function as precapillary sphincters, allowing vessel diameter to adapt to regulate blood pressure and, at the same time, blood flow to the capillaries.

Capillaries (**G**). The arterioles branch into capillaries, which have an average diameter of 5–15 μm and lack smooth muscle in their walls. Capillaries often form **networks** that are fed by numerous arteries. The capillary wall can be viewed as an endothelial tube (**H**). The *endothelial cells* (**H6**) are surrounded by a *basement membrane* (**H7**) and an outer covering of *pericytes*, both of which are identifiable by electron microscopy. Various **structural types** of the capillary wall can be distinguished by organ function: tightly sealed endothelia lacking fenestration and with a continuous basement membrane (**I**); endothelia with intercellular fenestration with a diaphragm (**II**) or with intracellular pores (**III**), but in either case with a continuous basement membrane; and endothelia with intercellular gaps and a discontinuous basement membrane (**IV**). (These are found, for instance, in: **I** skeletal muscles, **II** the gastrointestinal tract, **III** kidney glomeruli, **IV** liver sinuses.) A few organs such as the liver, bone marrow, spleen, and some endocrine organs, contain very wide capillaries. These are known as sinusoidal capillaries or **sinusoids**.

Vascular connections between arterioles and postcapillary venules (see p. 90) may bypass the capillaries. These are referred to as **arteriovenous anastomoses** and are most predominant in *acral regions* (nose, fingertips, etc.) and *cavernous bodies*.

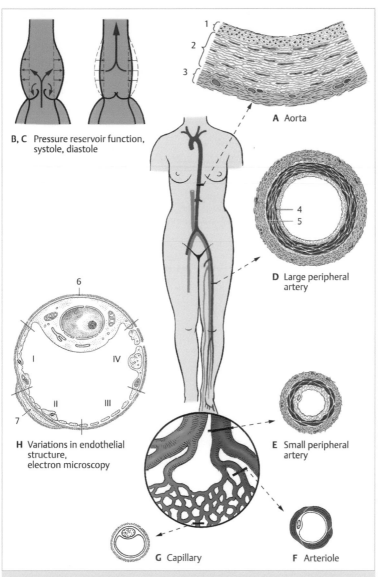

B, C Pressure reservoir function, systole, diastole

A Aorta

D Large peripheral artery

H Variations in endothelial structure, electron microscopy

E Small peripheral artery

G Capillary

F Arteriole

Fig. 2.42 Regional differences in vessel wall structure—arterial vessels.

Regional Variation in Vessel Wall Structure—Venous Vessels

Venules (**B**). On the venous side of the capillary bed, the vessels are continuous with venules. Venules can basically be divided into three segments. **Postcapillary venules** have a diameter of up to 30 μm, and their walls are still lacking smooth muscle cells. **Collecting venules** have a diameter of up to 50 μm and a *tunica media* consisting of fibrocytes and contractile cells. These are continuous with **muscular venules** (**B**), which have a diameter of up to 100 μm and contain irregularly arranged smooth muscle cells in the *tunica media* of their thin walls, which allows for adjustment of vessel diameter. In some organs, the venules are widened to form small "lakes," or blood reservoirs. These vessels are referred to as sinusoidal veins or **venous sinuses**.

Peripheral veins further from the heart (**C**). Blood flows from the venules into small peripheral veins. For the most part, the structure of their walls varies according to the vessel size and the respective region of the body. Veins generally have thinner walls than their companion arteries and it is often difficult to clearly discern the three layers.

In small veins, the *tunica intima* (**C1**) is poorly developed and lacks subendothelial connective tissue; the thin *tunica media* (**C2**) is composed of smooth muscle cells, lying in a flat, spiral arrangement, accompanied by connective tissue. The tunica media blends with the *tunica externa* (**C3**), which consists of collagen fibers, interwoven elastic fibers, and, with increasing vessel caliber, bundles of smooth muscle cells. Small veins give rise to **large peripheral veins** (**D**), the structure of which largely resembles that of the smaller veins. The number of smooth muscle cells in the *tunica externa* increases with increasing vessel caliber. Veins of the body wall and limbs contain **valves** (**DE**) formed by the *tunica intima*. The valves are thus composed of connective

tissue, and their surfaces are completely lined by endothelium. They resemble *pocket valves with two pockets.*

Functional anatomy. Although the veins of some organs do not contain any valves (e.g., brain, kidney, liver), valves are often present in the lower half of the body: in the lower limb, the walls of the veins are compressed by contracting skeletal muscle, which acts as a type of **"muscle pump"** directing blood through the pocket-shaped valves toward the heart. Venous return of blood to the heart is also facilitated by vascular bundles (**F**), usually consisting of two companion veins of a small or medium-sized artery, and bound to the arterial wall by connective tissue in such a manner that the arterial pulse wave narrows the lumen of the vein and propels the blood in the vein toward the heart.

Large veins near the heart. In the upper half of the body, the walls of veins contain scant smooth muscle bundles. The main trunk for the lower half of the body, the *inferior vena cava* (**G**), on the other hand, contains abundant smooth muscle cells: in the subendothelial connective tissue of the *tunica intima* (**G1**), there are longitudinally oriented muscle bundles; the thin *tunica media* (**G2**) contains a few circularly oriented bundles; and the extremely wide *tunica externa* (**G3**) has numerous bundles of longitudinally oriented muscle cells.

In general, veins collect large amounts of blood with minimal changes in pressure, hence the term **"capacitance vessels."**

> **Clinical note:** Enlargement of veins (usually in the lower limb) can lead to valve insufficiency and subsequent outpouchings in the wall of the vein called varices or **varicose veins**.

Lymphatic vessels. The structure of the walls of lymphatic vessels and trunks resembles that of the veins. Lymphatic capillaries consist of a layer of endothelial cells and often lack a basement membrane.

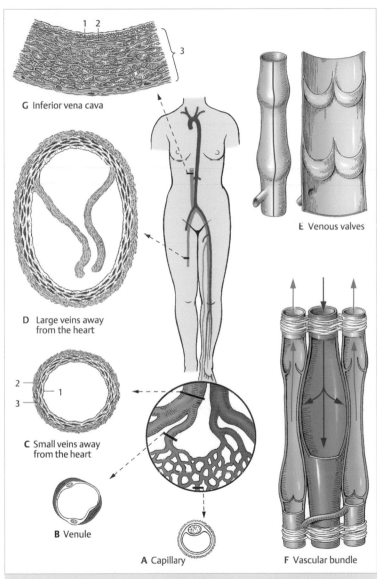

G Inferior vena cava

E Venous valves

D Large veins away from the heart

C Small veins away from the heart

B Venule

A Capillary

F Vascular bundle

Fig. 2.43 Regional differences in vessel wall structure—venous vessels.

3 Respiratory System

3.1 Overview

Anatomical Division of the Respiratory System

The primary task of the organs of respiration, or **respiratory apparatus**, is **"external respiration"**: extracting oxygen from the air and releasing carbon dioxide from the blood. The respiratory system is thus made up of surfaces for gas exchange and passages that conduct air. The **surfaces for gas exchange** consist of the combined surface area of all blind-ending *pulmonary alveoli*, which is very large, measuring 200 m². The pulmonary alveoli make up a significant portion of the *lungs* (**A1**). Inhaled air reaches the pulmonary alveoli through the **conducting airways**, which consist of the *nose* and *nasal cavity* (**A2**), *pharynx* (**A3**), *larynx* (**A4**), *trachea* (**A5**), and numerous levels of the *bronchial tree* (**A6**). Although the main bronchi lie outside the lungs, most of the branches of the bronchial tree are contained within them. On its way through the organs of the conducting airways to the alveoli, inhaled air is filtered, humidified, and warmed.

Along with **gas exchange**, the respiratory organs also serve other functions. These include a **filtering and protective function** of the entire respiratory apparatus; production of **sounds** and **vocalization** by the larynx and adjacent structures; and **olfactory perception** by the olfactory organ situated in the nose.

Clinical Division of the Respiratory System

In clinical practice, respiratory organs can be divided into upper and lower airways. The **upper airways** are chiefly contained in the *head* and include all structures located above the larynx, that is, the **nasal cavities**, adjacent **paranasal sinuses**, and **pharynx**. The paranasal sinuses are *pneumatized spaces* occupying the cranial bones connected to the nasal cavity. In the pharynx, the respiratory and alimentary passages intersect. The **lower airways** lie in the *neck* and *thorax* and consist of the **larynx**, **trachea**, and **bronchial tree**, including its branches as far as the gas-exchanging surfaces of the **alveoli**. Each lung is contained within the thorax in a *pleural cavity* (**A7**), which is lined by a serous membrane and borders medially with the *mediastinum*.

The respiratory organs are derived from the **part of the digestive tube located in the head**, which arises from the inner germ layer known as the **endoderm**, see respiratory system (p. 324).

Clinical Note: To understand the complex topography of the nasal cavities and paranasal sinuses, repeated study of the viscerocranium and its individual bones is recommended. The inferior nasal turbinate, maxilla, ethmoid bone, nasal bone, palatine bone, sphenoid bone, and vomer are involved in the structure of the nasal cavities and paranasal sinuses.

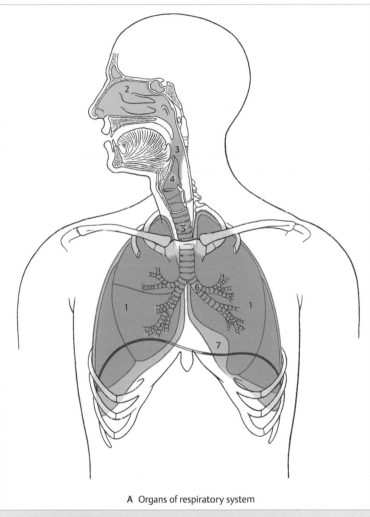

A Organs of respiratory system

Fig. 3.1 Anatomical and clinical organization of the respiratory system.

3.2 Nose

External Nose

The **external nose** (A) is unique to humans and consists of that part of the nose which protrudes from the face and is made up of an osseocartilaginous framework; it gives the human face its characteristic profile. The part of the framework formed by the **root of the nose** (A1) is made up of bone (B). It consists of the two *nasal bones* (B2) and the *frontal process of the maxilla* (B3) (see Vol. 1), which frame the *piriform aperture* (B4) anteriorly. The piriform aperture is completed by plates and rings of hyaline cartilage known as the *nasal cartilages* (C). The paired, triangular cartilaginous plate of the *lateral process* (C5) forms the foundation for the **lateral nasal wall** and the **dorsum of the nose** (AC6). It curves medially to become continuous with the cartilage of the *nasal septum* (see p. 100). The supporting framework of the **ala of the nose** (AC7) is formed on each side by the large, curved *major alar cartilage* (C8) and three or four small *minor alar cartilages*. The major alar cartilage surrounds the **nostrils** (C9), with the *lateral crus* (C8 a), which bounds them laterally, and the *medial crus* (C8 b), directed toward the septum. A small groove is formed at the **apex of the nose** (AD10), where the two major alar cartilages curve around from either side. The nasal cartilages are connected with each other and the surrounding bone by fibrous connective tissue. They lend the external nose a certain rigidity and ensure that the paired nasal cavity and nostrils remain open.

Around the nose there are numerous subcutaneous **mimetic muscles** (see Vol. 1), whose fibers mainly insert into the skin of the *ala of the nose* and *nasolabial groove* (A11). The mimetic muscles not only control the involvement of the *nose in facial expression*, they also serve to *dilate and* constrict the nostrils. Most of the external nose is covered by a thin layer of **skin**, which is thicker over the alae and apex. The skin of the nose contains numerous large *sebaceous glands*.

The **nostrils** (**nares**) (D), which are typically elliptical, form the entrance to the right and left **nasal cavity**; in front of each of these lies the *nasal vestibule* (D12). The lumen of the nasal vestibule is lined with *skin* and normally contains short, brushlike *hairs of the vestibule of the nose* (D13), which act like a weir to trap large particles from inhaled air. The openings of the nostrils lie in an approximately transverse plane.

Vessels, Nerves and Lymphatic Drainage

The external nose is supplied by the **angular artery**, which arises from the *facial artery;* the **posterior nasal artery** from the *ophthalmic artery;* and the **infraorbital artery** from the *maxillary artery.* Venous drainage is supplied by the **facial vein** and **superior ophthalmic vein** (see Vol. 1).

Sensory innervation of the skin of the external nose is supplied by branches of the **ophthalmic nerve** and **maxillary nerve** (see Vol. 1). Motor innervation of the mimetic muscles around the nose is provided by buccal branches of the **facial nerve**.

Lymph from the nose drains together with lymph from the upper and lower lip and cheek, to the *submandibular lymph nodes*.

Clinical note. The veins draining into the facial vein and ophthalmic vein anastomose between the medial angle of the eye and the root of the nose. In inflammation involving the lateral part of the face and external nose, bacteria can thus reach the deep venous sinuses of the cranial cavity and cause **venous sinus thrombosis**.

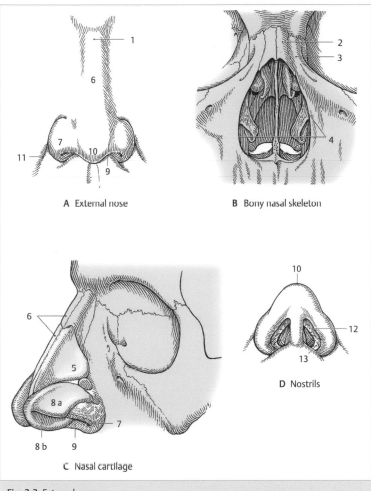

A External nose

B Bony nasal skeleton

C Nasal cartilage

D Nostrils

Fig. 3.2 External nose.

Nasal Cavity

The **nasal cavity** is divided into **right** and **left halves** by the **nasal septum**. The opening of the paired nasal cavity at the *external nostrils* is directed outward, anteriorly, and inferiorly. Each half of the nasal cavity opens posteriorly through an internal nasal aperture, the *choana,* into the continuation of the nasal cavity, the *nasopharynx.* Each half of the nasal cavity has a **floor**, a **roof**, and a **lateral** and **medial wall**. The floor of the nasal cavity is wider, and its roof consists of only a narrow ridge.

Lateral Wall

Bony structure (**A**). The bony lateral wall of the nasal cavity is formed anteriorly by the **maxilla** (**A1**), posteriorly by the **perpendicular plate of the palatine** (**A2**), and superiorly by the **ethmoid** (**A3**). The ethmoid contains numerous variously sized *ethmoidal cells* and forms the bony boundary between the nasal cavity and orbit. The two thin bony plates forming the **superior nasal concha** (**AB4**) and **middle nasal concha** (**AB5**) are also part of the ethmoid; the **inferior nasal concha** (**AB6**) is formed by a separate bone. Each of the conchae projects over a **nasal meatus** of the same name, into which the *paranasal sinuses* and *lacrimal duct* open (see p. 104). The small, superior nasal concha projects above the **superior nasal meatus**, into which the *posterior ethmoidal cells* open. Situated between the superior nasal concha, the adjacent body of the sphenoid (**A7**), and the nasal septum is the narrow **sphenoethmoidal recess** (**A8**), into which the *sphenoidal sinus* opens. Immediately below it is the **sphenopalatine notch** (**A9**), which leads to the *pterygopalatine fossa.* The large, middle nasal concha covers the **middle nasal meatus**, into which the *frontal sinus, maxillary sinus,* and *anterior ethmoidal cells open.* The inferior portion of the ethmoid forms the *uncinate process,* which projects into the middle nasal meatus and covers the orifice of the maxillary sinus. Bulging out over the uncinate process is a large anterior ethmoidal cell called the *ethmoidal bulla* (see p. 104). The thin, inferior nasal concha covers

the **inferior nasal meatus**, which contains the opening of the *nasolacrimal duct.*

Mucosal landmarks (**B**). The nasal mucosa can be divided into three parts: the anterior nasal vestibule, respiratory region, and olfactory region. The **nasal vestibule** forms the entrance to the nasal cavity. It lies within the nostrils and is lined with *skin* (stratified keratinized squamous epithelium). It is separated from the **respiratory region** by a curved ridge known as the *limen nasi* (**B10**). The respiratory region reflects the bony relief pattern of the lateral nasal wall, especially the protruding nasal conchae. Its mucosa is covered by *pseudostratified, ciliated epithelium* and contains numerous mixed glands, the *nasal glands.* The **olfactory region** is a circumscribed area on the lateral nasal wall above the superior nasal concha (**AB4**).

Neurovascular supply (**C**). The anterior and superior parts of the lateral nasal wall are supplied by branches from the **anterior** (**C11**) and **posterior** (**C12**) **ethmoidal arteries**, which arise from the *ophthalmic artery;* the posterior and inferior parts are supplied by branches of the **sphenopalatine artery** (**C13**), which arises from the *maxillary artery.* The veins draining the region run parallel to the course of the arteries, draining via the **ethmoidal veins** into the *ophthalmic vein;* through the sphenopalatine notch via the venous **pterygoid plexus**; and from the nasal vestibule via the **facial vein**. The anterior and superior portions of the nasal mucosa are supplied by sensory branches from the **ophthalmic nerve**; the posterior and inferior portions are supplied by branches of the **maxillary nerve**. The nerves take the same name as the arteries that they accompany. Innervation of the nasal glands is identical to that of the lacrimal glands (see Vol. 3).

Clinical note. The Kiesselbach (or Little) area is an area of mucosa about 1.5-mm wide, with a rich capillary supply at the junction between the nasal vestibule and the actual nasal cavity. This is a frequent site of nosebleeds.

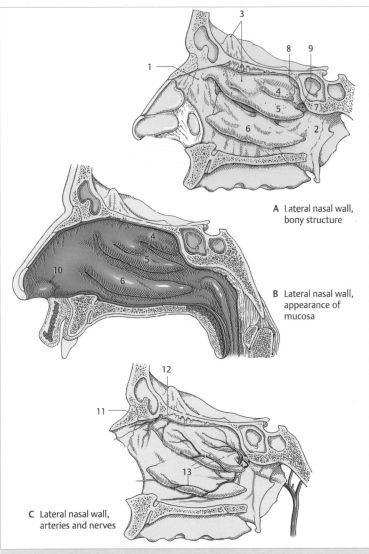

A Lateral nasal wall, bony structure

B Lateral nasal wall, appearance of mucosa

C Lateral nasal wall, arteries and nerves

Fig. 3.3 Nasal cavity.

Respiratory System

Nasal Cavity, cont.

Medial Wall

The **nasal septum** (A) extends slightly out of the nasal cavity into the external nose. Its posterior and inferior portions consist of a **bony part**, and its anterior portion consists of a **cartilaginous part** and **membranous part**.

Bony part (A). The upper part of the bony nasal septum is formed by the **perpendicular plate of the ethmoid** (A1), a sagittally oriented bony plate inserted into the bony roof of the nasal cavity. The anterior and superior parts of the bony roof of the nasal cavity are formed by the **nasal bone** (A2) and the **nasal part of the frontal bone** (A3); the central and superior parts are formed by the **cribriform plate of the ethmoid** (A4); and the posterior part is formed by the **body of the sphenoid** (A5). Articulating with the anteroinferior part of the perpendicular plate of the ethmoid is the **vomer** (A6). The caudal portion of this unpaired bone is inserted into the bony floor of the nasal cavity, which is formed by the **palatine process of the maxilla** (A7) and the **horizontal plate of the palatine bone** (A8). The posterosuperior part of the vomer articulates with the sphenoid. The free posterior margin of the vomer forms the medial boundary of the *choana* (A9).

Cartilaginous and membranous parts (A). Extending from the **cartilaginous part of the nasal septum** (A10), the thin, variably long *posterior process* (A11) is inserted into the gap between the two thin bony plates in the anterior part of the nasal septum. At the dorsum of the nose, the cartilaginous part of the nasal septum contributes to the formation of the external nose with the T-shaped *lateral process* (see p. 96). Inferiorly, the *medial crus* (A12) of the major alar cartilage attaches to the cartilaginous nasal septum. The *vomeronasal cartilage*, a thickened cartilaginous ridge, lies between the cartilaginous and bony parts of the nasal septum. In the adult, the nasal septum usually deviates from the midline at this site (*deviated septum*), so that the two sides of the nasal cavities are of unequal size.

Mucosa (B). The mucosa lying opposite the inferior and middle nasal conchae lines the **respiratory region**. It contains a well-developed cavernous plexus, the anterior part of which is usually identifiable as mucosal thickening and is the most frequent site of epistaxis. The **olfactory region** is located on the upper part of the nasal septum where it meets the *cribriform plate*.

Vessels, nerves, and lymphatic drainage (C). The anterior and superior portions of the nasal septum are similar to the lateral nasal wall, supplied by branches of the **anterior** (C13 a) and **posterior ethmoidal arteries** (C13 b), which are given off by the *ophthalmic artery*. The posterior portion is supplied by branches from the **sphenopalatine artery** (C14), given off by the *maxillary artery*. The sphenopalatine artery travels through the incisive canal (C15) in the hard palate, to anastomose with the *greater palatine artery*. Venous drainage of the nasal septum corresponds for the most part to that of the lateral nasal wall. Sensory innervation is provided by branches of the **ophthalmic nerve** and **maxillary nerve**. One of the terminal branches of the maxillary nerve to the nasal septum travels, as the *nasopalatine nerve* (C16), through the incisive canal to the inferior side of the palate.

Lymph from the **anterior** portion of the nose drains to the *submandibular lymph nodes* and the *superficial nodes of the front of the neck*. Lymph from the **posterior** portion drains to the *retropharyngeal* and *deep cervical lymph nodes*.

Histology of nasal mucosa. The mucosa of the **respiratory region** is lined by **pseudostratified, ciliated epithelium**. The *cilia* wave toward the pharynx, spreading the mucus produced by *goblet cells* and *small nasal glands* over the surface. The nasal mucosa contains veins that form the *cavernous plexus of conchae* in the walls of the conchae. **Olfactory epithelium** is composed of **olfactory cells**, **supporting cells**, and **basal cells**, and with a thickness of 400–500 μm, it is thicker than that of the respiratory region (see Vol. 3).

Clinical note. A severely **deviated septum** can impair nasal breathing on the affected side of the nose.

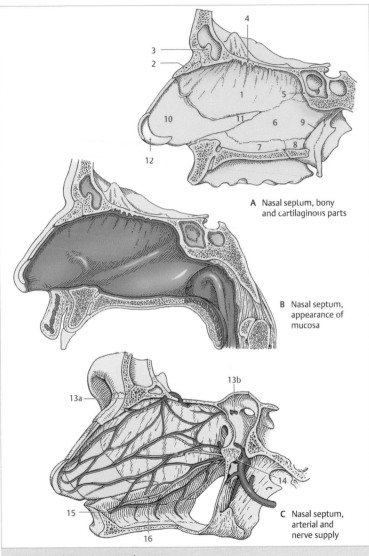

A Nasal septum, bony and cartilaginous parts

B Nasal septum, appearance of mucosa

C Nasal septum, arterial and nerve supply

Fig. 3.4 Nasal cavity, continued.

Paranasal Sinuses

The *paired* **paranasal sinuses** (**A–C**) are mucosa-lined *cavities within the bones adjacent to the nasal cavity.* They are connected to the nasal cavities by small ostia in the lateral nasal wall, through which the *respiratory epithelium* of the nasal cavity continues into the paranasal sinuses, where it is thinner and less well vascularized. The paranasal sinuses are rudimentary at birth and do not attain their full size until after eruption of the permanent teeth.

Frontal sinus (**AB1**). One frontal sinus lies on either side behind the *superciliary arch* (**AB2**) of the frontal bone. A variable **septum** (**A3**) separates the right and left frontal sinuses, typically dividing the irregular cavities asymmetrically, and often deviating from the midline. The **roof** and **posterior wall** of the frontal sinus border with the *anterior cranial fossa;* its **floor**, often a thin bony plate, borders with the *orbit* (**A4**). The frontal sinus is drained into the *middle nasal meatus.*

Ethmoidal cells (**AB5**). The ethmoidal cells are numerous cavities separated by thin, incomplete walls within the ethmoid, which collectively form the ethmoidal labyrinth. On each side, the ethmoidal cells are divided into **anterior, middle,** and **posterior** groups. The cells are highly variable. The largest cell, the **ethmoidal bulla,** is located on the lateral nasal wall above the *hiatus semilunaris.* The ethmoidal cells border **medially** with the upper part of the nasal cavity (**A6**) and **laterally** with the orbit, from which they are separated by only a paper-thin plate of bone. They are adjacent to the *anterior cranial fossa* **above** and the *maxillary sinus* **below**. Depending on their location, the groups of ethmoidal cells open into the *middle* or *superior nasal meatus.*

Maxillary sinus (**A–C7**). With a volume of 12–15 mL, the maxillary sinus is the largest of the paranasal sinuses, completely filling the *body of the maxilla.* Its **roof** forms the *floor of the orbit.* **Anteriorly** and **laterally**, the maxillary sinus is bounded by the *facial surface of the maxilla;* protruding from it **posteriorly** is the *maxillary tuberosity* (**B8**); **medially** it borders with the *nasal cavity.* The **floor** of the maxillary sinus extends into the *dental arch of the maxilla;* its lowest point is between the molar teeth and first premolar tooth. The maxillary sinus opens through its roof into the *middle nasal meatus.*

Sphenoidal sinus (**BC9**). The paired sphenoidal sinus lies in the body of the sphenoid behind the nasal cavity, from whose posterior portion it originally develops. A *septum* divides the variable right and left sphenoidal sinuses and may deviate to one side. The sphenoidal sinus borders **anteriorly** with the *ethmoidal cells;* anteriorly and superiorly with the *optic canal;* **posteriorly** and superiorly with the *hypophysial fossa* (**B10**), which houses the *pituitary gland* (**C11**); and **laterally** with the *carotid sulcus,* which has topographic relations to the *internal carotid artery* (**C12**) and *cavernous sinus* (**C13**). The sphenoidal sinus opens into the *sphenoethmoidal recess.*

Vessels, nerves, and lymphatic drainage. The arterial supply, as well as the venous and lymphatic drainage of the paranasal sinuses, corresponds to that of the nasal cavity.

Clinical note. Infections involving the nasal mucosa can spread to the paranasal sinuses through openings connecting them to the nasal cavity, causing sinusitis. Poorer circulation and unfavorably situated openings can cause impaired drainage of secretion from the paranasal sinuses and lead to **chronic inflammation**. Inflammation of the ethmoidal cells can spread to the orbit by penetrating the thin orbital plate of the ethmoid bone. Surgical approaches through the nasal cavity and sphenoidal sinus may be used to access the pituitary gland (**C**).

Respiratory System

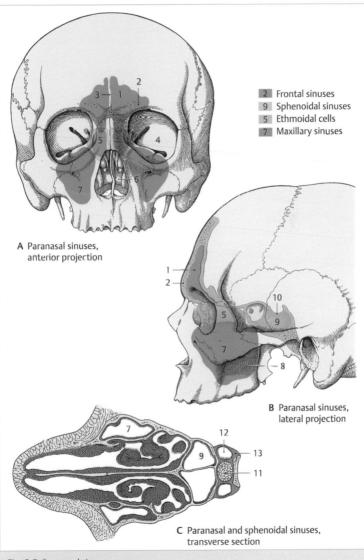

A Paranasal sinuses, anterior projection

2 Frontal sinuses
9 Sphenoidal sinuses
5 Ethmoidal cells
7 Maxillary sinuses

B Paranasal sinuses, lateral projection

C Paranasal and sphenoidal sinuses, transverse section

Fig. 3.5 Paranasal sinuses.

Respiratory System

Openings of Paranasal Sinuses and Nasal Meatuses

Between the posterior margin of the superior nasal concha (**A–C1**) and the anterior margin of the body of the sphenoid is the **sphenoethmoidal recess** (**A2**), into which the **sphenoidal sinus** opens (**AB3**). The bulging *posterior ethmoidal cells* (**A4**) cover the opening of the sphenoidal sinus, which is often difficult to access.

The **posterior ethmoidal cells** have 1–2 openings, which open below the superior nasal concha into the **superior nasal meatus** (**AC5**).

The complex relations of the **middle nasal meatus** (**A–C7**), situated below the middle nasal concha, are visible only after removal of the middle nasal concha. The middle nasal meatus contains the **hiatus semilunaris** (**AB8**), a curved crevice bounded inferiorly by a mucosal fold covering the *uncinate process* (**AC9**) and superiorly by the bulging *ethmoidal bulla* (**A10**). The **frontal sinus** (**AB11**) opens anteriorly and superiorly above the hiatus semilunaris; the **anterior ethmoidal cells** open behind the frontal sinus, and, at the lowest point, the **maxillary sinus** (**C12**) opens. The **middle ethmoidal cells** open above the ethmoidal bulla, which opens superiorly.

The anterior portion of the **inferior nasal meatus** (**AC14**), which lies below the **inferior nasal concha** (**A–C13**), contains the opening of the **nasolacrimal duct** (**A15**). The opening of the nasolacrimal duct is narrowed by a fold of mucosa.

The **nasopharyngeal meatus** (**A16**) extends from the posterior border of the nasal conchae to the choanae. It contains the **sphenopalatine foramen** (**A17**) at the level of the middle nasal concha.

Frontal Sections through the Nasal Cavity (C)

A frontal section between the **anterior** and **middle one-third** of the nasal cavity shows only the *inferior* (**A–C13**) and *middle* (**BC6**) *nasal conchae*, as well as the *uncinate process* (**AC9**). In this region, the *nasal septum* (**C18**) consists of cartilaginous and bony parts. The only identifiable paranasal sinus is the *maxillary sinus* (**C12**), with its opening into the *middle nasal meatus*.

A frontal section through the **posterior one-third** of the nasal cavity shows *all of the nasal conchae*. Here, the *nasal septum* consists entirely of bone. The paranasal sinuses visible in this section are the posterior portion of the *maxillary sinus* and the *posterior ethmoidal cells*.

The extensive venous plexus of the nasal conchae is of practical significance, as it acts as erectile tissue that can dilate or constrict the narrow openings of the paranasal sinuses, depending on stimulus.

C19 Ethmoidal cells

Clinical note. The middle nasal meatus is the access route for endoscopic surgery to treat chronic sinusitis of the frontal sinus, maxillary sinus, and ethmoidal cells.

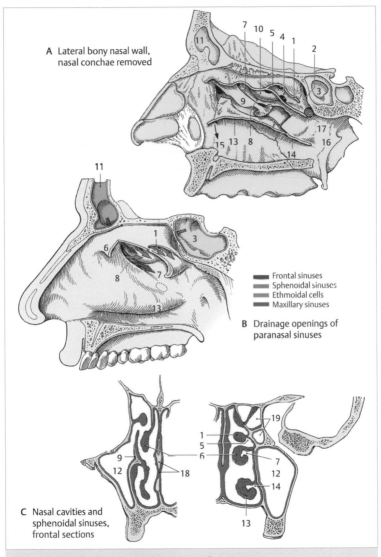

A Lateral bony nasal wall,
  nasal conchae removed

Frontal sinuses
Sphenoidal sinuses
Ethmoidal cells
Maxillary sinuses

B Drainage openings of
  paranasal sinuses

C Nasal cavities and
  sphenoidal sinuses,
  frontal sections

Fig. 3.6 Openings of the paranasal sinuses, nasal passages.

Posterior Nasal Apertures

Each of the nasal cavities opens through a posterior nasal aperture, the **choana**, into the upper portion of the pharynx, the *nasopharynx* (or epipharynx).

Bony margins (**A**). The bony **superior** margin of each choana is formed by the *body of the sphenoid* (**AC1**), which is continuous above and laterally with the root of the *medial plate of the pterygoid process* (**A2**). The latter is penetrated by the *pterygoid canal* (**A3**). The **medial** wall of the choana is formed by the *vomer* (**A4**), a sagittally oriented bony plate. The *ala of the vomer* (**A5**) is inserted superiorly into the roof of the choana. The vomer articulates **inferiorly** with the *posterior nasal spine* (**A6**) of the *palatine bone*. The *horizontal plate of the palatine bone* (**A7**) forms the inferior border of the choanae. The **lateral** border is formed by the *perpendicular plate of the palatine bone*, which further laterally articulates with the *medial plate of the pterygoid process*. The posterior view of the choanae allows visualization of the *inferior* (**A8**) and *middle* (**A9**) *nasal conchae*, as well as the *ethmoidal bulla* (**A10**) and *uncinate process* (**A11**).

A12 Basilar part of occipital bone, **A13** Petrous part of temporal bone

Mucosal landmarks (**B**). The mucosal structure differs according to the bony structures, as well as the muscles and tendons of the soft palate, which frame the posterior nasal apertures.

BC14 Cut edge of posterior wall of pharynx, **BC15** Uvula, **B16** Base of tongue, **B17** Soft palate

Nasopharynx

The following section addresses only the mucosal structure of the **nasopharynx** (**C**), which serves exclusively as a passageway for air (the pharynx is discussed with the alimentary system on p. 168).

The nasopharynx is continuous with the choanae. It is bounded **superiorly** by the *cranial base*, and **laterally** and **posteriorly** by the *pharyngeal wall*. The **inferior** boundary between the nasopharynx and the middle segment of the pharynx, the oropharynx, is formed by the *soft palate* (**BC17**) (see p. 146). In the dome of the **vault of the pharynx** (**C18**) and the upper portions of the posterior and lateral nasopharyngeal walls lies *lymphoid tissue*, which is collectively referred to as the *pharyngeal tonsil* (**C19**) (see p. 416). In the lateral wall 1–1.5 cm from the posterior border of the inferior nasal concha, the **pharyngeal opening of the auditory tube** (**C20**) is located, which leads into the *auditory tube* connecting the nasopharynx and middle ear. The opening of the tube is formed by the *cartilaginous part of the auditory tube*, which produces an elevation in the mucosa known as the *torus tubarius* (**C21**) in front of, above, and behind the opening. Behind the torus tubarius is the **pharyngeal recess** (**C22**). Below the pharyngeal opening of the auditory tube is a less prominent mucosal elevation known as the **torus levatorius** (**C23**), which is produced by the *levator veli palatini*, a muscle of the soft palate. If large masses of lymphoid tissue are present, the pharyngeal tonsil can extend as far as the region around the pharyngeal opening of the auditory tube, forming the *tubal tonsil* (see p. 416).

Clinical note. An enlarged pharyngeal tonsil can occur in children, displacing the choanae and impairing nasal breathing, or displacing the pharyngeal opening of the auditory tube, leading to abnormal ventilation of the auditory tube. A probe and catheter can be introduced through the inferior nasal meatus into the pharyngeal opening of the auditory tube. The torus tubarius and torus levatorius can serve as anatomical landmarks.

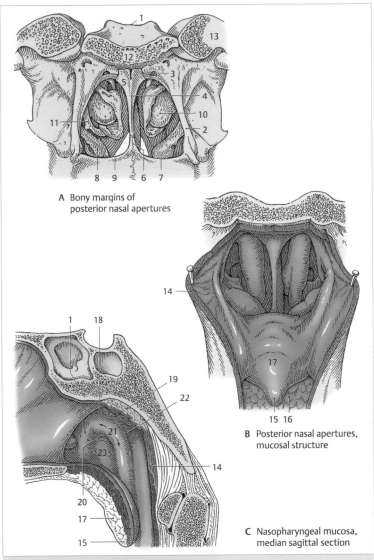

A Bony margins of
posterior nasal apertures

B Posterior nasal apertures,
mucosal structure

C Nasopharyngeal mucosa,
median sagittal section

Fig. 3.7 Posterior nasal apertures and nasopharynx.

Respiratory System

3.3 Larynx

The **larynx** is an **organ of the conducting airway** that extends from the inferior, *laryngeal part of the pharynx* to the *trachea* (**A**). The larynx has the important task of *closing off the lower airways from the pharynx.* In addition, it also contributes to the regulation of vocalization, or *phonation*. The larynx is located opposite C3–C6 in men, but is higher in women and children.

The supporting framework of the larynx, the **laryngeal skeleton**, consists of cartilages that are joined by ligaments and membranes and moved by muscle.

Laryngeal Skeleton

Thyroid cartilage (**B**). The thyroid cartilage consists of two four-sided hyaline cartilage plates known as the **right** (**B1**) and **left laminae** (**B2**). The inferior portions of the laminae unite anteriorly to form a midline wedge. Because of the shape of the plates, the upper part of the wedge projects furthest outward and is visible and palpable, especially in men, as the **laryngeal prominence** (**B3**), commonly known as the "Adam's apple." Above the laryngeal prominence there is a notch in the uppermost margin, the **superior thyroid notch** (**B4**). The laminae diverge posteriorly, and their posterior borders give rise to two narrow projections, the **superior horn** (**B5**), projecting superiorly, and the **inferior horn** (**B6**), projecting inferiorly. The latter bears an articular facet, the *cricoid articular surface* (**B7**), for articulation with the cricoid cartilage. The outer surface of each lamina has a ridge known as the **oblique line** (**B8**), which divides into an anterior and a posterior facet. The *anterior* facet gives rise to the *thyrohyoid* and the *posterior* facet gives attachment to the *sternothyroid* and *inferior constrictor muscle of the pharynx.*

Cricoid cartilage (**C**). The cricoid cartilage is composed of hyaline cartilage. It is shaped like a signet ring encircling the airway with a posterior lamina, the **lamina of the cricoid cartilage** (**C9**), and an anterior arch, the **arch of the cricoid cartilage** (**C10**). At the junction of the lamina and arch, on either side, there is a caudal articular facet known as the *thyroid articular*

surface (**C11**), which articulates with the inferior horn of the thyroid cartilage. The superior border of each lamina of the cricoid cartilage bears two articular facets, the *arytenoid articular surfaces* (**C12**), for articulation with the two arytenoid cartilages. In adults, the cricoid cartilage is at the level of C6.

Arytenoid cartilage (**D**). The two pyramid-shaped arytenoid cartilages, or arytenoids, consist mainly of hyaline cartilage. Each has **three surfaces** (*anterolateral, medial,* and *posterior*) as well as **three borders**, an apex, base, and two processes. The **apex of the arytenoid cartilage** (**D13**) is tilted medially and posteriorly and carries the *corniculate cartilage* (**D14**). The **base of each arytenoid cartilage** (**D15**) has an *articular surface* (**D16**) that is lined with cartilage and articulates with the cricoid cartilage. The base tapers into **two processes**: the laterally and posteriorly directed *muscular process* (**D17**) gives attachment to two *laryngeal muscles,* while the anteriorly projecting *vocal process* (**D18**) gives attachment to the *vocal ligament.*

Epiglottic cartilage (**E**). The leaf-shaped epiglottic cartilage is composed of elastic cartilage and is attached by its stem, the **stalk of the epiglottis** (**E19**), to the inner surface of the thyroid cartilage (see **A**). The convex **anterior surface** (**E20**) of the epiglottis faces the pharynx. It is lined with *nonkeratinized, stratified squamous epithelium.* The concave **posterior surface** faces the laryngeal inlet and is lined with *respiratory epithelium.* The epiglottic cartilage resembles a sieve, with perforations giving passage to *vessels* and *"packages" of glandular tissue.*

The hyaline cartilage of the laryngeal cartilages becomes mineralized and **ossifies** at the end of puberty in both sexes. Ossification occurs earlier and more extensively in boys than in girls. The elastic epiglottic cartilage undergoes regressive changes but does not ossify.

Clinical note. Perichondritis and periostitis can develop following trauma and radiotherapy. Fractures of the laryngeal skeleton lead to disorders of phonation and severe obstruction of the airways, with a risk of suffocation.

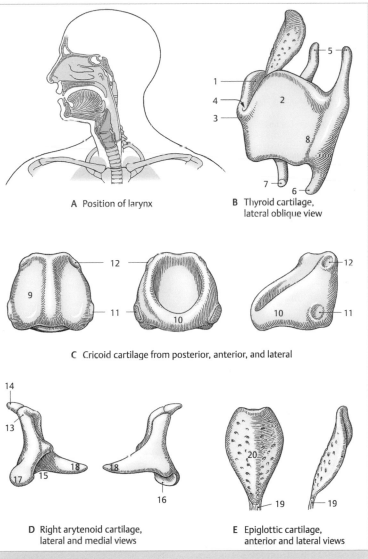

A Position of larynx

B Thyroid cartilage, lateral oblique view

C Cricoid cartilage from posterior, anterior, and lateral

D Right arytenoid cartilage, lateral and medial views

E Epiglottic cartilage, anterior and lateral views

Fig. 3.8 Laryngeal skeleton.

Structures Connecting the Laryngeal Cartilages

The laryngeal cartilages are connected to each other, the hyoid bone, and trachea, by ligaments, joints, and membranes.

Laryngeal Ligaments (A–C)

Stretched between the *superior border of the thyroid cartilage* (**A1**) and the *hyoid bone* (**A2**) is the *thyrohyoid membrane* (**AB3**). The thickened portion of the membrane forms a band of fibers that extends between the superior thyroid notch (**A4**) and the body of the hyoid bone (**A5**), known as the **median thyrohyoid ligament** (**A6**). The portion of the membrane lying lateral to it is thinner and perforated, to allow the passage of the *superior laryngeal vessels* and *internal branch of the superior laryngeal nerve* (**A7**). Another thickened portion of the membrane, the **lateral thyrohyoid ligament** (**A–C10**), passes between the superior horn of the thyroid cartilage (**A8**) and the posterior end of the greater horn of the hyoid bone (**AB9**). It contains a small cartilage known as the *triticeal cartilage* (**A–C11**). The *inferior border of the thyroid cartilage* is connected anteriorly with the *arch of the cricoid cartilage*, by the **median cricothyroid ligament** (**AC12**), which consists mainly of elastic fibers. This band is part of the **conus elasticus** (**AC13**). The *cricoid cartilage* is connected caudally to the *first tracheal cartilage*, by the **cricotracheal ligament** (**AC14**). The *stalk of the epiglottis* is connected by the **thyroepiglottic ligament** (**BC15**) to the *inner surface of the prowlike projection of the lamina of the thyroid cartilage*. The *epiglottis* is connected anterosuperiorly by the **hyoepiglottic ligament** (**C16**) to the *body of the hyoid bone*.

Laryngeal Joints (A–C)

The **cricothyroid joint** (**A–C17**) is a bilateral articulation formed between the *inferior horn of the thyroid cartilage* and the *posterior, lateral surface of the lamina of the cricoid cartilage*. It permits tilting of the cricoid cartilage against the thyroid cartilage, around a horizontal axis passing through both joints. This **tilting motion** changes the distance between the inner surface of

the prowlike projection of the lamina of the thyroid cartilage and the vocal processes.

The **cricoarytenoid joint** (**BC18**) is a bilateral articulation between the articular surfaces on the *base of the arytenoid cartilage* and the *superior border of the lamina of the cricoid cartilage*. The joint is loosely surrounded by a capsule that is reinforced posteriorly by the *cricoarytenoid ligament* (**C19**). The cricoarytenoid joints permit two different movements. The arytenoid cartilage allows **rotational and sliding movement**, whereby the vocal process glides medially or laterally. Rotational movement is accompanied by **tilting** of the arytenoid cartilages. **Gliding movement** allows the arytenoid cartilages to move toward or away from each other. Individual movements can be combined, permitting the vocal process a large radius of motion.

> **Clinical note.** Degenerative changes (arthrosis) occur in the cricoarytenoid joint at an advanced age.

Laryngeal Membranes (C, D)

The submucosal connective tissue of the larynx contains abundant elastic fibers, and is collectively referred to as the **fibroelastic membrane of the larynx**. The **upper portion** lies beneath the laryngeal mucosa, extends as far as the vestibular fold (see p. 114), and is composed of a thin **quadrangular membrane** (**D20**). The free inferior margin of the quadrangular membrane forms the *vestibular ligament* (**D21**). The **inferior portion** of the fibroelastic membrane of the larynx is thicker and is known as the **conus elasticus** (**D13**). It arises from the *inner surface of the cricoid cartilage* and is continuous with the *vocal fold*, whose thickened margin forms the bilateral *vocal ligament* (**CD22**). The anterior portion of the conus elasticus is tough and forms the *median cricothyroid ligament* (**AC12**), extending between the cricoid and thyroid cartilages.

> **Clinical note.** If a life-threatening closure of the rima glottidis occurs, an airway can be established by incision or puncture through the median cricothyroid ligament, which lies below the level of the rima glottidis. This procedure is known as **cricothyrotomy**.

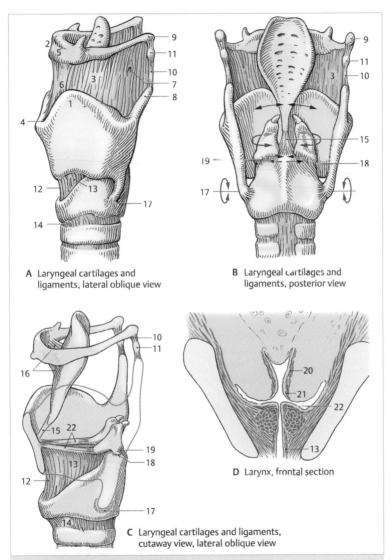

A Laryngeal cartilages and
   ligaments, lateral oblique view

B Laryngeal cartilages and
   ligaments, posterior view

C Laryngeal cartilages and ligaments,
   cutaway view, lateral oblique view

D Larynx, frontal section

Fig. 3.9 Connections of the laryngeal cartilages.

Laryngeal Muscles

The true laryngeal muscles act to *move the laryngeal cartilages against each other* and to influence the *position and tension of the vocal ligaments*. Depending on their position and origin, the muscles of the larynx can be divided into **extrinsic** and **intrinsic laryngeal muscles**. In addition, there are muscles that move the larynx as a whole (*infrahyoid muscles*, see Vol. 1; *suprahyoid muscles*; and *inferior constrictor muscle of pharynx*, see p. 168).

Extrinsic Laryngeal Muscles

The **cricothyroid** (**A1**) is the only extrinsic laryngeal muscle. It arises bilaterally, anterior to the *cricoid cartilage*, and consists of two portions, a **straight** (**internal**) **part** (**A1 a**) and an **oblique** (**external**) **part** (**A1 b**), which pass to the *inferior border of the thyroid cartilage* and to the *inner surface of the inferior horn of the thyroid cartilage*. If the thyroid cartilage is fixed, the cricothyroid tilts the cricoid cartilage posteriorly against the thyroid cartilage, tensing the vocal ligament.

The cricothyroid is the only laryngeal muscle that is innervated by the *external branch of the superior laryngeal nerve*.

The *inferior constrictor* and *thyrohyoid muscles* belong functionally with the extrinsic laryngeal muscles.

Intrinsic Laryngeal Muscles

The intrinsic laryngeal muscles are innervated by the *recurrent laryngeal nerve*, a branch of the *vagus nerve*. They are:

Posterior cricoarytenoid (**B–D2**). It originates bilaterally from the *posterior surface of the lamina of the cricoid cartilage* and extends to the lateral surface of the *muscular process of the arytenoid cartilage* (**B3**). It acts to draw the muscular process posteriorly, causing the vocal process to move laterally, thereby widening the rima glottidis. This is the **only muscle that opens the entire rima glottidis** for inspiration.

Lateral cricoarytenoid (**BD4**). This originates from the *superior border* and *outer*

surface of the arch of the cricoid cartilage and passes to the *muscular process of the arytenoid cartilage*, which it draws anteriorly. This causes the vocal process to move toward the mid line, closing the rima glottidis.

Vocalis (**B5**). This arises bilaterally from the *posterior surface of the thyroid cartilage* and passes to the *vocal process of the arytenoid cartilage*. It draws the thyroid cartilage toward the vocal process and completely closes the rima glottidis by becoming thicker as it contracts. The mostly isometric contraction of the muscle tenses the vocal fold and adjusts tension. The vocalis is continuous laterally with a broad, thin layer of muscle known as the *thyroarytenoid*.

Thyroarytenoid (**CD6**). The thyroarytenoid originates from the *inner surface of the thyroid cartilage* and attaches to the *lateral surface of the arytenoid cartilage*. Contraction of the thyroarytenoid draws the arytenoid cartilages forward, shortens the vocal fold, and closes the anterior, larger portion of the rima glottidis, the *intermembranous part*. Some of its fibers form the **thyroepiglottic part** (**D6 a**) of the thyroarytenoid, which passes to the epiglottis and assists in narrowing the laryngeal inlet.

Transverse arytenoid (**C7**). The transverse arytenoid is a single, unpaired muscle that originates from the *posterior surface of one side of an arytenoid cartilage* and passes to its *opposite side*. It draws the arytenoid cartilages toward each other and closes the posterior portion of the rima glottidis, the *intercartilaginous part*. It also tenses the vocal ligament.

Oblique arytenoid (**C8**). This muscle lies near the surface of the transverse arytenoid; it originates from the *posterior surface of the muscular process of an arytenoid cartilage on one side* and inserts into the *apex of the contralateral arytenoid cartilage*. It assists in narrowing the laryngeal inlet by drawing the *aryepiglottic folds* (**D9**), vocal folds lying between the arytenoid cartilages and epiglottis, closer together. The fibers of the **aryepiglottic part** of the oblique arytenoid have a similar function and continue into the *aryepiglottic fold*.

Respiratory System

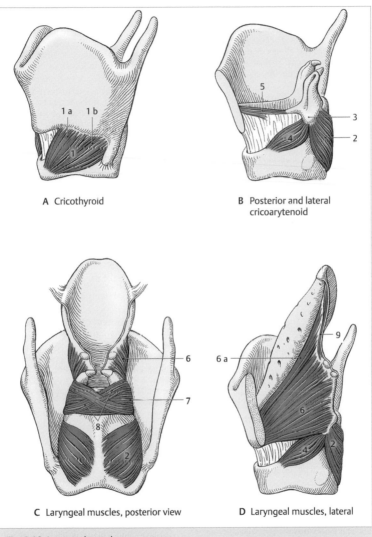

A Cricothyroid

B Posterior and lateral
   cricoarytenoid

C Laryngeal muscles, posterior view

D Laryngeal muscles, lateral

Fig. 3.10 Laryngeal muscles.

Laryngeal Cavity

The **laryngeal cavity** (**A**, **B**) is the mucosa-lined space between the *laryngeal inlet* and the *inferior border of the cricoid cartilage*. It is divided by two pairs of lateral folds, one above the other, into **upper**, **middle**, and **lower parts**.

Upper part. The obliquely oriented **laryngeal inlet** (**A1**) leads to the **laryngeal vestibule** (**I**), which extends as far as the **vestibular folds** (**AB2**). The laryngeal inlet is limited by the **epiglottis** (**A3**) and two mucosal folds known as the **aryepiglottic folds** (**A4**), both of which extend from the lateral margins of the epiglottis to the *corniculate cartilages* on the apex of the arytenoid cartilages. Each aryepiglottic fold also contains an additional small piece of cartilage, the *cuneiform cartilage*. These two cartilages produce the **corniculate tubercle** (**A5**) and *cuneiform tubercle* (**A6**). Between the two arytenoid cartilages is a posterior notch in the mucosa called the *interarytenoid notch*. On either side of the laryngeal inlet, that is, the aryepiglottic folds, is the inferior part of the *pharynx*, which contains a trench in the mucosa known as the *piriform recess* (**A7**) (see p. 168). This depression conveys fluid past the laryngeal inlet into the esophagus.

The **anterior wall** of the laryngeal vestibule is formed by the epiglottis, which is 4–5-cm long and connected by mucosal folds to the base of the tongue. The flat **posterior wall**, near the interarytenoid notch, lies at about the level of the vestibular folds.

Middle part. The **intermediate laryngeal cavity** (**II**) is the smallest part of the laryngeal cavity, extending from the **vestibular folds** (**AB2**) to the **vocal folds** (**AB8**). It is expanded on either side by a mucosal outpouching, the **laryngeal ventricle** (**BC9**). It is bounded above by the vestibular fold and below by the vocal fold and ends anterosuperiorly in a blind pouch called the *laryngeal saccule* (**C10**).

Lower part. The inferior portion of the laryngeal cavity, the subglottis or **infraglottic**

cavity (**III**), reaches from the **vocal folds** to the **inferior margin of the cricoid cartilage**. Becoming wider from cranial to caudal, it is continuous with the *trachea*. The wall of the infraglottic cavity is formed almost entirely by the **conus elasticus** (**C11**) and is lined by mucosa.

Histology. With the exception of the vocal fold, the mucosa of the laryngeal cavity is lined with **ciliated respiratory epithelium**. It contains numerous **mixed glands** in the laryngeal vestibule and vestibular folds.

Vestibular Folds and Vocal Folds (C)

Vestibular folds (**A2**) (**false vocal cords**). The vestibular folds contain the **vestibular ligament**, formed by the free inferior margin of the *quadrangular membrane* (**C12**), as well as numerous **glands** (**C13**). The vestibular folds do not protrude as far into the laryngeal cavity as the vocal folds. Thus, the space between the vestibular folds on either side, the *rima vestibuli* (**C14**), is wider than the space beneath it lying between the vocal folds, the *rima glottidis* (**C15**).

Vocal folds. The vocal folds (**AB8**) contain the **vocal ligament** (**C16**) and **vocalis** (**C17**) muscle. They bound the anterior part of the *rima glottidis*.

Histology. The vocal folds are covered with **nonkeratinized, stratified squamous epithelium**, which is firmly attached to the underlying vocal ligament. The vocal folds possess neither submucosa nor blood vessels, and so have a **white** appearance, which makes them readily distinguishable from the surrounding mucosa that has a shimmering red appearance.

Clinical note. The loose connective tissue in the mucosa of the laryngeal inlet permits the build-up of considerable amounts of fluid from the vascular system. Inflammation or insect stings can thus cause a life-threatening mucosal swelling, **laryngeal edema**, often incorrectly referred to as glottal edema.

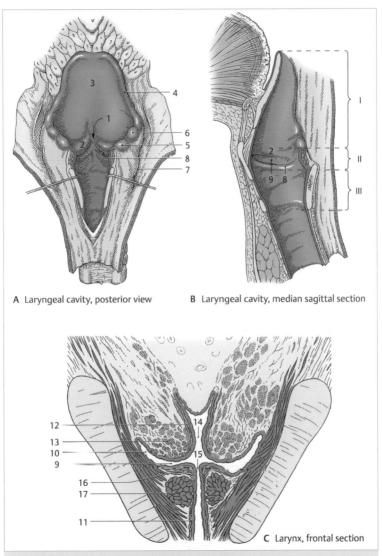

A Laryngeal cavity, posterior view

B Laryngeal cavity, median sagittal section

C Larynx, frontal section

Fig. 3.11 Interior of the larynx.

Glottis

The glottis (**A**) is the **part of the larynx involved in voice production**, consisting of the two **vocal folds** and **structures in their walls**. Each vocal fold contains in its long anterior part the *vocal ligament* (**A1**) and *vocalis* (**A2**). The shorter, posterior part contains the *arytenoid cartilage* (**A3**) and *vocal process* (**A4**). The **rima glottidis** (**AD5**) can similarly be divided into a long anterior and short posterior part. The anterior part consists of the *intermembranous part* (**A6**) and lies on top of the vocal ligament. The posterior, *intercartilaginous part* (**A7**) lies between the arytenoid cartilages. Both portions of the rima glottidis can be opened to various degrees.

> **Clinical note. Laryngoscopy** (**B**) is an examination in which a laryngoscope is introduced into the pharynx. The image is inverted: the anterior areas of the laryngeal inlet are at the top of the image and the posterior areas at the bottom.

Functional Anatomy

The shape of the **rima glottidis** changes according to function. During *quiet respiration* and *whispering*, the intermembranous part is closed, and the intercartilaginous part forms a triangular opening (**C**). With *progressively deeper breathing*, the anterior parts also open to the intermediate position (**D**). The rima glottidis reaches its maximum width (**E**) with deep breathing or upon coughing (opening explosively). **Phonation** occurs when the rima glottidis is first closed (**F**), and the vocal ligaments tensed. The rima glottidis is then opened by an expiratory stream of air, which causes the vocal folds to vibrate, producing sound waves. The *volume* of these sound waves depends on the *force of the stream of air*, while *pitch* depends on *vibration frequency*, which in turn varies by length, thickness, and tension of the vocal ligaments. Involuntary closure of the rima glottidis also occurs when a foreign body enters the airway; and the cough reflex causes it to reopen explosively.

D8 Epiglottis, **D9** Vocal fold, **D10** Aryepiglottic fold, **D11** Cuneiform tubercle, **D12** Corniculate tubercle, **C13** Interarytenoid notch

Vessels, Nerves, and Lymphatic Drainage

All laryngeal structures are supplied by the **superior laryngeal artery**, arising from the *superior thyroid artery*, and by the **inferior laryngeal artery**, arising from the *inferior thyroid artery*. Venous drainage is provided by the companion veins of the same name, which drain into the *internal jugular vein*.

The laryngeal mucosa is innervated as far as the vocal folds by the purely sensory *internal branch* of the **superior laryngeal nerve**. Below this level, it is innervated by the **inferior laryngeal nerve**. The *intrinsic* laryngeal muscles are all supplied by the **recurrent laryngeal nerve** (inferior). The only extrinsic laryngeal muscle, the *cricothyroid*, is innervated by the *external branch* of the superior laryngeal nerve.

> **Clinical note.** Unilateral injury of the **recurrent laryngeal nerve** results in paralysis of all intrinsic laryngeal muscles. The vocal fold on the affected side lies in an adducted, paramedian position. In patients with acute bilateral injury of the recurrent laryngeal nerve, the paralyzed vocal folds meet in the rima glottidis, causing stridor and shortness of breath, which may necessitate tracheostomy (see p. 120).

Lymphatic drainage from the *upper* part of the larynx as far as the vocal folds is to the **upper** group of *deep cervical lymph nodes.* Drainage from the *lower* half of the larynx, that is, from the level of the vocal folds downward, is to the **middle** and **lower** groups of *deep cervical lymph nodes* and to the *pretracheal* and *paratracheal lymph nodes.*

> **Clinical note.** The lymphatics form a superficial capillary network in the laryngeal mucosa, which drains to lymphatic vessels deep in the lamina propria. In advanced laryngeal cancer, the lateral cervical lymph nodes (superior deep nodes) are involved most frequently.

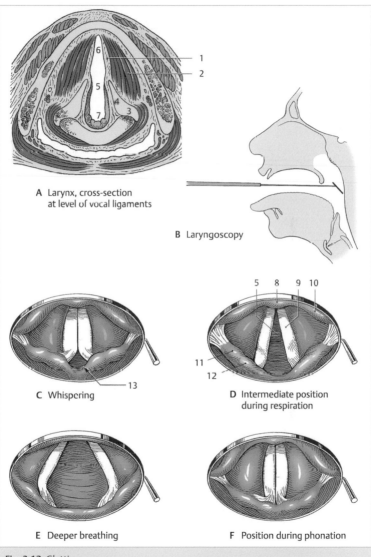

A Larynx, cross-section at level of vocal ligaments

B Laryngoscopy

C Whispering

D Intermediate position during respiration

E Deeper breathing

F Position during phonation

Fig. 3.12 Glottis.

Respiratory System

3.4 Trachea

Trachea and Extrapulmonary Main Bronchi

The **trachea** (**A**) consists of a flexible tube 10–12-cm long, extending from the *cricoid cartilage* to the *tracheal bifurcation*. It can be divided into a **cervical part** (**I**) and a **thoracic part** (**II**). The cervical part extends from C6 to C7 and the longer, thoracic part from T1 to T4.

The **wall** of the trachea (**B**) is made up of 16–20 horseshoe-shaped, hyaline cartilages known as the **tracheal cartilages** (**B1**), which reinforce the anterior and lateral walls of the trachea. The tracheal cartilages are linked together by the **annular ligaments** (**B2**). Along the posterior wall (**C**) of the trachea, the tracheal cartilages are closed to form a ring by the **membranous wall** (**C3**), a plate of connective tissue containing smooth muscle. At the asymmetrical **tracheal bifurcation** (**BC4**), the trachea divides into the **right** (**BC5**) and **left main bronchi** (**BC6**). The right main bronchus is the shorter of the two and its lumen is wider. It departs from the trachea at an angle of only 20° and thus continues in nearly the same direction as the trachea. The left main bronchus is longer and its lumen narrower. It departs from the trachea at an angle of about 35°.

At the **division** of the trachea (**D**), there is a sagittally oriented ridge overlying the cartilage, the **carina of trachea** (**D7**), which projects into the lumen and divides the airstream during inspiration. The transverse diameter of the trachea is greater than its sagittal diameter.

Microscopy. The walls of the trachea and main bronchi (**E**) are nearly identical in terms of structure and consist of three layers: an inner mucosal layer, the **mucosa** (**E8**), with stratified *respiratory epithelium* and mixed *tracheal glands;* a middle **fibromusculocartilaginous layer** (**E9**), which

is composed of the *tracheal cartilages* and *annular ligaments* anteriorly and laterally, as well as *connective tissue* containing *trachealis* smooth muscle posteriorly; and the **adventitia** (**E10**), an outer, sliding layer. The connective tissue in the tracheal wall, especially the annular ligaments, is rich in elastic fiber networks. Collagen and elastic fibers are thus integrated into the wall of the trachea in such a manner that the tracheal cartilages are under transverse and longitudinal tension.

Vessels, nerves, and lymphatic drainage. The *trachea* is supplied by tracheal branches of the **inferior thyroid artery**, and the *main bronchi* by the **bronchial branches**. Venous drainage is supplied by the respective companion veins. The *trachealis* consists of smooth muscle and is innervated by the **recurrent laryngeal nerve**, a branch of the **vagus nerve**, which is also responsible for sensory and secretory innervation. Lymphatic drainage is to the **paratracheal lymph nodes** lying along the adventitia of the trachea, and the **superior and inferior tracheobronchial lymph nodes** near the tracheal bifurcation.

Clinical note. Especially in children, **aspirated foreign bodies** are more likely to enter the more vertically oriented right main bronchus and consequently the right lung, where they may cause aspiration pneumonia.

The stratified respiratory epithelium has cilia on its surface, which beat to move inhaled particles and pathogens outward, thus forming an important part of the body's unspecific immune system. In heavy smokers, the respiratory epithelium is converted to stratified squamous epithelium (squamous metaplasia of the trachea). Smoking also leads to adhesion and immobilization of the cilia, so that mucociliary clearance of harmful substances can no longer be ensured. Impaired mucociliary clearance also leads to recurrent respiratory tract infections in mucoviscidosis patients.

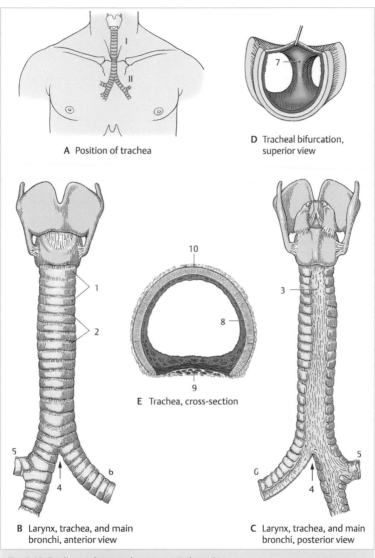

A Position of trachea

D Tracheal bifurcation, superior view

E Trachea, cross-section

B Larynx, trachea, and main bronchi, anterior view

C Larynx, trachea, and main bronchi, posterior view

Fig. 3.13 Trachea and extrapulmonary main bronchi.

Topography of the Trachea and Larynx

The **larynx** and **cervical part of the trachea** are component parts of the **neck viscera** and lie in the middle part of the anterior cervical region (**A**). The outer contour of this region is formed by the variously protruding *laryngeal prominence* (**A1**), since the part of the larynx located near the *thyroid cartilage* (**A2**) lies immediately beneath the skin. The laryngeal prominence, thyroid cartilage, and *cricothyroid ligament* (**A3**) can all be palpated beneath the skin. Distal to this point, toward the superior thoracic aperture, the viscera of the neck gradually move away from the outer surface of the neck, conforming to the curvatures of the vertebral column.

The viscera of the neck are embedded in the **visceral space of the neck** (**B**), situated between the middle and deep layers of the cervical fascia, the **pretracheal layer** (**AB4**), and the **prevertebral layers** (**AB5**) of the **cervical fascia**, and is continuous with the connective tissue spaces of the *head* and *thorax*. On its anterior side, the larynx is directly covered by the middle layer of cervical fascia, with the **superficial layer** (**B6**) lying almost directly over it. Posterior to the larynx is the *laryngeal part of the pharynx* (**A7**). The *trachea* is separated by the *thyroid gland* (**A–C8**), lying anterior to it from the middle and superficial layers of the cervical fascia. Lying behind the trachea is the *esophagus*.

Functional anatomy. The viscera of the neck are embedded in their surroundings, in such a fashion that they can be raised and lowered and are freely movable against each other. The larynx is suspended from the hyoid bone and indirectly from the basicranium above, and braced by the thoracic cage below via the pull of the elastic structures of the trachea and bronchial tree.

Movements of the larynx in the long axis of the body occur during *swallowing* (elevation of 2–3 cm), *vocalization*, and *deep breathing*. *Extension* of the head and cervical vertebrae elevates the larynx to about the next vertebral level, while *flexion* of the head and cervical vertebrae lowers the cricoid cartilage (**A10**) into the superior thoracic aperture. The total distance of possible up-and-down movement is up to 4 cm.

Clinical note. Life-threatening closure of the rima glottidis, for example, due to mucosal edema, can be managed by establishing the airway below it. An incision can be made through the median cricothyroid ligament (**cricothyrotomy**, red arrow), or in the trachea above the thyroid isthmus (**high tracheostomy**, black arrow), or below it (**low tracheostomy**, blue arrow).

Topography of Laryngeal Nerves (C)

Innervation of the larynx and trachea is provided by branches of the **vagus nerve** (**BC11**). The **superior laryngeal nerve** (**C12**) branches off the trunk of the vagus nerve below the inferior ganglion and passes medial to the *internal carotid artery* (**BC13**) and branches of the *external carotid artery* (**C14**). Near the level of the hyoid bone (**AC9**), it divides into an **external branch** (**C12 a**), a **motor branch** that supplies the cricothyroid (**C15**) and inferior constrictor muscle of the pharynx (**C16**), and an **internal branch** (**C12 b**), a **sensory branch** that pierces the thyrohyoid membrane (**C17**) and passes beneath the mucosa of the piriform recess, where it sometimes anastomoses with the *recurrent laryngeal nerve* (**BC18**). The internal branch supplies the laryngeal mucosa as far as the rima glottidis. The **recurrent laryngeal nerve** (**C19**) branches off the vagus nerve in the thorax. On the **left**, it loops around the *aortic arch* and, after giving off a branch, it passes back upward as the inferior laryngeal nerve in the groove between the esophagus and trachea to the larynx, distributing branches in its course. On the **right**, it loops around the *subclavian artery* (**C20**) and travels cranially alongside the trachea. On its way to the trachea, the recurrent laryngeal nerve courses behind the thyroid gland (**A–C8**). Its **terminal branch** (**BC18**) passes at the caudal border of the inferior constrictor muscle of the pharynx (**C16**) into the *interior of the larynx*. It divides into an **anterior and posterior branch** and provides *motor* innervation to all laryngeal muscles except the cricothyroid, and *sensory* innervation to the laryngeal mucosa below the level of the rima glottidis.

Clinical note. Thyroid surgery presents a risk of stretch injury or trauma to the recurrent laryngeal nerve (see also p. 116).

B21 Vertebral artery

Respiratory System

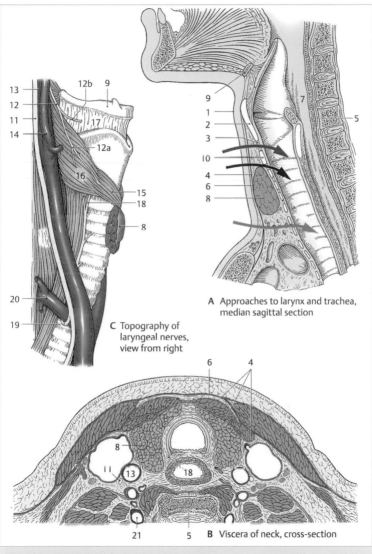

A Approaches to larynx and trachea, median sagittal section

C Topography of laryngeal nerves, view from right

B Viscera of neck, cross-section

Fig. 3.14 Topography of the larynx and trachea.

3.5 Lung

The paired **lungs** lie in the thorax, one on either side of the *mediastinum*, enclosed in a *pleural cavity* lined by a serous membrane (for position, see Overview of the respiratory system, p. 94).

Surfaces of the Lung

Each of the lungs is shaped like a *half cone*. In children, the surface of the lung is a pale pink color, but with advancing age it becomes slate gray as a result of deposits from pollutants in inhaled air.

External surface. The external surface of the lung conforms to its surrounding structures, that is, thoracic wall, diaphragm, and mediastinum. This can be especially well seen in the in situ lung. Each of the two lungs consists of a domelike **apex** (**AB1**), which projects a few centimeters above the *superior thoracic aperture* anteriorly. The **base of the lung** (**AC2**), or **diaphragmatic surface** (**AC3**), is *concave* and lies on the diaphragm. The outer surface of the lung resting against the ribs is *convex* and is known as the **costal surface** (**A, B**). The surface facing the mediastinum, the **mediastinal surface** (**C, D**) is divided by the *hilum of the lung* (**CD4**) into an anterior, *mediastinal surface* (**CD5**) and a posterior, *vertebral part* (**CD6**). Each of the mediastinal surfaces has an indentation produced by the heart, the *cardiac impression* (**CD7**). On the medial surface of the right lung are impressions produced by the *right subclavian artery* (**C8 a**), *azygos vein*, and *esophagus* (**C9**). The surface of the left lung is marked by visible grooves from the *aortic arch* (**D10 a**), *thoracic aorta* (**D10 b**), and *left subclavian artery* (**D8 b**).

Hilum of the lung. The **root of the lung** is formed by the collection of vessels and bronchi that enter and leave the lung in the center of its medial surface. These connect the lungs with the heart and trachea and are similarly arranged on the right and left sides.

The **pulmonary veins** lie anteriorly, the **bronchi** posteriorly, and the **pulmonary arteries** in the middle. The arrangement of these structures varies along the cranial–caudal axis.

On the **right** side, the cross section through the **superior lobar bronchus** (**C11**) is above the section through the **pulmonary artery** (**C12 a**) (*eparterial position*). Below this is the section through the **right main bronchus** (**C13 a**) (*hyparterial position*), and **inferior pulmonary veins** (**C14 a**). On the **left** side, the cross section through the **pulmonary artery** (**D12 b**) is furthest cranial, and the section through the **left main bronchus** (**D13 b**) is below it (*hyparterial position*), followed by horizontal sections through the **inferior pulmonary veins** (**D14 b**).

The structures that enter and leave the lung at the hilum are completely surrounded by a **reflection of pleura**, which extends caudally in front of the cardiac impression. The anterior and posterior folds are nearly directly adjacent, forming the **pulmonary ligament** (**CD15**). The pleural reflection separates the structures of the hilum of the lung from the pleural cavity. The hilum and the structures entering and leaving the lung are situated outside of the pleura and are directly connected with the connective tissue of the mediastinum.

Lung borders. The anterior and inferior surfaces of the lungs have thin, sharp borders. The *costal surface* and *mediastinal surface* meet anteriorly at the sharp **anterior border** (**A–D16**). On the left lung this border has a notch known as the *cardiac notch of the left lung* (**BD17**), which is produced by the *cardiac impression*. Between the *costal surface* and *diaphragmatic surface* is the **inferior margin** (**A–D18**).

Lung lobes and fissures. Each lung is divided into lobes by deep depressions, or fissures. The **right lung** normally has a **superior lobe** (**A19**), **middle lobe** (**A20**), and **inferior lobe** (**A21**). The *superior lobe* and *inferior lobe* are divided by the **oblique fissure** (**AC22**), which runs diagonally from posterosuperior to anteroinferior. The *superior lobe* and *middle lobe* are divided by the **horizontal fissure** (**A23**) lying anteriorly and laterally. The smaller **left lung** consists of only a **superior lobe** (**B19**) and **inferior lobe** (**B21**), which are also separated by an **oblique fissure** (**BD22**). The anteroinferior end of the superior lobe of the left lung usually has a tonguelike projection known as the *lingula* (**B24**). The facing surfaces between individual lobes are called *interlobar surfaces*.

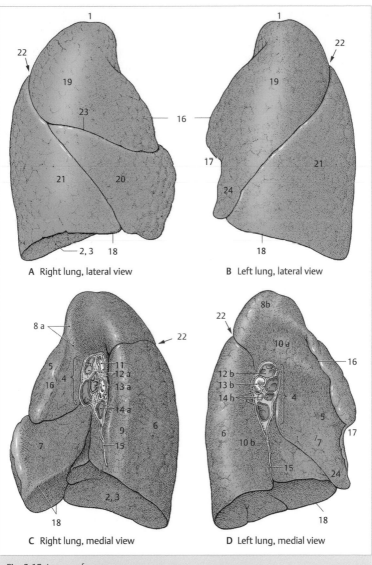

A Right lung, lateral view

B Left lung, lateral view

C Right lung, medial view

D Left lung, medial view

Fig. 3.15 Lung surface.

Divisions of the Bronchi and Bronchopulmonary Segments (A, B)

The right and left **main bronchi** divide on the *right side into three* and on the *left side into two* **lobar bronchi** (see below), 8–12 mm in diameter. On the **right** they branch off the main bronchus, as the *right superior lobar bronchus* about 1–2.5 cm from the tracheal bifurcation and as the *right middle* and *right inferior lobar bronchi* about 5 cm from the tracheal bifurcation. On the **left**, the main bronchus also divides about 5 cm from the bifurcation into the *left superior and inferior lobar bronchi*. The lobar bronchi divide on the right side into ten *and on the left side* into nine **segmental bronchi**. Proceeding from the **right** superior lobar bronchus are *segmental bronchi 1–3*; branching off the middle lobar bronchus are *segmental bronchi 4–5*; and from the right inferior lobar bronchus are *segmental bronchi 6–10*. On the **left** side, the left superior lobar bronchus divides into *segmental bronchi 1 and 2*, as well as *3–5*, and the left inferior lobar bronchus divides into *segmental bronchi 6–10*.

Bronchopulmonary Segments and Lobules

Bronchopulmonary segments. The bronchopulmonary segments are *subunits of the lung lobules* that are organized by segmental bronchi. Bronchopulmonary segments can be conceived of as **bronchoarterial units**: each contains a centrally located (i.e., *intrasegmental*) **segmental bronchus** and an accompanying branch of the **pulmonary artery**. Additional branches of a segmental bronchus are limited to the respective segment.

Branches of the pulmonary veins travel within the connective tissue on the surface of a segment, that is, they have an *inter*segmental course and demarcate the **boundaries between segments**. As they near the hilum, the branches converge to form the large *pulmonary veins*. Each of the bronchopulmonary segments forms a three-dimensional *wedge-shaped or pyramidal structural unit*, with its apex directed *toward the hilum*.

Lung lobules. The segmental bronchi divide in several steps into **medium-sized and small bronchi**, which subdivide into **bronchioles**. Each bronchiole supplies a **pulmonary lobule**. The lobules are *subunits of the bronchopulmonary segments*.

The lobules are not found throughout the lungs, but are mainly situated on their *surface*. They are identifiable as *polygonal regions* with sides measuring 0.5–3 cm, bounded by connective tissue, which can contain inhaled suspended solids. These give the borders of the lobules a blue or black appearance.

Each bronchiole situated within a lobule divides 3–4 times and ultimately subdivides into the terminal branches of the bronchial tree that bear the alveoli. The terminal branches consist of several generations of **respiratory bronchioles** and **alveolar ducts** containing **alveoli** in their walls for gas exchange.

Each lung contains two systems of connective tissue. **Peribronchial** or **periarterial connective tissue** surrounds the *branches of the bronchial tree and pulmonary artery* as far as the respiratory bronchioles and facilitates their movement against the surrounding gas-exchanging tissue of the lung. The second, external system consists of **subpleural connective tissue**, which lines the *surface of the lobes* and forms *septa* dividing the bronchopulmonary segments and lobules. The subpleural connective tissue acts as a sliding layer, but also protects against overexpansion.

Blue: Superior lobe, **Green:** Middle lobe, **Red:** Inferior lobe

I Right superior lobar bronchus, **I** Right middle lobar bronchus, **II** Right inferior lobar bronchus, **V** Left superior lobar bronchus, **IV** Left inferior lobar bronchus, **1** Apical segment and apical segmental bronchus (right lung only), **2** Posterior segment and posterior segmental bronchus (right lung only), **1 + 2** Apicoposterior segment and apicoposterior segmental bronchus (left lung only), **3** Anterior segment and anterior segmental bronchus, **4** Lateral segment and lateral segmental bronchus, **5** Medial segment and medial segmental bronchus, **6** Superior segment and superior segmental bronchus, **7** Medial basal segment and medial basal segmental bronchus, **8** Anterior basal segment and anterior basal segmental bronchus, **9** Lateral basal segment and lateral basal segmental bronchus, **10** Posterior basal segment and posterior basal segmental bronchus, **11** Tracheal bifurcation, **12** Right main bronchus, **13** Left main bronchus

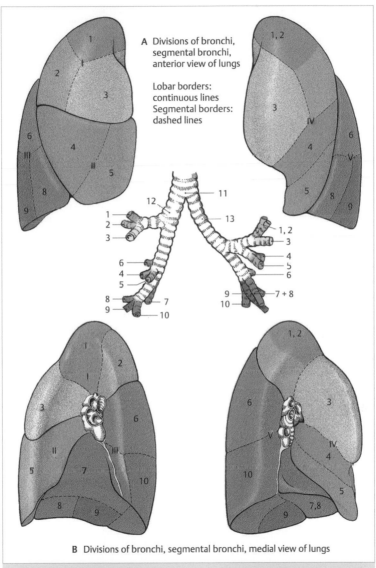

A Divisions of bronchi, segmental bronchi, anterior view of lungs

Lobar borders: continuous lines
Segmental borders: dashed lines

B Divisions of bronchi, segmental bronchi, medial view of lungs

Fig. 3.16 Bronchial divisions and bronchopulmonary segments.

Microscopic Anatomy

Lung tissue consists of *conducting* and *gas-exchanging portions of the bronchial tree*, as well as *pulmonary vessels, connective tissue*, and *smooth muscle*. As the bronchial tree and pulmonary vessels divide, their microscopic structure changes. The total transverse section of the bronchial tree enlarges with each division.

Conducting Portion

Intrapulmonary bronchi (**A**). The walls of the lobar and segmental bronchi have three layers, consisting of the mucosa (**A1**), musculocartilaginous layer (**A2**), and adventitia (**A3**). The **mucosa** is lined with *ciliated respiratory epithelium* (**A1 a**), which rests on a connective tissue *lamina propria* (**A1 b**) that is rich in elastic fibers. Unlike the extrapulmonary bronchi, below this is a **musculocartilaginous layer**, consisting of a nearly complete layer formed by a spiral arrangement of smooth muscle cells known as *spiral muscle* (**A2 a**). The irregularly shaped *bronchial cartilage* (**A2 b**), flat or curved cartilage plates in the bronchial wall, is composed of *hyaline cartilage* in the larger bronchi, but increasingly replaced by *elastic cartilage* in the smaller bronchi. Lying between the cartilage pieces are mixed seromucous *bronchial glands* (**A2 c**). In addition, the connective tissue of the musculocartilaginous layer contains a *venous plexus*. A narrow, connective tissue **adventitia** (**A3**) connects the bronchial wall to its surroundings and conveys the nutritive *bronchial branches* (**A3 a**) to the bronchus. The *bronchopulmonary lymph nodes* (**A3 b**) are often located at divisions of the bronchi. Accompanying each bronchus is a *branch of the pulmonary artery*.

Bronchioles (**B**). Arising from the small bronchi, the bronchioles have a diameter of 0.3–0.5 mm. Their walls consist of **mucosa**, a **muscular layer**, and **adventitia** and *do not contain cartilage*. The walls of the bronchioles possess a network of abundant *elastic fibers*, which prevent collapse of the noncartilaginous walls if the muscle becomes lax (**B**). The bronchioles end in the **terminal bronchioles** (**B4**). Smaller *branches of the pulmonary artery* accompany the bronchioles.

As far as the smallest bronchioles, the bronchial tree serves only as a conducting passageway for air to the lung, forming part of the **"anatomic dead space."** Its tasks consist of filtering, humidifying, and warming inhaled air.

Gas-exchanging Portion

Respiratory bronchioles and alveolar ducts (**B**). The terminal bronchioles branch into **respiratory bronchi** (**B5**), which may be viewed as connecting passages between the conducting and respiratory portions of the lung. The respiratory bronchi have an average diameter of 0.4 mm. Their walls are lined with *cuboidal epithelium* and contain *smooth muscle*. Interruptions in the wall in certain places form thin-walled outpouchings called *pulmonary alveoli*. The respiratory bronchioles are accompanied by *arterioles arising from the pulmonary artery*, and divide 3–6 times. They are continuous with the **alveolar ducts** (**B6**), whose walls are made up entirely of *alveoli* (**B7**), which in turn divide into blind-ending *alveolar sacs*. Traveling alongside the alveolar ducts are *precapillaries*, and accompanying the alveoli are *capillaries*.

Alveoli. Gas exchange takes place in the alveoli. Each lung contains about 300 million alveoli, with a total surface area of 140 m². Two adjacent alveoli share a thin wall called the **interalveolar septum**, containing *connective tissue* and *capillaries* and lined on either side with flat epithelium. The **alveolar epithelium** is made up of two types of cells. *Type I pneumocytes* make up more than 90% of epithelial cells *covering the surface* of the alveoli. The remaining 10% are *type II pneumocytes*, which produce *surfactant* (a factor in the reduction of surface tension) and act as *stem cells for type I pneumocytes*. The **blood–air barrier** describes that portion across which gas exchange occurs between the alveolar and capillary lumina. It is 0.3–0.7-μm thick and consists of *alveolar epithelium, fused basement membranes*, and *capillary epithelium*.

Clinical note. The bronchial connective tissue and alveolar septa also contain mast cells, which play an important part in allergic disorders of the airways (*bronchial asthma*).

Reduction or destruction of the alveoli and interalveolar septa leads to *pulmonary emphysema*, a condition in which air capacity is greatly limited. Conversely, an increase in the connective tissue in the alveolar septa leads to *pulmonary fibrosis*, with impaired diffusion in the lung.

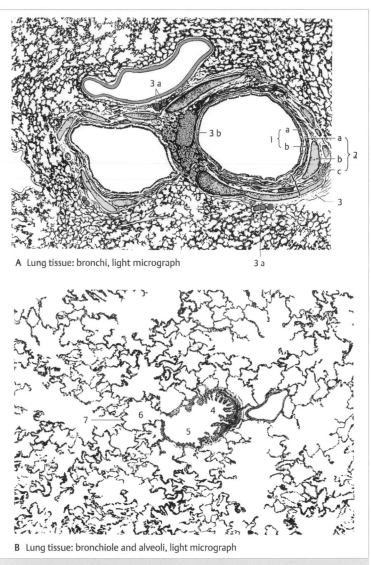

A Lung tissue: bronchi, light micrograph

B Lung tissue: bronchiole and alveoli, light micrograph

Fig. 3.17 Microscopic structure of the lung.

Vascular System and Innervation

Each lung has functional vessels, **pulmonary vessels**, which belong to the *pulmonary circulation*, as well as **nutritive vessels**, which arise from the *systemic circulation*.

Pulmonary vessels (A). Just below the tracheal bifurcation (**A1**), the **pulmonary trunk (A2)** divides into the two **pulmonary arteries**, which transport deoxygenated blood to the alveoli. The *right pulmonary artery* (**A3**) is longer and wider than the *left pulmonary artery* (**A4**). Both pulmonary arteries lie anterior to the main bronchi (**A5**) and ramify before reaching the hilum of the lung, giving off branches that further divide and parallel the bronchial tree. **Branches of the pulmonary artery** lie in close proximity (usually on the posterolateral side) to the bronchial tubes they accompany in the center of each bronchopulmonary segment. The pulmonary arteries and their large branches are *elastic arteries*. The smaller arterial branches accompanying smaller bronchi and bronchioles are *muscular arteries*.

Oxygenated blood is carried out of the lungs through **interlobular** and **intersegmental veins**, which travel toward the hilum and unite to form the **right and left pulmonary veins (A6** and **A7)**. At the hilum of the lung, the valveless pulmonary veins lie anterior and caudal to the arteries.

Lymphatic vessel system and regional lymph nodes. Similarly to the connective tissues of the lungs, the lymphatic vessel system can likewise be divided into two parts: the **deep** or **peribronchial lymphatic vessel system (B8)** extends along the *peribronchial connective tissue*. *Bronchopulmonary lymph nodes* (**B9**) form lymph node stations at divisions of the lobular bronchi into segmental bronchi. The next station is formed by the *inferior* (**A10**) and *superior tracheobronchial lymph nodes* (**A11**), located at the main bronchi and the bifurcation. The second set of lymphatic vessels, the **superficial** or **segmental lymphatic vessel system (B12)** begins with the *lymphatic capillaries in loose, subpleural connective tissue* and in the *interlobular*

and *intersegmental connective tissue septa*, which join to form lymphatic vessels following the pulmonary veins. The first lymph node stations are the *tracheobronchial lymph nodes*, which are continuous with the *paratracheal lymph nodes* situated along the trachea.

> **Clinical note.** Lymph nodes located in the hilum are referred to as **hilar nodes**. This term usually refers to bronchopulmonary lymph nodes at the divisions of the bronchi and along vessel branches. Hilar and paratracheal lymph nodes are the most important filtering stations in *tuberculosis* and *lung cancer*.

Bronchial vessels (C). Lung tissue is nourished by the **bronchial branches**, which arise from the *thoracic aorta* (**C13**). Usually two bronchial branches (**C14**) arise directly from the aorta and pass to the left lung. The right lung is supplied by a bronchial branch (**C15**) arising from the third or fourth *posterior intercostal artery*. The bronchial branches run in the peribronchial connective tissue and supply the walls of the bronchial tree and those of the accompanying arteries. Venous drainage is provided by the **bronchial veins**, which drain into the *azygos vein, hemiazygos vein*, and partly also into the *pulmonary veins*.

Innervation. The *vagus nerve* and *sympathetic trunk* form the **pulmonary plexus** (see Vol. 3) along the main bronchi, following the bronchi and vessels, supplying them as well as the visceral pleura.

Efferents of the vagus nerve cause contraction, while sympathetic efferents cause dilatation of the bronchial musculature and narrowing of vessels in the lung. **Afferent fibers** of the vagus nerve convey impulses from stretch receptors located along the trachea, bronchi, bronchioles, and visceral pleura. Sympathetic afferent fibers are predominantly pain fibers.

> **Clinical note.** In **bronchial asthma** there is abnormal innervation of smooth muscle in the small bronchi and bronchioles in response to stimuli, which leads to contraction and thus narrowing of the lumen during expiration.

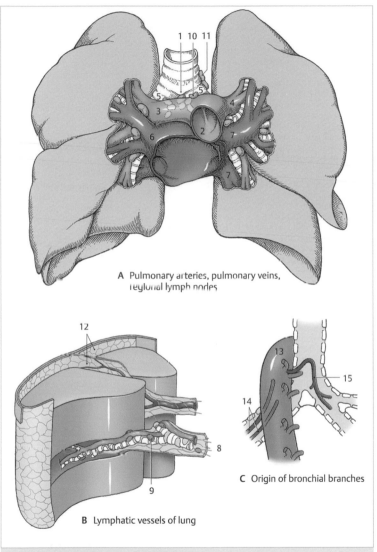

A Pulmonary arteries, pulmonary veins, regional lymph nodes

B Lymphatic vessels of lung

C Origin of bronchial branches

Fig. 3.18 Vascular system and innervation of the lungs.

Respiratory System

Pleura

The serous membrane covering the lung is referred to as the **pleura** (**A**, **B**). It consists of the visceral pleura (or **pulmonary pleura**) (**A1**) and **parietal pleura** (**A2**), which line the space on either side of the thoracic cavity that houses each lung. The visceral pleura and parietal pleura are continuous at the hilum of the lung. Between the two pleural layers is a cavity containing a capillary layer, which is known as the **pleural cavity** and contains a few milliliters of *serous fluid*. It acts to *reduce friction* and allow gliding movement of the lungs during respiration.

Visceral pleura. The visceral pleura covers the lung almost entirely and cannot be stripped from the *surface of the lung*. It also dips into the *interlobular fissures*, but does not cover those regions that are surrounded by the reflection of the visceral pleura onto the parietal pleura, that is, the hilum and the portion between the lung and pulmonary ligament.

Parietal pleura. The parietal pleura forms the peripheral wall of the pleural cavity and can be divided into parts according to the region it borders. The **costal part** (**AB3**) borders the *bony thoracic wall*; the **diaphragmatic part** (**AB4**) the *diaphragm*; and the **mediastinal part** (**AB5**) the *mediastinal connective tissue space*. The *pleural cupula* (**AB6**) is the continuation of the costal part, which protrudes anteriorly above the superior thoracic aperture and extends posteriorly to the head of the first rib. It is filled by the apex of the lung. Between the parietal pleura and the thoracic wall is a sliding layer of connective tissue, known as **endothoracic fascia**. Its thickened portion forms the *suprapleural membrane* at the pleural cupula, to which it is attached.

Pleural recesses. Pleural recesses are complementary spaces that develop at the junctions between the different parts of the pleura. Between the downward-sloping sides of the diaphragm and the thoracic wall, the *costal pleura* and *diaphragmatic pleura* bound the **costodiaphragmatic recess** (**AB7**), a space into which the lung can expand during deep inspiration. Another pocketlike space is located anteriorly between the thoracic wall and mediastinum. It is bounded by the *costal pleura* and *mediastinal pleura*, hence the name **costomediastinal recess** (**AB8**). On the left, it is wide at the level of the cardiac notch, but on the right, it is narrow.

Vessels, nerves, and lymphatic drainage. The pulmonary pleura forms an integral part of the lung, and its neurovascular supply and lymphatic drainage resemble that of the lung. The parietal pleura is supplied by the adjacent **arteries of the thoracic wall**, that is, branches of the *posterior intercostal arteries*, *internal thoracic artery*, and *musculophrenic artery*. Venous drainage is via the **veins of the thoracic wall**. The parietal pleura is highly sensitive to pain and is innervated by the **intercostal nerves** and **phrenic nerve**.

Lung and pleural borders. Sound knowledge of the surface projections of the lung and pleural borders (**A**) onto the thoracic wall is essential for clinical examination. The borders of the lung change during the phases of respiration, while those of the pleura do not. During normal respiration, the inferior margins of both lungs extend 1–2 intercostal spaces beyond the pleural borders (see table below).

> **Clinical note. Inflammation** can lead to build-up of serous fluid in the pleural cavity, elevated protein levels, or adhesion of the two pleural layers, restricting expansion of the lung.

	Sternal line	Midclavicular line	Axillary line	Scapular line	Paravertebral line
Lung borders	6th rib	6th rib	8th rib	10th rib	Spinous process of T10
Pleural borders	6th rib	7th rib	9th rib	11th rib	Spinous process of T11

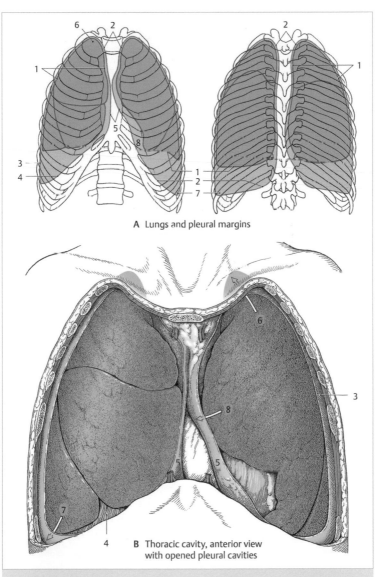

A Lungs and pleural margins

B Thoracic cavity, anterior view
with opened pleural cavities

Fig. 3.19 Pleura.

Cross-Sectional Anatomy

Sectional images available through modern imaging modalities and cadaveric cross sections of lung tissue can clearly demonstrate the course of large and medium-sized bronchi and vessels and their branches. Sections of the **pleural cupula** (A) and sections at the l**evel of the division of the main bronchi and arteries** (B) can enhance our understanding of topographical anatomy. The position of the nearly transverse planes is indicated in the illustrations of the lungs (see below).

Transverse Section at T2 (A)

This transverse section is through the *pulmonary apex* (**A1**) and *pleural cupula* (**A2**). Lateral to the pleural cupula, the section cuts through the *first rib* (**A3**). Anterolateral to it, the *middle scalene* muscle (**A4**) can be identified. Between the middle and *anterior scalene* (**A5**), that is, in front of the latter, is the *scalene space* (see Vol. 1), which gives passage to the *subclavian artery* (**A6**) and *brachial plexus* (**A7**). The close proximity of the subclavian artery to the apex of the lung explains why the artery produces an impression on the fixed anteromedial surface of the lung. The *subclavian vein* (**A8**) lies anterior to the artery and courses on the pleura and apex of the lung. Posteromedial to the section through the lung is the *sympathetic trunk* (**A9**).

A10 Trachea
A11 Esophagus
A12 Brachiocephalic trunk
A13 Internal jugular vein
A14 Thyroid gland
A15 Vagus nerve
A16 Common carotid artery
A17 Thoracic duct
A18 Recurrent laryngeal nerve

Transverse Section at the Level of T5 (B)

The section is below the level of the tracheal bifurcation and shows both *hila of the lungs*. On the right side, the course of the *right pulmonary artery* (**B19**) to the right hilum of the lung can be identified. Anterior to the artery, the section cuts through the *pulmonary vein* (**B20**). Posterior to the

artery, the section is through the *right main bronchus* (**B21**), after it has given off the *right superior lobar bronchus* further cranial. Branches of this bronchus can be identified in the tissue of the *right superior lobe* (**B22**). The right main bronchus is surrounded by *inferior tracheobronchial lymph nodes* (**B23**). On the left side, the *left main bronchus* (**B24**) can be seen at the bifurcation. Anterior to it, the *left pulmonary vein* (**B25**) is shown in the cross section. Its tributaries can be followed into the *left superior lobe* (**B26**). Posteriorly, the section cuts through the *left pulmonary artery* (**A27**), which parallels the bronchus and ramifies. The larger lymph nodes, situated at the hilum of the left lung, are the *inferior tracheobronchial lymph nodes* (**B23**). The smaller lymph node, located posteromedial to the artery at the *left inferior lobe* (**B28**), is a *bronchopulmonary lymph node* (**B29**).

B30 Superior vena cava
B31 Ascending aorta
B32 Subepicardial adipose tissue
B33 Pulmonary trunk
B34 Descending aorta
B35 Azygos vein
B11 Esophagus

Clinical note. The apex of the lung, which is not highly ventilated because of the relatively rigid construction of the pleural cupula (**A2**), can be percussed and auscultated in the *supraclavicular fossa*. Disease processes involving the lung apex can affect all adjacent structures. Infiltrating tumors of the apex of the lung, such as a *Pancoast tumor*, can surround the brachial plexus (**A7**) and cause severe pain in the arm.

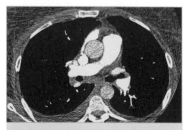
Fig. 3.20C Corresponding plane to Fig. 3.20B on CT.

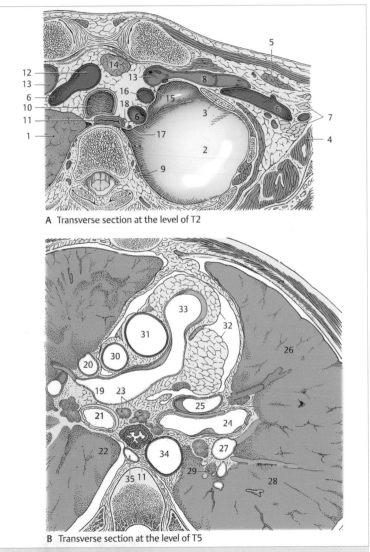

A Transverse section at the level of T2

B Transverse section at the level of T5

Fig. 3.20 Cross-sectional anatomy.

Respiratory System

Mechanics of Breathing

The exchange of gases between the pulmonary alveoli and the environment, that is, optimal aeration and ventilation of the alveoli, requires **pressure changes in the thorax**. These are generated by *active* and *passive* forces.

The **bony framework of the thoracic wall** is formed by the *ribs, thoracic vertebrae,* and *sternum*. The highly elastic ribs vary in shape, length, and position (see Vol. 1). The main **muscles responsible for movement of the bony thorax** are the *intercostal muscles* (see Vol. 1), situated between the ribs, and the *scalene muscles* (see Vol. 1). The *diaphragm* (see Vol. 1), which divides the abdominal and thoracic cavities, is another important respiratory muscle. The volume of the lung increases or decreases during inspiration or expiration, as the thoracic cavity expands or contracts (see below). Because it adheres to the thoracic wall, the surface of the lung follows the expansion of the thorax although, because of its own elasticity, the lung has a tendency to contract toward the hilum.

Inspiration (A). During inspiration, the thoracic cavity and lung volume enlarge. The ribs move upward, thereby increasing the transverse (**A1**) and sagittal (**A2**) diameter of the thorax and enlarging the epigastric angle (**A3**). This requires the action of the *scalene muscles* and/or *external intercostal muscles*. **Contraction of the diaphragm** (**A4**) causes the *central tendon of the diaphragm to descend,* the *domes of the diaphragm to flatten,* and the th*orax to expand caudally* (**A5**). The deeper the inspiration, the *flatter the costodiaphragmatic recess becomes,* allowing the inferior border of the lung to expand further into this supplementary space.

Expiration (B). During expiration, the thoracic cage and lung volume decrease again. During quiet respiration, the elastic thoracic cage returns to its original position, the *resting position of the thorax*. Its transverse (**B1**) and sagittal (**B2**) diameters decrease, in turn reducing the epigastric angle (**B3**). Contraction of the expiratory *internal intercostal muscles* can aid this process. The domes of the diaphragm (**B4**) move upward, decreasing the size of inferior portion of the thoracic cavity (**B5**). Deeper expiration is assisted by *intraabdominal pressure*, in which the *transverse abdominal muscles* in particular are active.

Thoracic and Abdominal Breathing

As may be presumed from the above description, in the healthy adult respiration involves the combination of two mechanisms.

Thoracic breathing involves changes in the volume of the thorax by movement of the ribs (**1–3**), while in **diaphragmatic breathing**, thoracic volume varies with displacement of the floor of the thoracic cavity (**4–5**).

Infants and older people rely chiefly on abdominal breathing, the former because of the horizontal position of the ribs and the latter because of diminished elasticity of the thorax.

Clinical note. An intact pleural cavity is necessary for normal breathing. If air enters it from outside or inside the body, negative pressure is lost and **pneumothorax** results. In the absence of capillary forces, the lungs cease to follow the movements of the thorax and the force of retraction of the elastic lung causes it to collapse to one-third of its original volume.

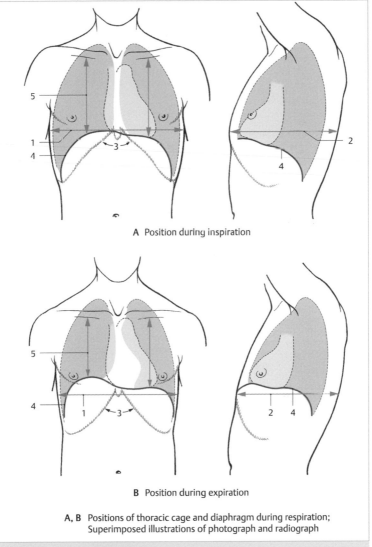

A Position during inspiration

B Position during expiration

A, B Positions of thoracic cage and diaphragm during respiration; Superimposed illustrations of photograph and radiograph

Fig. 3.21 Mechanics of respiration.

3.6 Mediastinum

The mediastinum is the **midline region of connective tissue in the thorax** lying between the two *pleural cavities* (for organization of structures, see p. 32). Contributing to the lateral wall of the mediastinum on either side is the *mediastinal pleura.* If the lung is removed from one half of the thorax and the *mediastinal pleura* is stripped, one can see all of the mediastinal structures in situ, in particular the structures making up the root of the lung.

Right View of the Mediastinum

Viewing the mediastinum from the right after removal of the right lung, it is evident that from craniad to caudad, the mediastinum forms a continuous connected space. The borders (see p. 32) dividing the superior and inferior mediastinum, as well as those further subdividing the inferior mediastinum, are purely descriptive in nature. They nevertheless serve as a guide for the following description of the topography of the mediastinum.

Superior mediastinum. Organs that can be observed in the superior mediastinum, the region above the heart, are the *esophagus* (**A1**) and *trachea* (**A2**). They are accompanied by the *right vagus nerve* (**A3**) and *paratracheal lymph nodes* (**A4**). Lying anterior to these organs is the *superior vena cava* (**A5**), which arises from the union of the *right* (**A6**) and *left brachiocephalic veins.* The right brachiocephalic vein covers the *brachiocephalic trunk* (**A7**), which arises from the aortic arch and gives rise to the *right subclavian artery* (**A8**). Looping around the right subclavian artery is the *recurrent laryngeal nerve* (**A9**), a branch of the vagus nerve. Anterior to the superior vena cava is the intrapericardial part of the *ascending aorta* (**A10**). The great vessels are covered anteriorly by *residual thymic tissue,* which is obscured from view in Figure A, as the overlying *mediastinal pleura* (**A11**) was not completely removed. Viewed from the

right, the boundary between the superior and inferior mediastinum is roughly demarcated by the course of the *azygos vein* (**A12**), which curves over and extends beyond the structures of the root of the right lung.

Inferior mediastinum. The **posterior part of the inferior mediastinum** contains the *thoracic duct* (**A13**), *esophagus* (**A1**), *right vagus nerve* (**A3**), and *greater splanchnic nerve* (**A14**). The wide **middle mediastinum** contains the *pericardium* (**A15**) and *heart,* as well as the intrapericardial portions of the *great vessels.* Running between the pericardium and removed mediastinal pleura is the *phrenic nerve* (**A16**), which accompanies the *pericardiacophrenic vessels* (**A17**). The middle mediastinum also houses the *right main bronchus* and its bronchi (**A18**), the *right pulmonary artery* (**A19**), and *right pulmonary veins* (**A20**), as well as the *tracheobronchial lymph nodes* (**A21**).

Between the sternum and pericardium lies the **anterior mediastinum**, which contains only *loose connective tissue,* a few *lymph nodes,* and branches of the *internal thoracic vessels.*

The medial surface of the right lung lies in close proximity to the esophagus and accompanying branches of the vagus nerve.

Posterior thoracic wall. The sympathetic trunk (**A22**) lies alongside the vertebral column on the posterior thoracic wall, which is partly visible in (**A**). At the inferior border of the ribs, the *intercostal nerves* (**A23**) accompany the *intercostal vessels* (**A24**). These structures lie within, or deep to, the *endothoracic fascia* and hence are not considered mediastinal structures. The endothoracic fascia merges with the *parietal pleura* at the posterior thoracic wall.

Clinical note. In clinical parlance, reference is often made only to the anterior and posterior mediastinum, with the trachea regarded as the boundary between them.

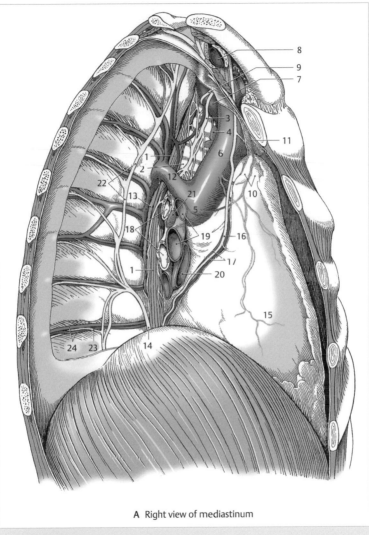

A Right view of mediastinum

Fig. 3.22 Mediastinum from the right side.

Respiratory System

Left View of the Mediastinum

Superior mediastinum. After removal of the left lung, the prominent *aortic arch* (**A1**) can be seen; it gives rise to the *left common carotid artery* (**A2**) and *left subclavian artery* (**A3**). Anterior to the aortic arch are the superficial parts of the *cardiac plexus* (**A4**), an autonomic plexus, and the *left vagus nerve* (**A5**), which branches into the *left recurrent laryngeal nerve* (**A6**). This nerve loops behind the aortic arch and *ligamentum arteriosum* (**A7**). Anterior to the aortic arch, the *left brachiocephalic vein* (**A8**) is visible before it disappears from view. Posterior to the aortic arch, the *esophagus* (**A9**) and *thoracic duct* (**A10**) are visible.

Inferior mediastinum. In the **posterior part of the inferior mediastinum**, the *esophagus* (**A9**) is accompanied by the *descending aorta* (**A11**). The plexus formed by the *left vagus nerve* passes between them caudally. The most posterior of the mediastinal structures on the left side are the *hemiazygos vein* (**A12**) and the *accessory hemiazygos vein* (**A13**).

The **middle part of the inferior mediastinum** is nearly entirely filled by the *pericardium* (**A14**) and *heart*. Passing across on the pericardium is the *left phrenic nerve* (**A15**), which accompanies the *pericardiacophrenic vessels* (**A16**). The structures of the *root of the lung*, which lie in the upper part of the middle mediastinum, are framed by the *aortic arch* and *thoracic part of the aorta*. Nestled

in the curvature of the aortic arch is the *left pulmonary artery* (**A17**), from which the *ligamentum arteriosum* (**A7**) extends to the inferior aspect of the aortic arch. Below the pulmonary artery lie the *left main bronchus* (**A18**) and *left pulmonary veins* (**A19**).

The few structures in the anterior part of the **inferior mediastinum** are not distinguishable in (**A**).

Pronounced impressions on the *medial surface* of the *left lung* are formed by the *aortic arch* and *thoracic part of the aorta*.

Clinical note. Inflammation involving the connective tissue spaces of the neck can spread unimpeded to the mediastinum. Modern imaging modalities such as computed tomography (CT) and magnetic resonance imaging (MRI) present a significant contribution and improvement over conventional radiography in the diagnosis of **mediastinal processes**. Mediastinal tumors arise from a variety of tissues. They are classified according to their location; tumors in the superior mediastinum include *restrosternal goiter, thymomas, lymphomas, hemangiomas, dermoid cysts,* and *teratomas* in children; lipomas are found in the anterior mediastinum; *hilar tumors, hilar lymph node metastases, bronchogenic cysts,* and *pericardial cysts* in the middle mediastinum; *esophageal tumors, lymphomas, neurinomas, fibrosarcomas,* and *ganglioneuromas* in the posterior mediastinum. **Mediastinoscopy** *allows direct visualization of the anterior superior mediastinum and therefore of the paratracheal and tracheobronchial regions of the mediastinum.*

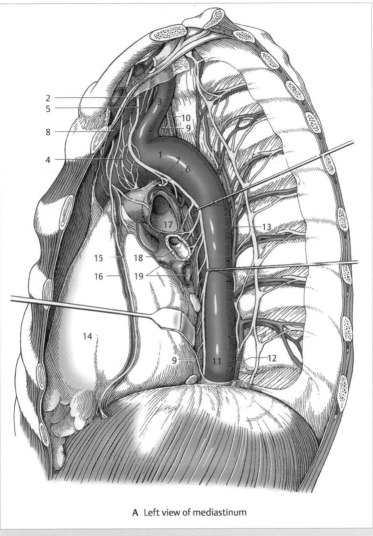

A Left view of mediastinum

Fig. 3.23 Mediastinum from the left side.

4 Alimentary System

4.1 Overview

General Structure and Functions

The main purpose of the **alimentary system** is to ingest food, break it down mechanically and enzymatically, and utilize its nutrients. Food supplies the human body with energy, mostly from proteins, fats, and carbohydrates, as well as providing vital nutritional supplements such as vitamins.

The human alimentary system can be divided into two parts, based on its tasks. The first part, consisting of the digestive organs contained in the **head**, is concerned with the ingestion and mechanical breakdown of food. In the second part, **beginning with the esophagus**, enzymes transform ingested food into nutrients, which are chemically broken down and absorbed, and wastes that are eliminated.

Mouth and pharynx (A). The initial part of the alimentary canal consists of the **oral cavity (A1)**, along with the major and minor **salivary glands**, and the **middle and lower portions of the pharynx (A2)**. In the first part of the digestive tract, food is ingested and broken down with the help of the *lips* (**A3**), *teeth* (**A4**), and *tongue* (**A5**). Saliva lubricates the food bolus, which is then swallowed in individual portions and transported into the pharynx.

Digestive tract proper. The second part of the alimentary system begins with the **esophagus (A6)** and includes the remainder of the alimentary canal, as well as the accessory digestive organs consisting of the **liver (A7)** and **pancreas (A8)**. The esophagus transports the bolus of food toward the **stomach (A9)**, where enzymatic breakdown of food into nutrients begins. Digestion is completed in the **small intestine (A10)**, where component nutrients are absorbed after being further broken down by secretions released from numerous glands. The main function of the **large intestine (A11)** is to absorb water and electrolytes from the intestinal contents, which are transformed by fermentation and decomposition into feces and transported to the **anus (A12)**.

Structure of the Walls of the Digestive Organs

The alimentary system is basically a **muscular tube lined with epithelium** and adapted regionally to the various functions of the digestive organs. The greater part of the epithelium-lined tube is derived from the endoderm (see p. 326).

Mouth and pharynx. Each of the organs of the initial part of the alimentary canal has a different function and thus structure. The tongue, for instance, is composed of striated muscle lined by highly differentiated and specialized epithelial cells. Also contained in the oral cavity are the teeth, which are composed of various hard tissues.

Organs of the digestive tract proper. Most of the organs making up the digestive tract proper are involved in *absorption* and have structurally similar **walls formed by several layers (B)**, consisting of a mucosa (**B13**), submucosa (**B14**), muscular layer (**B15**), serosa, and subserosa or adventitia (**B16**). The **mucosa** is composed of three layers: an *epithelial lining*, which varies regionally and is characteristic for each segment; a layer of connective tissue (*lamina propria*); and a muscular layer (*muscularis mucosae*). The **submucosa** consists of a layer of underlying connective tissue. The **muscular layer** contains two layers of smooth muscle: a *circular layer* and a *longitudinal layer*. On its outer surface, the intestinal canal is either covered by peritoneal **serosa** or embedded in the surrounding structures by the **adventitia**.

The entire intestinal canal is innervated by the **autonomic nervous system**. The **intrinsic**, or enteric, nervous system consists of intramural plexuses, that is, the **submucous plexus** (Meissner plexus) of the submucosa, and the **myenteric plexus** (Auerbach plexus) (see Vol. 3) between the layers of the muscular coat. The intramural plexuses are directly connected to the **extrinsic** (autonomic) nervous system located outside of the gut tube.

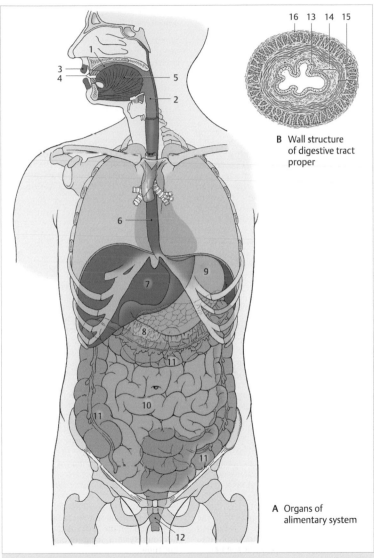

B Wall structure of digestive tract proper

A Organs of alimentary system

Fig. 4.1 General structure and functions of the digestive system.

4.2 Oral Cavity

General Structure

The **oral cavity** is the space lined by the **mucous membrane of the mouth**. It may be divided into three consecutive segments: the **oral vestibule** (**A1**), the **oral cavity proper** (**A2**), and the **fauces**. The **isthmus of fauces** (**A3**) forms the junction of the oral cavity with the pharynx.

Oral vestibule. The oral vestibule is bounded **anteriorly** by the *lips* (**A4**), **laterally** by the *cheeks* (**A5**), and **internally** by the *teeth* (**A6**) and *alveolar processes* (**A7**) of the maxilla and mandible. The *gingiva* (**CD8**) is the part of the mucous membrane that overlies the alveolar processes and is firmly attached to the bone. The gingival mucosa reflects on to the lips and cheeks, forming the *fornix* (**C9**), which has a freely movable mucous membrane. Each of the lips is attached at its midpoint to the gingiva of the maxilla or mandible by a fold of mucous membrane known as the *frenulum of upper lip* (**A10**) or *frenulum of lower lip* (**A11**). Numerous *minor salivary glands*, as well as the duct of the *parotid gland* (see p. 154) open into the oral vestibule. When the teeth are occluded, the only communication between the oral vestibule and the oral cavity proper is behind the third molar tooth.

Oral cavity proper. The **anterior** and **lateral** boundaries of the oral cavity proper are formed by the *alveolar processes, teeth*, and *gingiva*. It communicates **posteriorly** with the *isthmus of fauces*. The **roof** of the oral cavity, formed by the *hard palate* (**A12**) and *soft palate* (**A13**), separates it from the nasal cavity. Its **floor** is formed by the *muscular floor of the mouth* (see p. 152), on which the *tongue* (**ACD14**) rests.

A15 Palatoglossal arch, **A16** Palatopharyngeal arch, **A17** Palatine tonsil, **A18** Uvula

The boundary between the cheeks and the lips is demarcated on the face by the *nasolabial sulcus* (**B19**).

Lips. The upper lip extends to the base of the external nose and the lower lip to the *mentolabial sulcus* (**B20**). The **upper lip** (**B21**) and **lower lip** (**B22**), which meet at either side to form the **angle of the mouth** (**B23**) (labial commissure), surround the **oral fissure** (**B24**). Around the oral fissure, the skin of the face meets the mucous membrane of the mouth in a transition zone called the **vermilion border**. A thickening of the vermilion border on the upper lip forms a *tubercle*, from which a furrow in the skin called the *philtrum* (**B25**) passes toward the nose.

Histology. The lips are fibromuscular **folds** consisting of **facial skin and oral mucosa** overlying the **orbicularis oris** (**C26**), the muscle that forms their bulk, which is one of the muscles of facial expression. On their **outer** surface, the lips are covered by *epidermis*, as well as hair and sweat and sebaceous glands. The **transition zone**, or *vermilion border* (**C27**), where the orbicularis oris folds outwardly in the shape of a hook, is characterized by *lightly keratinized epithelium*. The **inner** surface of the vermilion border is continuous with the oral mucosa, which is lined by *stratified, nonkeratinized squamous epithelium* and contains seromucous *labial glands* (**C28**).

Cheeks (**D**). The principal muscle of the cheeks is the **buccinator** (**D29**), a sheet of muscle belonging to the muscles of facial expression. On its inner aspect, the buccinator is lined by the *mucous membrane of the mouth*, which contains small salivary glands called *buccal glands*. Lying on its outer aspect is the *buccal fat pad* (Bichat fat pad) (**D30**), followed by the masseter muscle (**D31**).

Vessels, nerves, and lymphatic drainage. The cheeks and lips are supplied by branches of the **facial artery**. Venous drainage is through the facial vein. **Sensory** innervation of the upper lip is provided by the *infraorbital nerve* (a branch of the maxillary nerve); that of the lower lip by the *mental nerve* (a branch of the mandibular nerve); and that of the mucous membrane of the cheek by the *buccal nerve* (a branch of the mandibular nerve). **Lymph** from the upper lip drains to the submandibular lymph nodes and the upper group of cervical lymph nodes. Lymph from the lateral portion of the lower lip drains to the submandibular lymph nodes, and lymph from the middle of the lower lip to the submental lymph nodes.

D32 Platysma, **D33** Geniohyoid, **D34** Mylohyoid

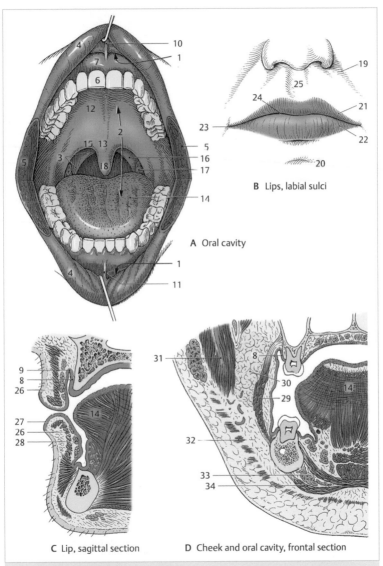

A Oral cavity

B Lips, labial sulci

C Lip, sagittal section

D Cheek and oral cavity, frontal section

Fig. 4.2 General structure of the oral cavity.

Palate

Hard palate (A). The anterior two-thirds of the roof of the oral cavity are formed by the hard palate. The **skeletal** framework of the hard palate consists of the *palatine process of the maxilla* and the *horizontal plate of the palatine bone* (see Vol. 1). The bones of the hard palate are covered by **periosteum** and a **thick mucosa** that is firmly attached to the periosteum and is continuous anteriorly with the *gingiva*. In the midline, there is a mucosal ridge known as the **palatine raphe (A1)**, a tissue elevation that overlies the bony median palatine suture and ends anteriorly in a small eminence known as the *incisive papilla* (**A2**). On either side of the palatine raphe, the mucosa forms flat, transverse ridges called **palatine rugae (A3)**. When food is ingested, the tongue presses it against these ridges and grooves. Lying to the right and left of the midline, in the posterior portion of the mucosal lining of the hard palate, are small mucus-secreting **palatine glands (A4)**, which produce saliva that lubricates ingested food.

Soft palate (B). The posterior one-third of the roof of the oral cavity is formed by the **soft palate**, a musculotendinous structure that extends obliquely backward from the hard palate like a sail. Hanging down from the middle of the posterior border of the soft palate is the **uvula (A–C5)**, a small conical mass of tissue. On either side from the uvula, two **palatine arches** extend downward, diverging as they pass caudally. The two folds of each side surround a niche containing the **palatine tonsil (B6)**. The anterior of the two, the **palatoglossal arch (B7)**, passes to the lateral margin of the tongue, while the posterior arch, the **palatopharyngeal arch (B8)**, extends into the wall of the pharynx. The narrowed portion of the fauces produced by the two arches, the **isthmus of fauces**, forms the entrance to the pharynx and can be closed by muscular action. The mucosa and glands of the hard palate are continuous with those of the soft palate.

Palatine Muscles

The palatine muscles insert into the firm, fibrous **palatine aponeurosis (C9)**, a continuation of the periosteum, which contributes to formation of the soft palate.

Tensor veli palatini (C10). The tensor muscle of the soft palate arises as a thin, triangular sheet of muscle from the *cranial base* and the *wall of the auditory tube*. It passes downward and ends in a tendon that passes around the pterygoid hamulus (**C11**) and continues horizontally to merge with the *palatine aponeurosis*. The tensor veli palatini tenses and elevates the soft palate until it lies in the horizontal plane, thereby opening the orifice of the auditory tube. It is innervated by a branch from the *mandibular nerve*.

Levator veli palatini (C12). The levator veli palatini arises at the *cranial base* posterior and medial to the tensor veli palatini and the *torus tubarius*. It passes obliquely forward, downward, and medially, to insert into the *palatine aponeurosis*. It elevates and retracts the soft palate. Innervation is by the *pharyngeal plexus* (vagal nerve and glossopharyngeal nerve).

Along with the superior constrictor muscle of the pharynx, the tensor veli palatini and levator veli palatini contribute to the formation of the lateral wall of the pharynx.

Palatoglossus (B13). The palatoglossus muscle lies in the *anterior* palatine arch. It arises from the *palatine aponeurosis* and passes into the *lateral margin of the base of the tongue*. It acts to constrict the isthmus of fauces by elevating the root of the tongue or lowering the soft palate and is innervated by the *glossopharyngeal nerve*.

Palatopharyngeus (B14). The palatopharyngeus lies in the *posterior* palatine arch. It also arises from the *palatine aponeurosis* and is one of the muscles that elevate the pharynx. Innervation is by the *glossopharyngeal nerve*.

Musculus uvulae (B15). The musculus uvulae is a paired muscle that arises from the palatine aponeurosis and sometimes from the bony *hard palate*. It inserts behind the levator veli palatini into the *aponeurosis of the uvula*, extending within the uvula to its tip. It shortens the uvula and is innervated by the *pharyngeal plexus*.

Clinical note. Cleft palate interferes with the function of the soft palate and hence with ventilation of the middle ear via the auditory tube.

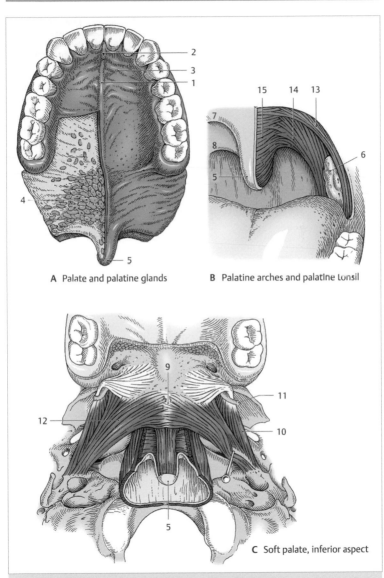

A Palate and palatine glands

B Palatine arches and palatine tonsil

C Soft palate, inferior aspect

Fig. 4.3 Palate.

Tongue

The **tongue** is a **strong muscular organ** that can change its shape and has a highly differentiated **mucous membrane**. It can be divided into a **body**, a **tip** (**apex**) (**A1**), and a root which attaches it to the surrounding bony structures. The convex surface of the tongue, the **dorsum of the tongue** (**A2**), is divided into two portions by a V-shaped furrow known as the **terminal sulcus** (**A3**). At the tip of the terminal sulcus is the *foramen cecum* (**A4**), from which the thyroid precursor is derived.

About two-thirds of the tongue lie in front of the sulcus. This part forms the oral tongue, also known as the **anterior part** or **presulcal part** (**A5**). Posterior to the sulcus, the remaining one-third forms the pharyngeal part, also known as the **posterior part** or **postsulcal part** (**A6**). This part of the tongue lies behind the palatoglossal arch in the oropharynx and is nearly vertical. The anterior and posterior parts of the tongue differ in terms of mucosal structure, innervation, and embryological origin.

Anterior part. The oral tongue lies on the floor of the mouth. The dorsum of the anterior part of the tongue is in contact with the palate, the tip touches the incisor teeth, and the *margin of the tongue* (**A7**) touches the premolar teeth. The dorsum of the tongue is continuous at its margin with the *inferior surface of the tongue* (see p. 152). The **mucous membrane** covering the dorsum of the tongue is composed of *stratified, nonkeratinized squamous epithelium* and is firmly attached to the underlying sheet of connective tissue known as the *lingual aponeurosis*. The mucous membrane covering the oral tongue presents a midline groove known as the **median sulcus of the tongue** (**A8**). The mucosal structure of the dorsum of the tongue is given its characteristic appearance by the various macroscopically visible **papillae of the tongue** (**A9**, **B–E**) which consist of a connective tissue core with an epithelial covering.

Papillae of the tongue. The lingual papillae may be divided into **four types** according to shape: **filiform papillae** (**B10**, **C**) are threadlike papillae that have projections composed of keratinized epithelium and are split at their tips. They are distributed over most of the dorsum of the tongue and

mainly transmit *tactile information*. They do not contain taste buds. **Fungiform papillae** (**B11**, **D**) are mushroom-shaped epithelial projections with a smooth surface that are mostly located on the margin of the tongue. They contain *taste buds* as well as mechanoreceptors and thermoreceptors. Their main function is to perceive dissolved flavors. **Foliate papillae** (**A12**) are leaf-shaped papillae arranged in rows along the posterior margin of the tongue that have abundant *taste buds*. There are 7–12 **vallate papillae** (**B13**, **E**), lying anterior to the terminal sulcus. They are surrounded by a deep narrow circular sulcus with a raised wall, and contain numerous *taste buds* (see Vol. 3). The ducts of the serous secreting glands (Ebner glands) open in the base of the sulcus.

Posterior part. The postsulcal, pharyngeal part of the tongue (also referred to as the base or root of the tongue) forms the *anterior wall of the oropharynx*. The base of the tongue is continuous laterally with the *palatine tonsil* (**A14**) and the *lateral wall of the pharynx*. Three mucosal folds extend from the posterior part of the tongue to the epiglottis: the **median glossoepiglottic fold** (**A15**) in the midline and a **lateral glossoepiglottic fold** (**A16**) from each side. Between these folds are two depressions known as the **epiglottic valleculae** (**A17**). The irregular and bumpy surface of the base of the tongue is formed by subepithelial lymphoid follicles known as **lingual follicles** (**AB18**). The lingual follicles collectively form the **lingual tonsil** (see p. 416). There are no papillae here.

Innervation of the mucous membrane of the tongue. General sensory innervation of the **presulcal part** is provided by the *lingual nerve* (arising from the mandibular nerve). Innervation of sensory receptor organs, with the exception of the vallate papillae, is by the *chorda tympani* (arising from the intermediate nerve, part of the facial nerve). The **postsulcal part**, with the exception of the epiglottic valleculae, receives sensory innervation from the *glossopharyngeal nerve*. The epiglottic valleculae are innervated by the *vagus nerve*. Sensory afferent fibers from the taste buds on the posterior one-third of the tongue also travel via the *glossopharyngeal nerve*, and those from the region around the epiglottic valleculae travel via the *vagus nerve*.

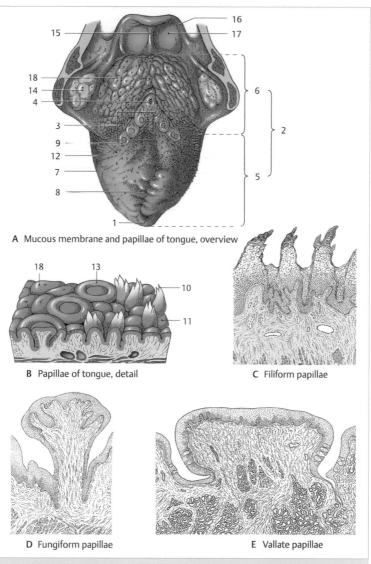

A Mucous membrane and papillae of tongue, overview

B Papillae of tongue, detail

C Filiform papillae

D Fungiform papillae

E Vallate papillae

Fig. 4.4 Tongue.

Alimentary System

Muscles of the Tongue

The **muscles of the tongue** are divided into **extrinsic** muscles, which arise from skeletal structures, and **intrinsic** muscles, which are located only inside the tongue and are not attached to bone.

Extrinsic Muscles of the Tongue

The extrinsic muscles of the tongue include the genioglossus, hyoglossus, styloglossus, and palatoglossus. For information on the palatoglossus, see the discussion of the muscles of the soft palate (see p. 146).

Genioglossus (**AB1**). The genioglossus is a paired muscle that arises from the *mental spine* of the mandible above the geniohyoid. It fans out posteriorly and superiorly from the tip of the tongue into the *body of the tongue*, where its fibers attach to the lingual aponeurosis and merge with those of the intrinsic tongue muscles. The genioglossus moves the tongue forward and draws it toward the floor of the mouth. The genioglossus is covered laterally by the hyoglossus.

Hyoglossus (**A2**). The hyoglossus arises as a thin, four-sided sheet of muscle from the *greater horn of the hyoid bone* (**A3**) and the *body of the hyoid bone* (**A4**). It passes almost vertically to radiate into the *tongue* laterally to the genioglossus. If the hyoid bone is fixed, the hyoglossus draws the tongue backward and upward.

Styloglossus (**A5**). The styloglossus arises from the styloid process and radiates to the tongue in the posterior palatine arch. Its fibers pass anteriorly in the lateral border of the tongue to the *apex of the tongue*. The styloglossus draws the tongue backward and upward.

Vessels and nerves. With the exception of the palatoglossus, the extrinsic muscles of the tongue are innervated by the **hypoglossal nerve** (**A6**). The hypoglossal nerve lies on the hyoglossus muscle, giving off a small branch to its anterior border, which passes forward into the geniohyoid. It also gives rise to a thick, ascending branch to the genioglossus and intrinsic tongue muscles. The ascending terminal branch of the hypoglossal nerve crosses below the duct of the submandibular gland (**A7**) and the lingual nerve (**A8**). Blood supply to the tongue muscles is from the **lingual artery** (**A9**), which runs from posterior and passes deep under the hyoglossus, distributing its terminal portions, the *deep lingual artery* and *sublingual artery*, beneath the muscle.

AB10 Geniohyoid, **A11** Palatoglossus, **A12** Palatopharyngeus, **A13** Superior constrictor muscle of pharynx

Intrinsic Muscles of the Tongue

The intrinsic muscles of the tongue consist of groups of fibers that run in each of the three principal planes and are attached to the connective tissue framework of the tongue. The connective tissue framework consists of the *lingual septum*, a median, vertically fibrous tissue septum dividing the tongue incompletely into two halves, and the *lingual aponeurosis* (**C14**), a tough sheet of connective tissue on the dorsum of the tongue between the mucous membrane and muscles of the tongue. On either side of the lingual septum are the following fiber bundles.

Superior and inferior longitudinal muscles (**B15**). These superior and inferior longitudinal muscles are well-defined bundles that pass near the dorsum of the tongue under the lingual aponeurosis and the inferior surface of the tongue from its *tip* to its *base*.

Transverse muscle of tongue (**C17**). The transverse muscle of the tongue is a powerful muscle consisting of transverse fibers, some of which radiate into the *lingual septum*, *lingual aponeurosis*, and *lateral margin of the tongue*. A small number of fibers cross over the septum.

Vertical muscle of tongue (**C18**). The vertical muscle of the tongue is composed of vertical fibers that pass in a slight curve from the *surface of the tongue* to the *lingual aponeurosis*.

The intrinsic muscles **alter the shape of the tongue**. Two muscles usually act as agonists, forcing the third to relax. The intrinsic muscles of the tongue are innervated by the **hypoglossal nerve**.

Clinical note. Disorders of the hypoglossal nerve can lead to paralysis of one half of the tongue. The unaffected half moves toward the affected half, with the tip of the tongue pointing toward the side affected by paralysis. The surface of the tongue on the affected half appears wrinkled, as a result of atrophy of the intrinsic muscles.

BC19 Mylohyoid, **C20** Platysma

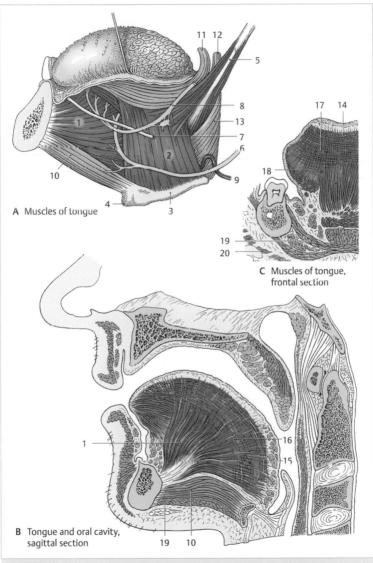

A Muscles of tongue

C Muscles of tongue, frontal section

B Tongue and oral cavity, sagittal section

Fig. 4.5 Muscles of tongue.

Alimentary System

Inferior Surface of the Tongue (A)

The inferior surface of the tongue rests on the floor of the mouth and can only be observed when the tongue is lifted. The mucosa on the inferior surface of the tongue is thin and adheres loosely to the body of the tongue. In the midline, the mucosa forms the **frenulum of the tongue** (**A1**), a mucosal fold that extends to the gingiva of the mandible. On either side of the frenulum of the tongue, the thick, blue **deep lingual vein** (**A2**) can be seen shimmering through the mucosa. The fringed **fimbriated fold** (**A3**) usually lies lateral to it and is a rudiment of the sublingua, which is present in animals. Near the tip of the tongue, a small sublingual gland may produce a mucosal elevation on each side. On the floor of the oral cavity, the mucosa contains a narrow longitudinal fold on either side, known as the **sublingual fold** (**A4**), which conceals the sublingual gland (see p. 154). At the anterior end of the fold is a wartlike prominence known as the **sublingual caruncle** (**A5**), where the ducts of the large sublingual gland and submandibular gland open together or near each other.

Clinical note. Some drugs can be absorbed rapidly through the thin mucosa of the floor of the mouth and inferior surface of the tongue (*sublingual administration*), for example, glyceryl trinitrate to treat the symptoms of angina.

Floor of the Mouth

The floor of the oral cavity lies between the anterior portions of the rami of the mandible. It is formed by a sheet of muscle known as the **diaphragma oris**, which is mainly formed by the mylohyoid muscles.

Mylohyoid (**B6**). The mylohyoid muscle originates from the *mylohyoid line* (**B7**) on the mandible and passes downward, medially, and backward to a median *raphe* and to the *hyoid bone* (**B8**). Innervation of the mylohyoid is supplied by the *nerve to the mylohyoid* (arising from the mandibular nerve).

Geniohyoid (**B9**). The geniohyoid lies on either side of the midline of the floor of the oral cavity and reinforces it from the inside.

It arises at the *mental spine* on the body of the mandible and passes to the body of the *hyoid bone*. Innervation is provided by the anterior rami of the *first and second cervical nerves* (cervical plexus), via fibers traveling in the hypoglossal nerve.

Digastric. The digastric muscle consists of two bellies. Its **posterior belly** arises from the *mastoid notch* of the temporal bone and is continuous at the level of the body of the hyoid bone with an intermediate tendon; innervation is provided by the *facial nerve*. Its **anterior belly** originates from the *digastric fossa* of the mandible and is continuous with the intermediate tendon, which is attached to the *hyoid bone* by a connective tissue loop (see Fig. **A** of the major salivary glands, p. 155). Innervation of the anterior belly is provided by the *nerve to the mylohyoid*.

Stylohyoid. The stylohyoid muscle originates from the *styloid process* and inserts into the *body and greater horn of the hyoid bone*. Its tendon of insertion divides to encircle the intermediate tendon of the digastric. The stylohyoid is innervated by the *facial nerve*.

The muscles discussed above, all of which are located above the hyoid bone, are referred to as the **suprahyoid muscles**. The suprahyoid muscles are involved in active opening of the mouth and raising the hyoid bone upward and forward during swallowing.

B10 Hyoglossus, **B11** Stylohyoid, **B12** Lingual artery, **B13** Genioglossus

Clinical note. Diffusely spreading and poorly demarcated inflammation due to *staphylococcal* and *streptococcal* infection can develop in the loose tissue of the floor of the mouth, leading to **oral cellulitis**. It may be caused by dental caries, stomatitis, or a local lymph node abscess. Painful infiltration produces palpable swelling of the floor of the mouth, difficulty swallowing, and general symptoms of sepsis.

Alimentary System

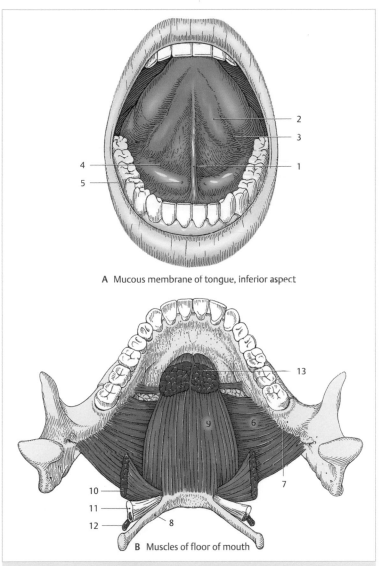

A Mucous membrane of tongue, inferior aspect

B Muscles of floor of mouth

Fig. 4.6 Undersurface of the tongue and floor of the mouth.

Salivary Glands

The ducts from numerous small salivary glands known as the **minor salivary glands** as well as those from the three paired **major salivary glands** drain into the oral cavity and vestibule.

Minor Salivary Glands

The minor salivary glands include the *"packages" of glandular tissue lying in the mucosa of the lips, cheeks, tongue, and palate* containing mucous secretory units (see p. 156), as well as the *anterior lingual glands*, which are located in the tip of the tongue, sometimes on the underside of its apex. On top of the papillae of the tongue are small glands known as *cleansing glands* that contain only serous secretory units (see p. 156). The main function of the minor salivary glands is to **moisten the oral mucosa**.

Major Salivary Glands

Parotid gland (**A1**). The **purely serous** parotid gland ("parotid" for short) is the largest of the salivary glands. It is enclosed in the tough **parotid fascia** and lies in front of and below the *external acoustic meatus* on the posterior part of the masseter (**A2**). It covers the temporomandibular joint and is divided by the branches of the *facial nerve* into a **superficial part** and a **deep part**. The parotid gland extends superiorly to the *zygomatic arch* (**A3**), inferiorly to the *angle of the mandible* (**A4**), and deeply, behind the ramus of the mandible in the *retromandibular fossa* (see Vol. 1), to the wall of the pharynx. The 3–4-mm thick **parotid duct** (**A5**) projects from the anterior border of the gland and passes parallel to the zygomatic arch over the masseter and buccal fat pad, penetrating the buccinator obliquely (**A6**) and opening in the *oral vestibule* at the level of the upper second molar tooth on the **parotid papilla**. A small **accessory parotid gland** (**A7**) often lies adjacent to the duct. The production and release of glandular secretions are regulated by the autonomic nervous system. Preganglionic **parasympathetic**

fibers travel in the *glossopharyngeal nerve* (see Vol. 3), synapse in the *otic ganglion*, and are distributed to the gland in *branches of the facial nerve*.

Sympathetic fibers arise from the *external carotid plexus* and accompany vessels to the gland.

Submandibular gland (**AB8**). The **predominantly serous** submandibular gland lies in the *submandibular triangle* below the floor of the mouth (see Vol. 1), which is bounded by the mandible and the anterior (**A9**) and posterior (**A10**) bellies of the digastric muscle. The body of the gland is enclosed in a capsule and lies under the *mylohyoid* (**A11**), extending deeply to the *hyoglossus* (**B12**) and *styloglossus*. The **submandibular duct** (**B13**) is accompanied by a hook like process of glandular tissue. It travels along the superior surface of the posterior border of the mylohyoid, then passes forward, medial to the sublingual gland (**B14**), to open on the **sublingual caruncle** (**B15**). The preganglionic **parasympathetic** fibers to the submandibular gland arise from the *chorda tympani*, a branch of the facial nerve (see Vol. 3), pass to the *submandibular ganglion*, and leave it as the postganglionic fibers that innervate the gland. **Sympathetic** fibers reach the gland via adjacent blood vessels.

Sublingual gland (**B14**). The **predominantly mucous** sublingual gland lies on the *mylohyoid* and *produces the sublingual fold* (**B16**). It extends laterally as far as the *mandible* and medially to the *genioglossus* (**B17**). The duct of the **principal gland** of the sublingual gland complex, the **major sublingual duct**, opens on the **sublingual caruncle** beside the frenulum, alone or after uniting with the submandibular duct. The numerous **minor sublingual glands** have short ducts that open along the *sublingual fold* directly into the oral cavity. **Parasympathetic** fibers reach the sublingual gland by the same route as those to the submandibular gland. **Sympathetic fibers** travel to it via the vascular plexus along the lingual artery.

B18 Hypoglossal nerve, **B19** Lingual artery

Alimentary System

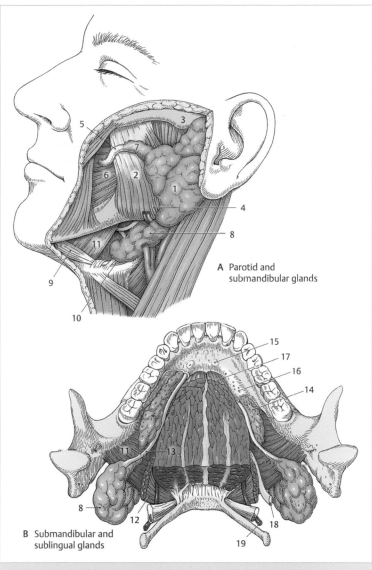

A Parotid and submandibular glands

B Submandibular and sublingual glands

Fig. 4.7 Salivary glands.

Microscopic Anatomy of the Salivary Glands

The salivary glands are **exocrine glands** that secrete **saliva** through their ducts into the oral cavity. Saliva increases the slipperiness of chewed food, has bactericidal properties, and contains an enzyme that breaks down carbohydrates. A total of 0.5–2.0 L of saliva are secreted daily in response to stimulation of chemoreceptors in the mouth, as a result of chewing movements, and due to psychological stimuli. The **composition** of saliva depends on the gland from which it is secreted and its functional status. Saliva can be in the form of *watery, serous saliva* containing the enzyme α-amylase, or it can be *viscous, mucous saliva* containing *mucopolysaccharides* and *glycoproteins*. Microscopic features of individual salivary glands vary accordingly. Each gland consists of groups of exocrine cells that make up the **secretory unit** (**I**) and a **system of ducts** (**II**). *Secretory units* may consist of only *serous cells* (**A–C1**), only *mucous cells* (**ACD2**), or *mixed cells* in various proportions (**D**).

Secretory unit. Serous cells typically form a secretory unit (end-piece) called an **acinus**, which is shaped like a berry and contains a small lumen (**A1**). Acinar cells are tall and pyramidal in shape, have finely granulated cytoplasm, and a round, centrally located nucleus.

Mucous cells tend to form secretory units consisting of a small **tubule** with a wide lumen (**A2**). Tubular cells are tall, their cytoplasm has a honeycomb appearance, and their flattened nuclei lie near the base of the cells. Lying between the mucous cells and their basement membranes are **myoepithelial cells**, contractile cells that are believed to facilitate the secretion of saliva.

Excretory duct system. The duct system proceeds from the secretory units and is composed of various portions, some of which are not present in every gland. The **intercalated duct** (**A3**), which has a small diameter and is lined by low epithelium, drains the secretory unit. This segment is followed by a **secretory** (**striated**) **duct** (**A–C4**).

Secretory ducts have a large diameter and are lined by a simple epithelium consisting of tall prismatic cells with basal striations. These striations are produced by infoldings of the plasma membrane with columns of vertically arranged mitochondria between them. The secretory ducts open into progressively larger **excretory ducts** (**A5**), which have a wide lumen containing simple or pseudostratified epithelium consisting of stratified tall prismatic cells.

Salivary glands are subdivided by connective tissue into lobes and lobules. The *secretory units, intercalated ducts,* and *secretory ducts* are **intralobular** structures situated within the lobules of the gland. The *excretory ducts* lie in the connective tissue between the lobules and thus are **interlobular** structures.

The **parotid gland** (**B**) is a **purely serous** gland which contains all of the components of the duct system. Fat cells and plasma cells are often found in the interlobular connective tissue.

The **submandibular gland** (**C**) is a **mixed, predominantly serous** gland, some of whose intercalated ducts are converted into mucous tubules. The crescent-shaped tubules rest atop the serous secretory units. The submandibular gland also contains all other components of the duct system.

The **sublingual gland** (**D**) is a **mixed, predominantly mucous** gland with virtually no intercalated or secretory ducts.

Clinical note. Stones (sialoliths) can form in the large ducts, owing to deposition of calcium phosphate or calcium carbonate, causing blockage and painful swelling of the gland. Dental tartar is also a product of saliva.

Mumps (epidemic parotitis) is an infection caused by the mumps virus, which can cause typical swelling of the parotid gland(s). Chewing movements are very painful because the tough capsule enclosing the parotid gland is unable to stretch. Mumps is the most common cause of unilateral early childhood deafness. Mumps orchitis may also occur, with a risk of testicular atrophy and infertility.

Alimentary System

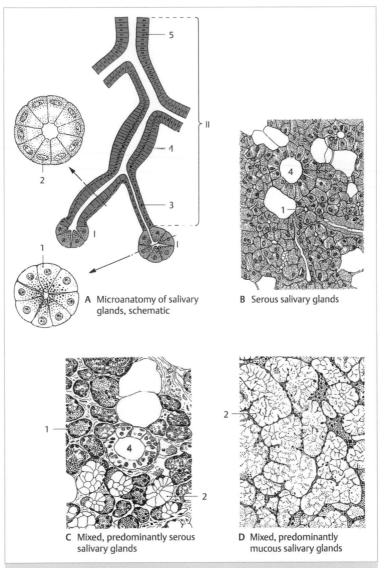

A Microanatomy of salivary glands, schematic

B Serous salivary glands

C Mixed, predominantly serous salivary glands

D Mixed, predominantly mucous salivary glands

Fig. 4.8 Microscopic structure of the salivary glands.

Alimentary System

Teeth

In human dentition, the **teeth** are contained in the bony sockets of the mandible and maxilla, without any space (*diastema*) between adjacent teeth. Humans have **heterodont** dentition, that is, individual teeth are shaped differently according to function. In the human dental arcade, one set of teeth replaces another, that is, humans are **diphyodont**. The first set of teeth consists of the *deciduous teeth*, which are later replaced by the *permanent teeth*.

Tooth segments. Each tooth can be divided into three segments: a **crown** (**A1**), a **neck** (**A2**), and a **root** (**A3**). The root is the part of the tooth that lies in the bony socket and is secured by the periodontium. The neck of the tooth describes the narrow junction between the crown and root; it projects above the socket but is covered by the gingiva. The neck corresponds to the dentinoenamel junction.

Crown. The crown is the part of the tooth that is visible above the gingiva. Several surfaces may be distinguished: the **occlusal surface** (**B4**), which has contact with the tooth in the opposing dental arcade; the **vestibular surface** (**B5**) facing the *lips* (**B5 a**) or *cheeks* (**B5 b**); the **lingual surface** (**B6**) or **palatal surface** (**B7**), namely the inner surface; and the **approximal surface** (**B8**) facing the adjacent tooth. The approximal surface is subdivided into a *mesial surface* (**B8 a**), which faces anteriorly or medially, and a *distal surface* (**B8 b**), which faces posteriorly or laterally.

Dental arcades. The teeth of the maxilla and mandible are arranged in dental arches known as the **upper** and **lower dental arcades**.

The maxillary dental arcade is shaped like a half of an ellipse, while the mandibular dental arcade is shaped like a parabola. With normal **occlusion**, the teeth thus do not meet exactly; the incisor teeth of the maxilla overlap those of the mandible; that is, the dental arcades are not congruent. If the dental arcade is divided in half along the median plane, the teeth of one half are arranged in the mirror image of those of the other half. The permanent teeth are ordered according to function. From mesial to distal

they are: the two **incisor teeth** (**B9**), followed by one **canine tooth** (**B10**), then two **premolar teeth** (**B11**), and finally **three molar teeth** (**B12**) (4 × 8 = 32 teeth).

Functional anatomy. The **incisor teeth** are used for *biting* and have a chisel-shaped crown with a horizontal cutting edge. There is usually an eminence on the lingual or palatal surface known as the *tubercle of the tooth* (**B13**). The incisor tooth has a single, long, conical root. The **canine teeth** are used for *tearing* and *grasping*. Each canine tooth has two cutting edges, a cusp tip, and a single, very long root. The **premolar teeth** are used for *grinding* food. Each premolar tooth has two *cusps* on its occlusal surface, which end in an *apex of the cusp*. The roots of the *upper premolar teeth* are divided, while the *lower premolars* have simple roots. The **molar teeth** are responsible for the *bulk of chewing*. Their occlusal surfaces have four or five cusps each (**B14**). The molar teeth of the maxilla have three roots each and those of the mandible have two roots each.

Tooth sockets, alveoli. The teeth are housed in the bony sockets of the alveolar processes of the maxilla and mandible. Individual sockets are separated from each other by **interalveolar septa** (**B15**). Sockets that hold teeth possessing multiple roots are subdivided within the socket by **interradicular septa** (**B16**).

Dental formulae (**permanent dentition**). Various numbering systems are used to identify teeth and these often differ internationally. The Federation Dentaire Internationale (**FDI**) has introduced a computerized system for numbering teeth by quadrants, beginning from the upper right quadrant with 1–4 (first digit) and then numbering the teeth from mesial to distal as 1–8 (second digit).

Right maxillary quadrant: 11, 12, 13, 14, 15, 16, 17, 18

Left maxillary quadrant: 21, 22, 23, 24, 25, 26, 27, 28

Left mandibular quadrant: 31, 32, 33, 34, 35, 36, 37, 38

Right mandibular quadrant: 41, 42, 43, 44, 45, 46, 47, 48

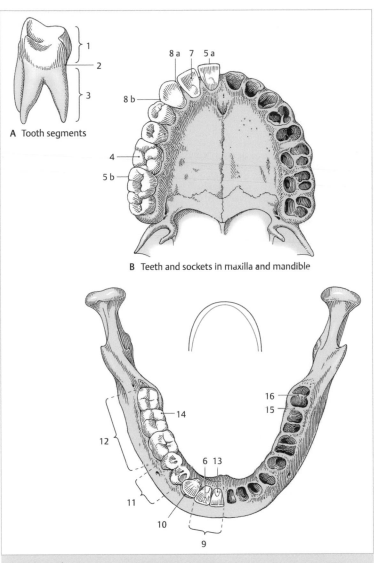

A Tooth segments

B Teeth and sockets in maxilla and mandible

Fig. 4.9 Teeth.

Alimertary System

Alimentary System

Parts of the Tooth and the Periodontium

The bulk of the tooth consists of **dentin** (**AB1**) surrounding a **pulp cavity** (**AB2**) filled with loose connective tissue known as **dental pulp**. The pulp cavity consists of the *pulp cavity of the crown* (**B2 a**), the *root canal* (**B2 b**), and the *apical foramen* (**B2 c**), an opening at the tip of the root. The portion of the dentin in the tooth crown is surrounded by **enamel** (**AB3**) and the dentin of the tooth root is covered by a substance that resembles woven bone, called **cement** (**AB4**). The enamel and cement meet at the neck of the tooth. The tooth in the bony socket is held by a fibrous **periodontal ligament** (**B5**) that connects the root to the alveolar bone and permits slight mobility. Together, the *periodontal fibers, cement, gingiva,* and *alveolar wall* are collectively known as the **periodontium**. The **gingiva** (**B6**), which projects above the border of the alveolus, is lined on its surface facing the tooth by epithelial cells that form a *junctional epithelium* (**B7**). The junctional epithelium overlies the dentinoenamel junction of the neck of the tooth and lines the *gingival sulcus* (**B8**), a furrow between the tooth and gingival margin.

Microscopic Anatomy of the Tooth and Periodontium

The dentin, enamel, and cement of the tooth are all composed of hard tissue that resembles bone. They contain the same chemical components as bone, but in different proportions.

Dentin. Dentin, which is yellowish in color, is formed by **odontoblasts** lying in epithelial formation adjacent to its inner surface. Odontoblasts send projections of cytoplasm called *odontoblastic processes* (*Tomes' fibers*) into the **dental canaliculi** (**B9**), which extend to the dentinoenamel or

cementodentinal junction, giving dentin its characteristic radial striping (**B10**). The dental canaliculi are walled in by **ground substance**, which, similar to bone, consists of *organic matrix, collagen fibrils,* and *calcium salts*. There are no blood vessels in the dentin. Odontoblasts constantly synthesize new predentin on the inner surface of the pulp cavity even after tooth eruption (**B11**).

Enamel. Enamel, the *hardest substance in the human body,* consists of about 97% inorganic material, 90% of which is hydroxyapatite. Enamel is acellular and contains no vessels or nerves; it is composed of **enamel prisms**, which are produced by cells of the inner enamel epithelium following differentiation to *enameloblasts* (adamantoblasts), and joined by a calcified organic interprismatic matrix.

Cement. Cement, produced by cementoblasts, contains **few cells and resembles woven bone**. It is connected by collagen fibers to the dentin and alveolar wall. The collagen fibers (Sharpey fibers) in the periodontal ligament (**B5**) run between the cement and bony socket and are anchored in both of these hard tissues.

Dental pulp. Dental pulp fills the dental cavity with **loose connective tissue**. It is well vascularized and contains myelinated and unmyelinated nerves. The *odontoblasts* are arranged like a palisade at the dentine junction and continue to produce dentin, even in old age.

Clinical note. Deepening of the gingival sulcus leads to formation of pockets, leaving the neck of the tooth exposed. In clinical usage, the part of the tooth projecting above the gingiva is referred to as the **clinical crown**, and the part below the gingival margin as the **clinical root**. **Periodontitis** is a condition in which the gingiva separates from the tooth. Colonization of bacteria in periodontal "pockets" can ultimately lead to inflammation and damage to the periodontium (periodontal disease).

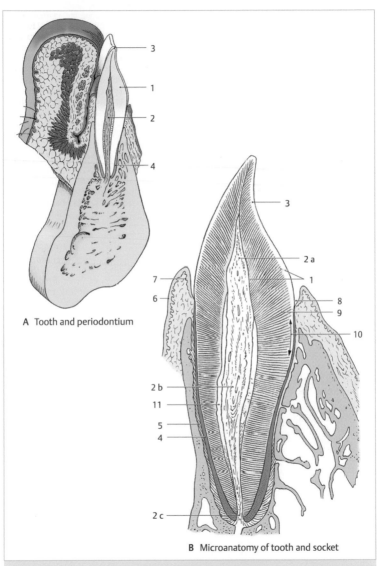

A Tooth and periodontium

B Microanatomy of tooth and socket

Fig. 4.10 Tooth and periodontium components.

Deciduous Teeth

The **deciduous** (**primary**) teeth are a light bluish color and have a translucent appearance, similar to that of porcelain. The entire dental arcade contains a total of **20** teeth, with each half of the dental arch holding **two incisor teeth** (**A1**), **one canine tooth** (**A2**), and **two primary molars** (**A3**). The shape of the primary teeth resembles that of the permanent teeth. The dentin is thinner and less durable than that of the permanent teeth.

The primary and permanent teeth develop in two phases. The germs of the primary teeth begin forming during the 2nd month of embryonic development at the site of the future maxilla and mandible (see p. 164, Development of the Teeth).

Dental formula for deciduous teeth. Based on the **FDI** system (see p. 158), primary dentition is numbered as follows: the first digit (5–8) corresponds to the quadrants from upper right to lower right, and the second digit (1–5) identifies the teeth from mesial to distal:

Right maxillary quadrant: 51, 52, 53, 54, 55.
Left maxillary quadrant: 61, 62, 63, 64, 65.
Left mandibular quadrant: 71, 72, 73, 74, 75.
Right mandibular quadrant: 81, 82, 83, 84, 85.

Eruption of the Primary and Permanent Dentition

Eruption of the **primary dentition** begins postnatal between *months 6 and 8* and is completed by *age 2*. The incisor teeth are the first to appear, followed by the first primary molar and canine teeth, and finally the second primary molar tooth. Deciduous teeth erupt after the crown has been completely formed, at which point the root formation is still incomplete, and the root canal is wide. Before eruption, the gingiva around the site of the emerging tooth becomes swollen and discolored. The white apex of the tooth appears beneath the gingival epithelium, which it soon perforates. Following eruption, the tooth root grows considerably, and differentiation of the tissue of the periodontal ligament starts. The enamel cuticle covering the crown of the erupted tooth is gradually resorbed.

The crowns of the **permanent teeth** (**B**) lie below the primary teeth. In the maxilla they are mostly situated at the future site of development of the maxillary sinus. The premolar teeth lie between the roots of the primary molar teeth. Distal to the primary molars are the tooth germs of the three true molar teeth. Although they erupt later, they are considered part of the primary dentition, and are thus also called "accessional teeth" (**B4**). By contrast, the incisor teeth, canine teeth, and primary molar teeth are replaced by permanent teeth.

> **Clinical note.** The primary teeth serve as placeholders for the permanent teeth. In the event of damage, they should be retained as long as possible, in order to ensure proper positioning of the permanent teeth. Premature loss of primary teeth has a serious impact on the permanent teeth, as these can move into the resulting gaps unobstructed and usually misdirected. The resulting abnormal tooth positions often lead to inhibition of jaw growth, with a discrepancy between the upper and lower jaws. Orthodontic treatment is then required.

Table 4.1 Order and Age at Eruption of Primary and Permanent Teeth

Teeth	Month (primary dentition)	Year (permanent dentition)
Incisor tooth 1	6–8	7–8
Incisor tooth 2	8–12	8–9
Canine tooth	16–20	11–13
Premolar tooth	12–16	9–11
Premolar tooth	20–24	11–13
Molar tooth 1		6–7
Molar tooth 2		12–14
Molar tooth 3		17–40

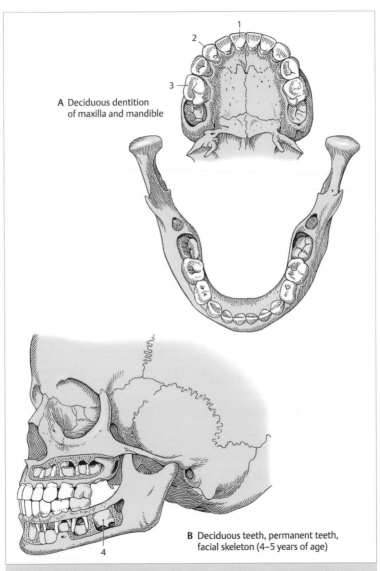

A Deciduous dentition
of maxilla and mandible

B Deciduous teeth, permanent teeth,
facial skeleton (4–5 years of age)

Fig. 4.11 Deciduous teeth.

Alimentary System

Alimentary System

Development of the Teeth

Two germ layers are involved in the development of each tooth: *ectoderm*, which produces the enamel, and *mesoderm*, which forms the dental pulp, predentin, and dentin. The developmental processes of the deciduous and permanent teeth are identical, but occur in two separate stages.

Development of the Tooth Germ (A)

During the 2nd month of embryonic development, a curved band of epithelium, the **dental lamina** (**A2**), forms in the deeper connective tissues (**A3**) at the sites of the future maxilla and mandible. The dental lamina produces 10 nodular epithelial **dental organs** on its labial surface, which initially assume a *cap* or *bell* shape and eventually form the 10 deciduous teeth. The bell-shaped dental organ has a bilayered wall, consisting of an external layer of *outer enamel epithelium* (**A4**) and an internal layer of *inner enamel epithelium* (**A5, B8**), which forms the basic shape of the future crown. The bell surrounds a condensation of *mesenchymal connective tissue* that forms the **dental papilla** and is a precursor of the **dental pulp** (**AB6**). The dental organ and dental pulp are enclosed in the **dental sac**, consisting of highly *cell-rich connective tissue*. In the 4th month of prenatal development, the first hard tissues arise. **Enamel** is formed by the *inner enamel epithelium*, and dentin and cement by the *odontoblasts in the dental pulp*. The connection between the dental lamina and the tooth germ and oral epithelium is lost during the 4th month of fetal life, and the dental lamina later gradually disintegrates. Lingual to the tooth germs of the deciduous teeth, the successional tooth germs of the permanent teeth develop from portions of the dental lamina.

Microscopic Anatomy of the Tooth Germ (B)

Enamel formation. The dental organ can be divided into the **outer enamel epithelium**, which forms the boundary with the surrounding mesenchymal dental sac; the **enamel pulp** (**B7**) inside the organ; and the **inner enamel epithelium** (**B8**). The cells of the inner enamel epithelium undergo differentiation into enamel-producing **ameloblasts** (enameloblasts), which secrete first *organic enamel matrix* (**B9**), and later *calcium* and *phosphate*. Enamel begins to form soon after dentin, starting at the crown of the tooth near the future occlusal surface.

In the process of later development, the dental organ is reduced to only a small number of cells (see below).

Dentin formation. Formation of dentin begins near the site of the future crown of the tooth. Dentin is produced by **odontoblasts** (**B10**), which arise from differentiation of the *mesenchymal cells of the dental pulp* (**B6**). The **matrix components of dentin** are secreted at the apical pole of the odontoblasts. Together with collagen fibrils extending from the odontoblasts, the matrix forms **predentin** (**B11**), **uncalcified dentin**, which mineralizes to become **dentin** (**B12**). As the predentin zone thickens, the odontoblasts extend elongated, radicular processes, which are walled in by predentin. These give rise to the *radially arranged dentinal tubules* containing the odontoblast processes known as **Tomes' fibers** (**B13**). Odontoblasts can continue to form uncalcified predentin throughout life.

Root formation and tooth eruption (**C**). Once the crown has formed, the roots of the tooth begin to develop. **The margin of the inner enamel epithelium** starts to grow toward the **outer enamel epithelium** (**C14**) and begins forming sheaths for the corresponding number of roots. New odontoblasts accumulate on the inner aspects of the root sheaths, elongating the dentine. Before eruption, the dental organ degenerates, and the remaining cells are later involved in formation of the junctional epithelium (**C15**). Elongation of the tooth root causes eruption, which destroys some of the tissue located above the crown (oral cavity epithelium and enamel epithelium).

Supporting tissues of the tooth. The *cement, periodontal ligament,* and *alveolar bone* arise from the **dental sac**, and their development coincides with that of the tooth root; that is, they develop later than the structures forming the crown. The development of the tooth root and supporting tissues (periodontium) is not completed until the eruption is complete.

The formation of **cement** is similar to the process of *intramembranous ossification* (see Vol. 1). Cement is formed by cementoblasts, cells arising from the side of the dental sac facing the tooth germ. The **alveolar bone** arises from the outer layer of the dental sac and also undergoes intramembranous ossification. The **fibers of the periodontal ligament** develop from the middle portion of the dental sac.

Alimentary System

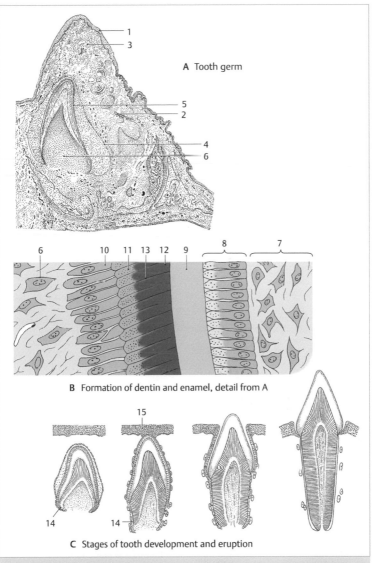

A Tooth germ

B Formation of dentin and enamel, detail from A

C Stages of tooth development and eruption

Fig. 4.12 Tooth development.

Alimentary System

Position of the Teeth in the Dental Arcades

In normal occlusion, or **eugnathia**, the crowns of the maxillary incisors are angled slightly outward toward the oral vestibule and the crowns of the mandibular teeth slightly inward toward the tongue (**A**). This enables the incisal edges of the upper and lower incisor teeth to move past each other like the blades of a pair of scissors. When the jaws are closed, the incisal edges of the upper incisor teeth lie anterior to those of the lower incisors in **neutral occlusion** (**scissors bite**).

The outer chewing surfaces of the upper premolar and molar teeth overlap those of the lower teeth, while the inner chewing surfaces of the lower teeth extend beyond those of the upper teeth (**B**). Interdigitation of opposing mandibular and maxillary teeth allows each tooth to articulate with two opposing teeth: the **main antagonist**, the tooth with which it is has the most contact, and the **secondary antagonist** (**C**). The lower first incisor tooth and the upper third molar tooth have only one antagonist each.

Articulation refers to movement of the maxillary teeth and mandibular teeth against each other. In the rest position, or **terminal occlusion**, the teeth meet in the **occlusal plane**. A tooth that is lacking an antagonist can grow beyond the occlusal plane. Over a lifetime, the teeth are worn down by physiological processes that assist in maintaining terminal closure.

> **Clinical note.** Dysgnathia is an abnormality of the teeth involving the jaws, as a result of due maldevelopment. Protrusion of the jaw is called **prognathism**, while **progenia** is a prominent chin due to an overdeveloped mandible. Such anomalies can interfere with swallowing, nasal breathing, and speech.

Vessels, Nerves, and Lymphatic Drainage

Arterial supply. The teeth, alveolar processes, and gingiva of the maxilla and mandible are supplied directly and indirectly by branches of the maxillary artery.

In the posterior part of the **maxilla**, the teeth and gingiva are supplied by the **posterior superior alveolar artery** (**C1**), and in the anterior portion they are supplied by the **anterior superior alveolar arteries** (**C2**), which spring from the infraorbital artery. Both maxillary arteries course in the wall of the maxillary sinus and are interconnected, giving off the dental and peridental branches. The mandible is supplied by the **inferior alveolar artery** (**C3**), which travels in the mandibular canal, where it distributes *dental branches* (**C4**) to the teeth and *peridental branches* to the gingiva and periodontal ligaments. The terminal branch of the inferior alveolar artery emerges from the mental foramen as the *mental branch*, to supply the skin of the chin and lower lip.

Veins. Venous blood from the maxilla and mandible is drained by veins that parallel the course of the arteries, and mostly flows to the **pterygoid plexus**.

Innervation. Nerve supply is provided by the second and third divisions of the trigeminal nerve (**V**), namely the **maxillary nerve** (**V2**) and the **mandibular nerve** (**V3**). The **infraorbital nerve** (division of **V2**) gives rise to several *posterior superior alveolar branches*, a *middle superior alveolar branch*, and a few *anterior superior alveolar branches*, which unite on the floor of the maxillary sinus to form the **superior dental plexus** (**C5**) and supply the teeth and gingiva of the maxilla. The teeth of the mandible are supplied by the **inferior alveolar nerve** (**C6**) (branch of V3), which accompanies the inferior alveolar vessels in the alveolar canal. An inferior alveolar nerve block can anesthetize the nerve at its entrance to the alveolar canal.

Lymph from the maxilla and mandible drains to the submental, submandibular, and deep cervical lymph nodes.

> **Clinical note.** The close proximity of the maxillary sinus, nerves, and tooth roots near the upper molar teeth is extremely important in clinical practice and should be taken into consideration in any **inflammation** affecting this area.

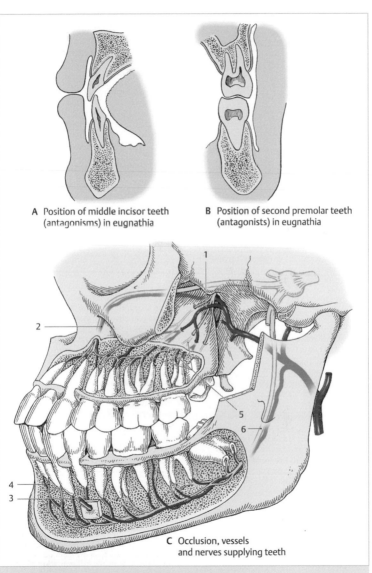

A Position of middle incisor teeth (antagonisms) in eugnathia

B Position of second premolar teeth (antagonists) in eugnathia

C Occlusion, vessels and nerves supplying teeth

Fig. 4.13 Position of the teeth, vessels, and nerves.

Alimentary System

4.3 Pharynx

Organization and General Structure

The pharynx is a 12–15-cm long **muscular tube** that extends from its attachment at the *base of the cranium* to the level of the *cricoid cartilage* (**A1**), where it becomes continuous with the esophagus (**A2**). Its posterior and lateral walls form a continuous surface without any openings. Anteriorly, it communicates with the *nasal cavity*, *oral cavity*, and *larynx*, and can thus be divided into the following three portions: the **nasopharynx** (**I**) (epipharynx), which communicates with the *nasal cavity* through the nasopharyngeal meatus at the *choanae;* the **oropharynx** (**II**) (mesopharynx), which is continuous at the *isthmus of fauces* with the *oral cavity*. The passageways for air and food intersect near the oropharynx; the **laryngopharynx** (**III**) (hypopharynx), which opens anteriorly into the *larynx* at the *laryngeal inlet*.

Structure of the Laryngeal Wall

The wall of the larynx is composed of four layers: the mucosa, the submucosa, the muscular layer, and the connective tissue adventitia. There is no muscularis mucosae.

Mucosa. The mucosa lining the nasopharynx is continuous with the **ciliated respiratory epithelium** of the nasal cavity. The mucosa that lines the oropharynx and laryngopharynx is continuous with that of the oral cavity and consists of **stratified, nonkeratinized squamous epithelium**, whose surface is lubricated by the saliva secreted by numerous mucus-producing *pharyngeal glands*. The **subepithelial connective tissue** contains abundant *elastic fibers*, allowing the pharyngeal wall to stretch and recoil. At the junction with the esophagus, the mucosa is cushioned against the laryngeal skeleton in front, and the vertebral column behind, by *connective tissue* and rich *venous plexuses*.

Mucosal landmarks. The mucosal structure of the **nasopharynx** (see p. 106) is chiefly produced by the *opening of the auditory tube* (**A3**), the *torus tubarius* (**A4**), and the *torus levatorius*. The **oropharynx** is bounded by the *base of the tongue* (**AB5**) and laterally

by the *palatine arches* and *tonsillar fossa* (**A6**), that is, the structures of the *isthmus of fauces* (see p. 144). Lying in the laryngopharynx, lateral to the laryngeal inlet where the larynx projects up into the pharynx, is a trench called the *piriform recess* (**B7**).

Muscular layer. Two striated muscle systems can be distinguished; those that act to constrict and those that elevate the pharynx. The three **constrictor muscles of the pharynx** consist of posteriorly ascending fibers that overlap like shingles and join in the midline to form a tough connective tissue raphe known as the **pharyngeal raphe** (**C8**), which attaches to the *pharyngeal tubercle* (**C9**) on the base of the cranium. The horizontal fibers of the upper border of the superior constrictor muscle are attached to the base of the cranium by a tough connective tissue membrane known as the *pharyngobasilar fascia* (**C10**). Most of the fibers of the **superior constrictor muscle of the pharynx** (**C11**) originate from the *pterygoid process* and *pterygomandibular raphe* (a tendinous band extending between the pterygoid hamulus and mandible). The fibers of the **middle constrictor muscle of the pharynx** (**C12**) mainly originate from the *hyoid bone* (**C13**) and those of the **inferior constrictor muscle of the pharynx** (**C14**) from the *thyroid* and *cricoid cartilages*. The constrictor muscles of the pharynx act to narrow the pharynx and elevate the larynx and hyoid bone. The **muscles that elevate the pharynx** are poorly developed muscles that include the *stylopharyngeal muscle* (**C15**), *palatopharyngeal muscle* (**B16**), and *salpingopharyngeal muscle*. Bundles of muscle fibers radiate upward into the wall of the pharynx.

Peripharyngeal space. The peripharyngeal space is a peripheral layer of connective tissue that allows for free movement of the pharynx against the vertebral column and other adjacent structures. It can be divided topographically into a **retropharyngeal space**, which lies between the posterior pharyngeal wall and the prevertebral layer of cervical fascia, and a **parapharyngeal space** lateral to the pharynx. The two connective tissue spaces communicate with the *mediastinum*, at their caudal ends. Covering the muscular layer of the entire pharynx is a thin fascia known as the **buccopharyngeal fascia**.

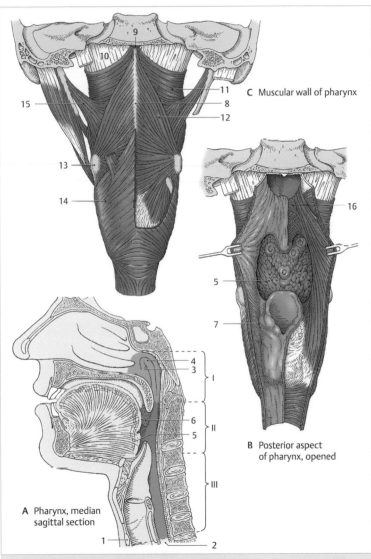

C Muscular wall of pharynx

B Posterior aspect of pharynx, opened

A Pharynx, median sagittal section

Fig. 4.14 Organization and general structure of the pharynx.

Vessels, Nerves, and Lymphatic Drainage

The **arterial supply** of the pharynx is mainly derived from the *ascending pharyngeal artery*, which arises from the external carotid artery, and from *pharyngeal branches* arising from the inferior and superior thyroid arteries. **Venous blood** drains to the *pharyngeal plexus* lying posterior to the pharynx. The muscles and mucosa of the pharynx receive **innervation** from branches of the *glossopharyngeal nerve* (IX) and *vagus nerve* (X), which form a nerve plexus on the outside of the pharynx known as the **pharyngeal plexus of the vagus nerve**. The regional **lymph nodes**, draining the pharynx are the *retropharyngeal lymph nodes*, which in turn drain to the *deep cervical lymph nodes*.

The Act of Swallowing

In the adult, the laryngeal inlet is located in the food passageway (**A**). In order to prevent ingested food from entering the larynx or airways during swallowing (deglutition) (**B**), the larynx must close briefly and be sealed shut. This process can be divided into the following phases:

1. Voluntary initiation. During the voluntary phase of swallowing, the floor of the mouth (**AB1**) contracts and the tongue (**AB2**) presses the food bolus against the soft palate (**AB3**). Subsequent events are initiated by stimulation of sensory receptors located in the mucosa of the palate.

2. Reflexive sealing of the airways. The soft palate is elevated, tensed, and pressed against the posterior wall of the pharynx. The superior constrictor muscle of the pharynx contracts, forming a prominence called the *Passavant ridge* (**B4**). The soft palate and upper portion of the posterior pharyngeal wall are pressed together, sealing the *upper* airways from the food passageways. Contraction of the muscles of the floor of the mouth (the mylohyoid and digastric muscles), assisted by the thyrohyoid muscles (**AB5**) (see Vol. 1), visibly

and palpably elevates the hyoid bone (**AB6**) and larynx (**AB7**). The laryngeal inlet approaches the epiglottis (**AB8**), which in turn is lowered by the muscles of the base of the tongue (**AB9**) and the aryepiglottic muscles. At the same time, the rima glottidis closes, and respiration is briefly interrupted: the *lower* airways are now also sealed from the food passageway.

3. Transport of the food bolus through the pharynx and esophagus. When the larynx is elevated, the pharynx expands anteriorly and superiorly. The tongue is drawn posteriorly by the styloglossus and hyoglossus, propelling the food bolus through the isthmus of the fauces into the enlarged pharynx. Most of the food travels through the piriform recess, and part slides over the epiglottis. Contraction of the constrictor muscles propels the food bolus through the wide-open esophagus into the entrance of the stomach.

Fluids reach the pharynx via a flattened portion of the tongue that forms a type of channel. In upright posture, rapid contraction of the floor of the mouth propels liquid into the cardial orifice, with the tongue acting like the plunger of a syringe.

The **swallowing reflex** is maintained during sleep. The swallowing center is located in the medulla oblongata (see Vol. 3) above the respiratory center. Efferent and afferent fibers involved in the swallowing reflex are carried by a number of cranial nerves, ensuring that the swallowing reflex is maintained.

In **neonates** and **infants**, the high position of the larynx and the projection of the epiglottis beyond the base of the tongue allow liquids to pass through the piriform recess into the esophagus, without endangering the airway. Infants thus can drink and breathe simultaneously.

Clinical note. If the soft palate is paralyzed, for example, owing to diphtheria, food can get into the nasal cavity. **Pharyngitis** causes pain on swallowing, with soreness, burning, and dryness in the throat; the pharyngeal mucosa is reddened.

Alimentary System

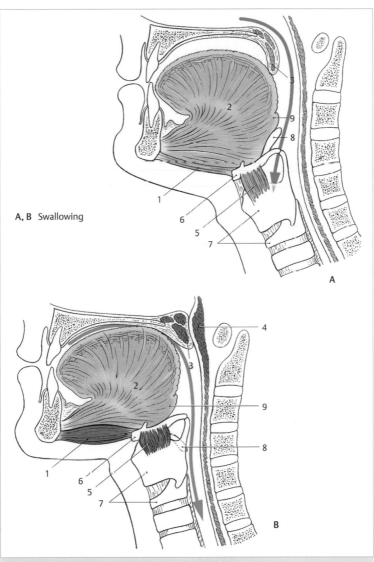

A, B Swallowing

Fig. 4.15 Swallowing.

4.4 Topographical Anatomy I

Cross-Sectional Anatomy of the Head and Neck

The sectional anatomy of the head and neck is complicated by the presence of numerous structures within a limited space. In the following sections through the head and neck regions, structures are discussed purely in terms of topography rather than their relation to organ systems. This is useful in successfully employing and interpreting modern diagnostic imaging methods.Neurocranium

In the upper portion of the section, the *temporal bone* (**A1**) is visible on either side in the region of the *middle cranial fossa* which supports the *temporal lobes of the brain* (**A2**). In the center of the image, the *body of the sphenoid* and the posterior end of the *sphenoidal sinus* (**A3**) are shown. The body of the sphenoid contains a depression that receives the *pituitary gland* (**A4**). On either side of the depression, the portion of the *internal carotid artery* traveling in the *carotid canal* (see Vol. 3) can be seen.

Viscerocranium

In the region around the viscerocranium, the section cuts through the *rami of the mandible* (**A5**) on either side, as well as the anterior end of the *head of the mandible* (**A6**) and the *temporomandibular joint capsule* (**A7**). The lateral aspect of the ramus of the mandible is covered by the *parotid gland* (**A8**). Between the mandible and the parotid gland, the section cuts through the *external carotid artery* (**A9**) and *retromandibular vein* (**A10**). The *medial* (**A11**) and *lateral pterygoid muscles* (**A12**), muscles of mastication, insert on the medial side of the ramus of the mandible. The section cuts through several of the veins forming the *pterygoid plexus* (**A13**), which lies in the niche between the two muscles. On the left-hand side of the image, the *mandibular nerve* (**A14**) is visualized as it emerges from the foramen ovale medial to the lateral pterygoid and gives rise to the *masseteric nerve* (**A15**), a motor nerve that travels laterally. The lumen of the *nasopharynx* (**A16**) is in the center of the image, with the lateral walls of the *opening of the auditory tube* (**A17**) on either side of it. The opening of the auditory tube is surrounded above by the *cartilaginous part of the auditory tube* (**A18**) and below by the *levator veli palatini* (**A19**). Below the lumen of the pharynx, fibers from the *levator veli palatini* and *tensor veli palatini* (**A20**) can be identified as they radiate to either side of the *soft palate* (**A21**). Beneath this, the insertion of the *styloglossus* (**A22**) into the tongue is visible. Intrinsic muscles of the tongue that can be seen in this section include the *transverse* (**A23**) and *vertical muscles of the tongue* (**A24**). Lying below the tongue is the *hyoid bone* (**A25**). Its lateral surface affords attachment to the *mylohyoid* (**A26**), and its caudal surface attaches to the *infrahyoid muscles* (**A27**). Lateral to the mylohyoid, the section cuts through the *submandibular gland* (**A28**) and the *facial artery* (**A29**) lying lateral to it. The *platysma* (**A30**), one of the muscles of facial expression, can be identified within the subcutaneous tissue. Structures around the palatopharyngeal arch and tonsillar fossa cannot be differentiated in this section.

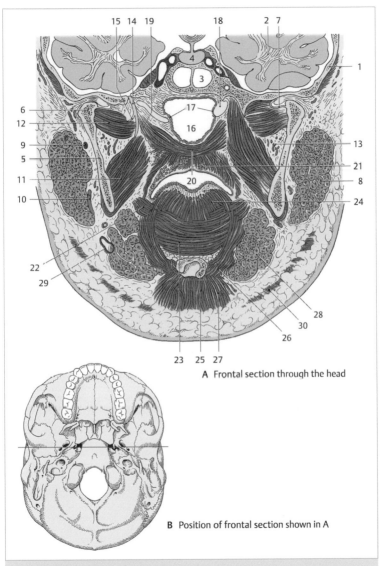

A Frontal section through the head

B Position of frontal section shown in A

Fig. 4.16 Cross-sectional anatomy of the head and neck.

Alimentary System

Cross-Sectional Anatomy of the Head and Neck, cont.

Transverse Section at the Level of the Atlas (A)

The section is through the posterior part of the *atlantoaxial joint* (**A1**). The structures visible in this section are discussed from posterior to anterior.

This section cuts through the *foramen transversarium of the atlas* (**A2**) and the *vertebral artery* (**A3**) emerging from it. Situated in front of the vertebral column are the *deep muscles of the neck* (**A4**), with the neurovascular bundle of the neck, consisting of the *internal jugular vein* (**A5**), *internal carotid artery* (**A6**), and *vagus nerve* (**A7**), lying lateral to them. The lumen of the *pharynx* (**A8**) can be seen anterior to the deep neck muscles. The section is at the level of the *oropharynx*, the posterior wall of which is formed by the *middle constrictor muscle of the pharynx* (**A9**). Its lateral wall contains the *tonsillar fossa*, *palatopharyngeus* (**A10**), *palatine tonsil* (**A11**), and *palatoglossus* (**A12**). Posterolateral to the tonsillar fossa, the transverse section cuts through the *styloid process* (**A13**), as well as the *external carotid artery* (**A14**) and *retromandibular vein* (**A15**) running lateral to it. In this section both vessels are visible adjacent to the *parotid gland* (**A16**). Inside the gland, the large lumen of the *parotid duct* (**A17**) can be seen. The parotid gland surrounds the posterior border of the *ramus of the mandible* (**A18**) like a forceps, extending deeply from its superficial location in the subcutaneous tissue to the *retromandibular fossa*. Within the ramus of the mandible, the section shows the *mandibular canal*, with the *mandibular nerve* (**A19**) and *inferior alveolar artery* (**A20**) running through it. The medial and lateral aspects of the ramus of the mandible are surrounded by the muscular sling formed by the *medial pterygoid* (**A21**) and *masseter* (**A22**) muscles. Anterior to the medial pterygoid, the section depicts the *lingual nerve* (**A23**) and adjacent *submandibular ganglion*. Along the anterior border of the masseter, the *facial vein* (**A24**) and *facial artery* (**A25**) are visualized. The section cuts through the *body of mandible* at the level of the inferior

border of the alveolar process, which still contains the roots of the *canine teeth* (**A26**) and is covered on its outer aspect by the *muscles of facial expression* (**A27**). Along the inner side of the mandible, the narrow cavity of the *oral vestibule* (**A28**) can be observed. The floor of the section, just above the floor of the mouth, enables visualization of the *sublingual gland* (**A29**), *sublingual caruncle*, and *opening of the submandibular duct* (**A30**). Posterior to it, a portion of the tortuous course of the thick *sublingual vein* (**A31**) is visible. The intrinsic muscles of the tongue that are visible in this section are the *genioglossus* (**A32**) and, especially, the *transverse muscle of the tongue* (**A33**) and *inferior longitudinal muscle*.

Transverse Section through the Neck at C5 (B)

This section cuts through the posterior portion of the neck at the level of the bilateral *intervertebral foramina* (**B34**), from which the *spinal nerves* (**B35**) emerge. Nearby, the *vertebral artery* (**B3**) and *vertebral vein* (**B36**) course anterior to the cervical vertebrae, passing outside of the *foramina transversaria* between consecutive vertebrae. The *deep muscles of the neck* (**B4**) are again depicted in front of the vertebral column, as in the previous section. Lateral to the deep neck muscles are the muscles of the *scalene group* (**B37**), and, lying on their anterior aspect, the neurovascular bundle of the neck containing the *common carotid artery* (**B38**), *internal jugular vein* (**B5**), and *vagus nerve* (**B7**). Accompanying the neurovascular bundle, which runs under cover of the *sternocleidomastoid* (**B39**), are the *deep cervical lymph nodes* (**B40**). The anteromedially situated viscera of the neck are covered on their anterior surfaces by the *infrahyoid muscles* (**B41**). The viscera consist of the *laryngopharynx* (**B42**), whose lumen is reduced to a narrow space, and the *larynx*, seen below the level of the rima glottidis. The *thyroid cartilage* (**B43**), *arytenoid cartilages* (**B44**), and parts of the *intrinsic laryngeal muscles* (**B45**) are also visible. The external aspect of the lateral wall of the larynx is covered on either side by the upper poles of the *thyroid gland* (**B46**).

Alimentary System

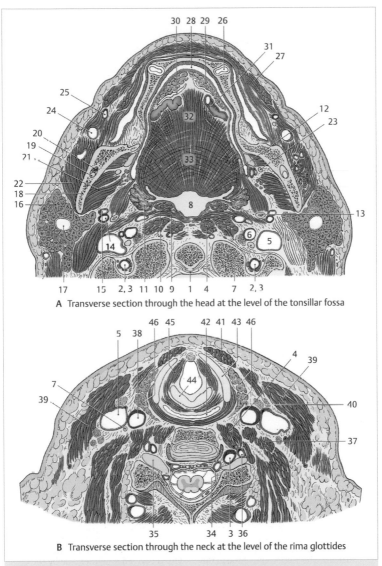

A Transverse section through the head at the level of the tonsillar fossa

B Transverse section through the neck at the level of the rima glottides

Fig. 4.17 Cross-sectional anatomy of the head and neck.

4.5 Esophagus

General Organization and Microscopic Anatomy

The esophagus is a pliable muscular tube that transports food from the *pharynx* (**AB1**) to the *stomach* (**A2**). It is about 25-cm long, beginning at the *inferior border of the cricoid cartilage* (**A3**) in front of C6/C7 and opening at the level of T10/T11 into the *cardial orifice* (**A4**). The esophagus may be divided into three parts based on the respective regions of the body through which it passes:

Cervical part (**A5**). The posterior wall of the short cervical part of the esophagus rests against the vertebral column, and the anterior wall rests against the trachea (**B8**).

Thoracic part (**A6**). During its course, the 16-cm long thoracic part of the esophagus gradually moves away from the vertebral column. It runs parallel to the trachea in front of it, as far as the tracheal bifurcation (**B9**) at the level of T4. At this point, the aortic arch (**B10**) crosses over it. The thoracic aorta initially passes along the left side of the esophagus, but as it continues distalward it courses further behind it. The left atrium of the heart rests directly against the thoracic part of the esophagus (see Fig. B Thoracic part, p. 179).

Abdominal part (**A7**). The abdominal part of the esophagus is very short, only 1–3 cm. It extends from the *esophageal hiatus* of the diaphragm (**B11**), to which it is connected by loose connective tissue that allows movement to the cardial orifice of the *stomach.*

Esophageal constrictions. The esophagus has three constrictions: **the first or upper constriction** (**I**), the **pharyngoesophageal constriction**, is located *behind* the *cricoid cartilage* (**AB3**) and is produced by the circular fibers of esophageal muscle. This is the narrowest of the three constrictions, and its lumen is just a horizontal slit with a maximum diameter of about 14 mm when open. The **second or middle constriction** (**II**), the bronchoaortic constriction, is located near the *crossing of the aortic arch over* the esophagus, about 10–cm distal from the first constriction. The **third or lower constriction**, (**III**), the **diaphragmatic constriction**, is at the *esophageal hiatus of the diaphragm.* This narrowing is produced by the spiral arrangement of muscle fibers in

the wall of the esophagus and venous plexuses beneath the mucosa, both of which serve to seal the cardial orifice.

Layers of the esophageal wall and microanatomy (**C**). The structure of the esophageal wall shares the basic structure found in the rest of the alimentary canal (see p. 142). Its **mucosa** (**C12**) is lined by *stratified, nonkeratinized squamous epithelium* (**C12 a**). Beneath the connective tissue (*lamina propria*) (**C12 b**), it contains a prominent *muscularis mucosae* (**C12 c**). In the resting state, the mucosa has 5–8 longitudinal folds, which give the lumen a stellate appearance. The stratified, nonkeratinized squamous epithelium of the esophagus ends abruptly at the junction with the cardial orifice and is replaced by the *columnar epithelium of the gastric mucosa*. The **submucosa** (**C13**) consists of a layer of loose connective tissue containing *vessels*, that is, *venous plexuses* and *nerves* (Meissner submucous plexus), as well as scattered mixed glands known as the *esophageal glands* (**C13 a**).The **muscular layer** (**C14**) is composed of an *inner layer of circular muscle* (**C14 a**), which helps propel the bolus toward the stomach by means of wavelike muscular contractions, and an *outer longitudinal layer* (**C14 b**), which is responsible for longitudinal tension and for shortening segments of the esophagus. In the upper two-thirds of the esophagus, the muscular layer contains striated muscle fibers from the pharyngeal muscles; in the lower one-third, it is composed entirely of smooth muscle. The Auerbach myenteric plexus is located between the circular and longitudinal muscle layers. The esophagus is connected to its surroundings by the **adventitia** (**C15**).

Functional anatomy. The esophagus is stabilized within its surroundings by longitudinal tension, which also helps to transport the bolus during swallowing. The upper constriction of the esophagus opens briefly to allow solids or liquids to pass to the stomach. Solids are conveyed within about 3 seconds, by peristaltic waves to the stomach, and liquids are propelled into the cardial orifice within a few tenths of a second. The total distance from the incisor teeth to the cardial orifice is about 40 cm.

Clinical note. The wall of the esophagus contains a thin area that represents a weak point (*Laimer triangle*) in the muscle between the inferior constrictor muscle of the pharynx and the circular layer of muscle. This weakness can give rise to **diverticula**, outpouchings in the esophagus wall.

Weakening of the connective tissue of the esophageal hiatus of the diaphragm can result in a **hiatal hernia**, in which the abdominal part of the esophagus as well as parts of the stomach, protrude into the thoracic cavity.

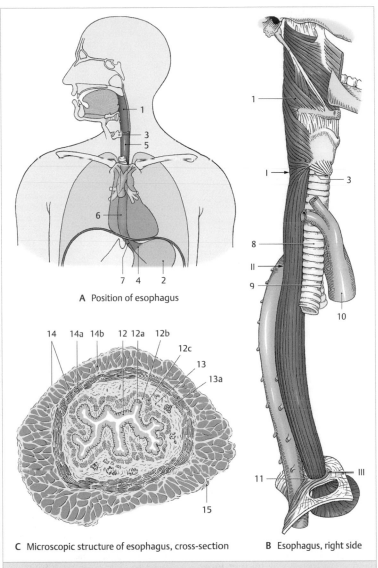

A Position of esophagus

C Microscopic structure of esophagus, cross-section

B Esophagus, right side

Fig. 4.18 General organization and microscopic structure.

Topographical Anatomy of the Esophagus and the Posterior Mediastinum

Cervical Part

The short cervical part of the esophagus (**A–C1**) lies *behind the trachea* (**AC2**) (see also Topography of the Trachea and Larynx, p. 120) and in front of the vertebral column, slightly to the left of the midline. The cervical esophagus is thus in direct contact with the *thyroid lobe* (**AC3**), as well as the *inferior thyroid artery* (**A4**). The left lobe of the thyroid covers the groove between the esophagus and trachea, where the recurrent laryngeal nerves ascend to the larynx. The supplying branches of the inferior thyroid artery pass anteroposteriorly to the esophageal wall. The left *recurrent laryngeal nerve* (**A5**) travels alongside and then nearly anterior to the esophagus. Its posterior aspect is separated from the deep muscles of the neck by the *prevertebral layer of the cervical fascia*.

Thoracic Part

The thoracic part of the esophagus lies slightly to the left of the superior mediastinum and then hidden in the *posterior part of the inferior mediastinum* (**B**). This is the longest part of the esophagus and it is positioned in relation to the *trachea* (**AC2**) in front, the *left subclavian artery* (**A6**) on the left, and the *brachiocephalic trunk* (**A7**) on the right. The *thoracic duct* (**B8**) crosses behind it. Below the level of the *tracheal bifurcation*, the esophagus curves to the right posterior to the *pericardium* of the left atrium. Also known as the *retropericardial part*, this segment is positioned in relation to the *descending aorta* (**B9**) on the left and the *azygos vein* (**B10**) on the right. Initially, it lies adjacent to the vertebral column (see also **C**), but gradually moves further away from it as it courses caudally; in some individuals, the *parietal pleura* (**B11**) can slide in between the esophagus and aorta from the right. Behind the esophagus, the *thoracic duct* (**B8**) ascends through the posterior mediastinum between the aorta and azygos vein. The greater part of the esophagus is located to the right of the midline; it does not lie on the left of center until it reaches the level of the *aortic arch* (**B12**). Lying along the posterior aspect of the esophagus are parts of the autonomic *esophageal plexus* and *posterior vagal trunk* (**B13**). Running along either side of the vertebral column are the thoracic *sympathetic trunk* (**B14**) and the *greater splanchnic nerve* (**B15**). The close proximity of the esophagus (**A–C1**), pericardium, and left atrium (**C16**) can be clearly seen in a paramedian sagittal section (**C**) through the thorax. In clinical practice, the close proximity of these structures is useful for transesophageal echocardiography.

C17 Left atrium of heart, **C18** Aortic arch, **C19** Left pulmonary artery, **C20** Brachiocephalic vein, **C21** sternum, **C22** Diaphragm

Clinical note. Epibronchial traction diverticula of the esophagus occur at the level of the tracheal bifurcation. These account for about 20% of esophageal diverticula and are usually asymptomatic.

Alimentary System

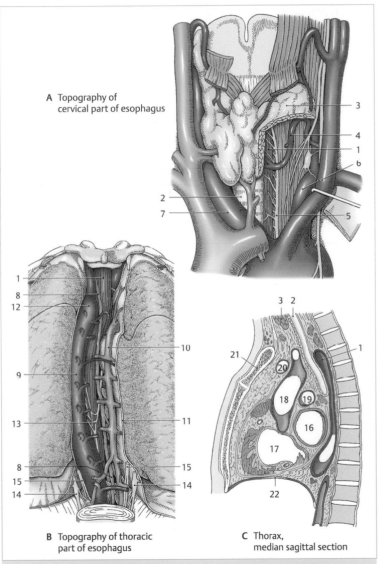

A Topography of cervical part of esophagus

B Topography of thoracic part of esophagus

C Thorax, median sagittal section

Fig. 4.19 Topographical anatomy of the esophagus and posterior mediastinum.

Alimentary System

Vessels, Nerves, and Lymphatic Drainage

Arteries. The *cervical part* of the esophagus is supplied by branches from the **inferior thyroid artery**; the *thoracic part* by the segmental **esophageal branches** arising from the aorta; and the *abdominal part* by the **inferior phrenic and left gastric arteries**.

Veins. Blood from the esophagus ultimately drains to the **superior vena cava** (**A1**) *above* and the **hepatic portal vein** (**A2**) *below*. Blood from the *cervical part* drains to the **inferior thyroid vein** (**A3**) and, via the brachiocephalic vein (**A4**), to the superior vena cava. Esophageal veins from the *thoracic part* empty directly into the **azygos vein** (**A5**) and **hemiazygos vein** (**A6**), which in turn drain into the superior vena cava. Blood from the *abdominal part* flows into the **left gastric vein** (**A7**), which runs along the upper margin of the stomach and drains via the superior mesenteric vein (**A8**) or directly into the hepatic portal vein.

The esophageal veins form **rich venous plexuses** lying in the adventitia and submucosa. These can form anastomoses connecting the systemic and portal circulations.

> **Clinical note.** A pathological rise in portal venous pressure (portal hypertension) can result in a retrograde flow of blood in the veins that drain the inferior portion of the esophagus. Blood from regions normally drained by the hepatic portal vein instead flows via the left gastric vein, through the esophageal veins to the azygos and hemiazygos veins. This leads to increased pressure in the esophageal venous plexuses and development of **esophageal** varices, which can rupture and cause massive, life-threatening hemorrhage.

Nerves. Parasympathetic innervation is provided by the **vagus nerve** (**B9**). The *cervical part* of the esophagus and the *upper portion of the thoracic part* are innervated by branches of the **recurrent laryngeal nerve**. In the portion of *thoracic part* below the tracheal bifurcation, the right and left

vagus nerves form a plexus in the adventitia called the **esophageal plexus** (see Vol. 3). Arising from this plexus is the *anterior vagal trunk* (**B10**), which lies in front of the esophagus, and the *posterior vagal trunk*, along its posterior wall, both of which travel with the esophagus into the abdominal cavity. **Postsynaptic sympathetic innervation** of the esophagus arises from the **cervicothoracic ganglion** (stellate ganglion), **thoracic sympathetic trunk**, and **abdominal aortic plexus**. The sympathetic and parasympathetic nerves are directly connected to the **enteric nervous system** of the esophagus, which, as elsewhere in the intestinal wall, consists of a *myenteric plexus* and *submucous plexus*.

Lymphatic drainage. Lymph from the part of the esophagus located *above the level of the tracheal bifurcation* flows cranially and is mainly drained by the **lower group of deep cervical lymph nodes** and **paratracheal lymph nodes** (**C11**). Lymph from the parts of the esophagus lying *below the tracheal bifurcation* mostly drains to the **tracheobronchial lymph nodes** (**C12**) and **prevertebral lymph nodes** (**C13**). Lymph from the abdominal part of the esophagus drains to the adjacent **perigastric** and **subphrenic lymph nodes**.

> **Clinical note.** The shared autonomic innervation of the esophagus and heart is responsible for the fact that both cardiac and noncardiac (esophageal) chest pain can have identical clinical symptoms, despite their different origin.
> **Connections between** esophageal and tracheobronchial innervation explain the reflex cough caused by passage of gastric acid into the esophagus ("acid reflux"). Approximately 5% of gastrointestinal malignant tumors involve the esophagus and are 2–3 times more common in men than in women. They are classified according to their location: cervical esophagus (15%), close to the tracheal bifurcation (50%), and below the tracheal bifurcation (35%). **Esophageal cancer** (squamous epithelial or undifferentiated carcinoma) typically grows longitudinally within the wall of the esophagus initially. Early lymphatic metastasis to the cervical, paraesophageal, and mediastinal lymph nodes occurs. Increasing *dysphagia* is the classic symptom of esophageal cancer.

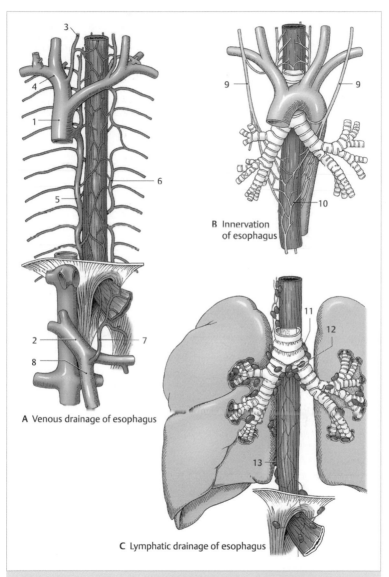

A Venous drainage of esophagus

B Innervation of esophagus

C Lymphatic drainage of esophagus

Fig. 4.20 Vessels, nerves, and lymphatic drainage of the esophagus.

Alimentary System

4.6 Abdominal Cavity

General Overview

The organs described in the following section lie in the **abdominal cavity**, which will be discussed before the individual organs are presented.

Boundaries (A). The **superior** boundary of the abdominal cavity is formed by the *domes of the diaphragm* (**A1**), which separate it from the thoracic cavity. Its **posterior** boundary is formed by the *lumbar vertebral column* (**A2**), the *sacrum*, and the *posterior abdominal muscles* (see Vol. 1). The **lateral and anterior** boundaries are formed by the *lateral and medial groups of the abdominal muscles* and their *aponeuroses* (see Vol. 1). The upper portion of the muscular wall of the abdominal cavity is reinforced by the *costal margin* and *sternum* (**A3**), and the lower and lateral parts by the *bony alae of the ilium*. The **inferior** boundary of the abdominal cavity is formed by the *pelvic diaphragm* (see Vol. 1).

Peritoneal cavity and connective tissue spaces (B). The abdominal cavity contains the **peritoneal cavity** (green), a space lined by peritoneum; the **retroperitoneal space** (yellow), an area bounded by connective tissue situated in front of the vertebral column; and the **subperitoneal space**, located in the lesser pelvis beneath the peritoneum. The peritoneal cavity is completely surrounded by a lining of *parietal peritoneum* (**B4**). The parietal peritoneum covers the anterior aspect of the retroperitoneal space, dividing it from the peritoneal cavity. Below the *linea terminalis* (see Vol. 1), the parietal peritoneum covers portions of the pelvic viscera, including parts of the *rectum* (**B5**), *uterus* (**B6**), and *urinary bladder* (**B7**). Its reflection onto the *anterior abdominal wall* (**B8**) divides the subperitoneal space from the true peritoneal cavity. The retroperitoneal space is continuous with the subperitoneal space; both contribute to the **extraperitoneal space**.

The abdominal cavity houses most of the organs of digestion. Their **relations to the peritoneum** (**C**) vary: **intraperitoneal** organs lie *in the peritoneal cavity* and are lined by *visceral peritoneum* (**C9**) (e.g., the stomach, **C10**), while **retroperitoneal** organs lie on the posterior wall of the peritoneal cavity, that is, *behind the parietal peritoneum*, which covers their anterior surface. Organs that initially lie intraperitoneally during prenatal development, but are later positioned on the posterior abdominal wall where they grow behind the parietal peritoneum, are considered **secondary retroperitoneal** organs (e.g., the pancreas, **C11**). An **extraperitoneal** organ is one that has no relation to the peritoneum (e.g., the prostate).

In the peritoneal cavity, as in all other serous cavities, the **parietal** and **visceral layers** of the peritoneum are continuous at the **site of reflections** or **folds**. The reflections consist of *sheets of connective tissue* that are lined on both sides *by peritoneum* and are thus called *peritoneal folds*. These double layers of peritoneum form **mesenteries** or **peritoneal ligaments**. A mesentery or ligament **connects an intraperitoneal organ to the abdominal wall** and conveys vessels embedded in connective tissue to the respective organ.

Intraperitoneal abdominal organs lying *above the umbilicus* are attached by both *anterior* and *posterior mesenteries* to the anterior and posterior abdominal walls. *Below the umbilicus*, intraperitoneal parts of the intestine are suspended by just a *posterior mesentery* from the posterior abdominal wall (see p. 329).

Microanatomy of **the peritoneum**. The **serosa** of the peritoneum is composed of flat, simple squamous epithelial cells with a brush border. Beneath this is the loose connective tissue known as the **subserosa**. Only the parietal peritoneum receives sensory innervation.

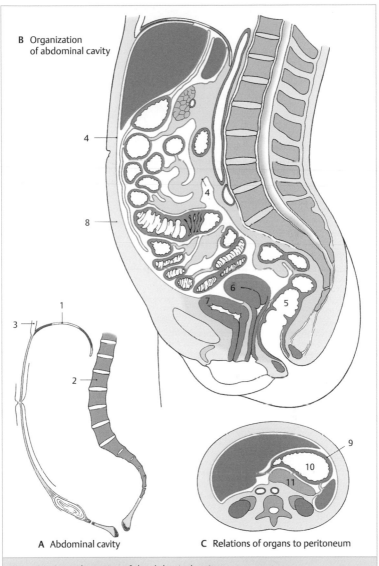

B Organization of abdominal cavity

A Abdominal cavity

C Relations of organs to peritoneum

Fig. 4.21 General overview of the abdominal cavity.

Alimentary System

Topography of the Opened Abdominal Cavity

The opened abdominal cavity can be divided into different parts: a **supracolic part** (**I**), an **infracolic part** (**II**), and a **pelvic part**. The **horizontal boundary** dividing the first two is at the **mesocolon** of the **transverse colon** (**A1**), at about the level of L1. Attached to the anterior surface of the transverse colon is the *greater omentum* (**A2**), which hangs down like an apron covering the intestinal loops, leaving visible only parts of the large intestine, that is, the *ascending colon* (**A3**) and *descending colon* (**A4**). The colon frames the loops of the small intestine.

Supracolic Part

The supracolic part contains the **liver** (**AB5**), **gallbladder** (**AB6**), **stomach** (**AB7**), superior part of the **duodenum** (**B8**), **pancreas**, and **spleen** (**AB9**).

Opened abdominal cavity (**A**). In the opened abdominal cavity, the **inferior border** of the **right lobe of the liver** (**A10**) and the **fundus of the gallbladder** (**AB6**) can be seen protruding below the right costal margin. The **inferior border** of the **left lobe of the liver** extends into the area between the costal margins known as the *epigastrium*. The **falciform ligament** (**A11**) passes between the right and left lobes of the liver to the anterior abdominal wall. Its free inferior margin is thickened to form the **round ligament of the liver** (**AB12**) containing the *obliterated umbilical vein* (see p. 8). Depending on the distention of the stomach, a part of the **anterior surface of the stomach** (**AB7**) may be visible below the left costal margin and between it and the right costal margin. Extending between the inferior border of the stomach, known as the *greater curvature of stomach* (**B13**), and the *transverse colon* (**A1**) is a peritoneal fold called the **gastrocolic ligament** (**AB14**).

Raised liver (**B**). The upper abdominal organs and the **lesser omentum** (**B15**)

can be visualized after lifting the liver. The **quadrate lobe of the liver** (**B16**) and much of the **visceral surface of the left lobe of the liver** are visible. Between the right and left lobes, the round ligament continues as the *fissure for the round ligament* (**B17**). The parts of the **gallbladder** that rest in the *fossa for the gallbladder* of the liver, that is, the *fundus* (**B19**), *body* (**B20**), and *neck of the gallbladder* (**B21**), can be seen in their entirety. Parts of the **anterior wall of the stomach**, that is, the *cardia* (**B22**), *fundus of the stomach* (**B23**), *body of the stomach* (**B24**), and *pyloric part of the stomach* (**B25**), are visible. To the left of the stomach, the *superior border* (**B26**) of the *spleen* (**B9**) can be seen. The **lesser omentum** (**B15**) extends in a near-frontal plane between the liver and stomach. Its free right margin is thickened to form the **hepatoduodenal ligament** (**B27**), which extends between the liver and the intraperitoneally situated beginning part of the duodenum (**B8**). It contains the *bile duct, hepatic portal vein,* and *hepatic artery proper.* The adjacent part of the lesser omentum extending between the liver and the upper border of the stomach, that is, the lesser curvature of the stomach (**B28**), is the **hepatogastric ligament** (**B29**). Shimmering through the middle part of the ligament is the **caudate lobe** (**B30**) of the liver. Behind the lesser omentum is the **omental bursa** (to which the arrow is pointing), a saclike cavity forming a smaller part of the peritoneal cavity. The narrow entrance to the omental bursa is located behind the free margin of the lesser omentum, that is, posterior to the hepatoduodenal ligament, and is known as the **omental foramen** (formerly known as the *epiploic foramen* and still referred to in clinical practice as the *foramen of Winslow*) (arrow).

Clinical note. The levels of the peritoneal cavity are not separate but are broadly connected. Infections in one part can therefore spread throughout the cavity, leading to **peritonitis**. Increased accumulation of fluid in the peritoneal cavity caused by a variety of diseases is called **ascites**.

Alimentary System

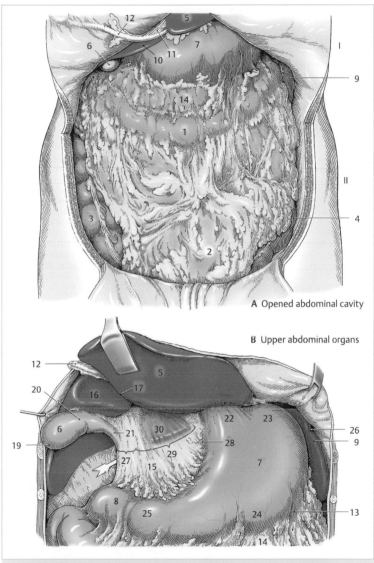

A Opened abdominal cavity

B Upper abdominal organs

Fig. 4.22 Topography of the opened abdominal cavity.

186 Alimentary System

Topography of the Opened Abdominal Cavity cont.

Infracolic Part

The organs of the infracolic part of the abdomen, which include the **small** and **large intestines**, are located below the transverse colon, lying between its mesentery and the linea terminalis. In the opened abdomen, the lower abdominal organs are mostly covered by the *greater omentum* (see p. 185 **A**).

View in (A). After *reflecting the greater omentum* (**AB1**) and *the transverse colon* (**AB2**), and moving the *loops of the small intestine to the left side*, almost all of the organs of the infracolic part are visible. The **small intestine** consists of the **duodenum** (**AB3**), **jejunum** (**AB4**), and **ileum** (**AB5**). Except for its initial (superior) part, the duodenum is a *secondarily retroperitoneal* organ and can be seen shimmering through the parietal peritoneum (**AB3**). The *intraperitoneal* jejunum and ileum are attached to the posterior abdominal wall by a wide **mesentery** (**AB6**). The **root of the mesentery** (**A7**) is 15–18-cm long and passes obliquely from the upper left (at the level of L2) downward to the right iliac fossa. In the right iliac fossa, the ileum becomes continuous with the initial part of the large intestine known as the **cecum** (**AB8**), which is followed by the **ascending colon** (**A9**). Near the junction of the intraperitoneal ileum and the often *secondarily retroperitoneal* cecum, there are *peritoneal folds* and *peritoneal recesses*. Above the ileocecal junction is the **superior ileocecal recess** (**A10**) produced by the **vascular fold of the cecum** (**A11**), which contains vessels. Almost all of the **typical characteristics of the colon** are apparent on the cecum and ascending colon: the *haustra of the colon* (**A12**), evenly spaced sacculations in the colon wall; one of the *teniae coli* (**A13**), a thickened part of the longitudinal muscle layer; and the *omental appendices* (**A14**), fatty appendages covered by peritoneum. At the **right colic flexure** (**A15**), the ascending colon becomes continuous with the intraperitoneal **transverse colon** (**AB2**), which is attached to the

posterior abdominal wall by the **transverse mesocolon** (**AB16**).

The remaining segments of the large intestine (descending and sigmoid colon) are covered by the loops of the small intestine that have been moved to the left side.

View in B. After *moving the small intestine loops and their mesentery to the right side*, the junction of the duodenum (**AB3**) and the jejunum (**AB4**), as well as the descending part of the colon, are easily visible. The secondarily retroperitoneal part of the duodenum transitions at the **duodenojejunal flexure** (**B17**) into the jejunum. Similar to the ileocecal junction, there are also peritoneal folds and recesses near the duodenojejunal flexure. The **superior duodenal fold** (**B18**) covers the **superior duodenal fossa** (**B19**); and the **inferior duodenal fold** (**B20**) covers the **inferior duodenal fossa** (**B21**). Since the small intestine loops have been moved to the right, the blind-ending **cecum** (**AB8**) and its appendage, the **vermiform appendix** (**B22**), can be observed. This small intraperitoneal appendage is attached by the **mesoappendix** (**B23**) to the posterior abdominal wall. The **transverse colon** (**AB2**) and **transverse mesocolon** (**AB16**) are visible almost as far as the **left colic flexure** (**B24**), that is, to the junction with the **descending colon** (**B25**). The descending colon is secondarily retroperitoneal; its anterior surface is covered with parietal peritoneum. It is continuous in the left iliac fossa, where it lies on the iliacus muscle, with the intraperitoneal **sigmoid colon** (**B26**). The sigmoid colon is attached to the posterior abdominal wall by the **sigmoid mesocolon** (**B27**), the root of which may contain a peritoneal recess called the **intersigmoid recess** (**B28**).

Clinical note. Loops of small intestine or parts of the greater omentum can enter these recesses to produce internal hernias. They are not visible externally and are usually only discovered at operation. Incarceration of the loops of the intestine causes abdominal pain, nausea, vomiting, and problems with digestion. Intestinal obstruction (ileus) occurs rarely. The numerous pockets and recesses between the loops of the small and large intestine can contain up to half a liter of free fluid, which may escape detection clinically and by ultrasound examination.

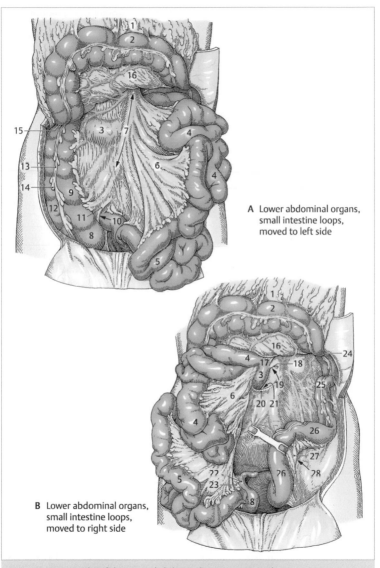

A Lower abdominal organs, small intestine loops, moved to left side

B Lower abdominal organs, small intestine loops, moved to right side

Fig. 4.23 Topography of the opened abdominal cavity, continued.

Parietal Peritoneum: Relations

Posterior abdominal wall. After *removal of the intraperitoneal organs* (the liver, stomach, spleen, jejunum, ileum, transverse colon, and sigmoid colon), the posterior wall of the peritoneal cavity, including the lines of attachment of the peritoneal folds and the attachment sites of the liver, as well as the retroperitoneal organs, can be seen (A). Near the **bare area** (**A1**) of the liver, which lacks a peritoneal covering, the organ is attached to the diaphragm. This area is surrounded by the reflection site of the visceral peritoneum of the liver onto the parietal peritoneum of the diaphragm, known as the **coronary ligament** (**A2**). The coronary ligament continues laterally, with its pointed margins forming the *right triangular ligament* (**A3**) and *left triangular ligament* (**A4**). The part of the right coronary ligament that is attached to the right kidney bed (**A5**) is known as the *hepatorenal ligament* (**A6**). The anterior and superior surfaces of the **falciform ligament** (**A7**) are in contact with the parietal peritoneum of the diaphragm. Posterior to the liver, the retroperitoneal **inferior vena cava** (**A8**) and the aorta (**A9**) can be identified. On the left side of the aorta is the cut edge through the cardial orifice (**A10**). Passing from the cardial orifice to the diaphragm is the **gastrophrenic ligament** (**A11**), which continues as the **gastrosplenic ligament** (**A12**), between the greater curvature of the stomach and the spleen. Below the inferior pole of the spleen, a peritoneal fold known as the **phrenicocolic ligament** (**A13**) extends between the diaphragm and the descending colon. The root of the **transverse mesocolon** (**A14**) is cut at the center of the posterior abdominal wall. Above it, the parietal peritoneum covering the posterior wall of the omental bursa (see p. 222) can be seen behind the pancreas (**A15**). At the superior border of the duodenum (**A16**), the **hepatoduodenal ligament** (**A17**) is cut. Lying behind it is the **omental foramen** (**A18**). In the infracolic part of the abdomen, the posterior abdominal wall is subdivided by the diagonally running **root of the mesentery** (**A19**) and the **sigmoid mesocolon** (**A20**). The sigmoid mesocolon continues downward into the lesser pelvis, where the sigmoid colon joins the rectum (**AB21**). Lying at either side of the posterior abdominal wall are the ascending colon (**A22**) on the right and the descending colon (**A23**) on the left.

Pelvis. The peritoneum of the posterior abdominal wall extends downward past the linea terminalis into the lesser pelvis (**B**), as the **urogenital peritoneum**. The peritoneum covers a part of the anterior and lateral surfaces of the rectum (**AB21**) and in the female pelvis reflects onto the female internal genitalia arranged in the frontal plane and consisting of the uterus (**B24**), uterine tubes (**B25**), and ovaries (**B26**). Between the uterus and rectum is a deep depression known as the **rectouterine pouch** (**B27**), the deepest point in the peritoneal cavity. Passing from either of the lateral walls of the uterus to the wall of the lesser pelvis is a peritoneal fold called the **broad ligament of the uterus** (**B28**). The shallower **vesicouterine pouch** (**B29**) is formed by a reflection of the peritoneum from the posterior wall onto the posterior surface of the urinary bladder (**B30**). In men, the peritoneum covers the rectum and urinary bladder, as well as the seminal vesicle lying behind the urinary bladder. Thus, there is only a peritoneal pocket, the **rectovesical pouch**, between the rectum and urinary bladder. Laterally, the parietal peritoneum lines the wall of the pelvis, covering the internal iliac vessels and ureters.

Anterior abdominal wall. The inner surface of the anterior abdominal wall is lined by the **anterior parietal peritoneum**, which has a characteristic surface architecture. Extending in the midline of the abdominal wall to the umbilicus is the **median umbilical fold** (**B31**), a peritoneal fold that contains the *obliterated urachus*, which connects the primordial bladder to the allantois in the embryo. Passing lateral to the median umbilical fold on either side is the **medial umbilical fold** (**B32**), which contains the *obliterated umbilical artery*. The area bounded by the three folds and the urinary bladder is the **supravesical fossa** (**B33**). Lying on the lateral part of the anterior abdominal wall is the **lateral umbilical fold** (**B34**), which contains the *inferior epigastric vessels* and flattens out as it passes cranially. Near its inferior end, between it and the medial umbilical fold, is a small depression known as the **medial inguinal fossa** (**B35**), which corresponds to the *superficial inguinal ring*. Lateral to the lateral umbilical fold is the **lateral inguinal fossa** (**B36**), corresponding to the *deep inguinal ring* beneath it.

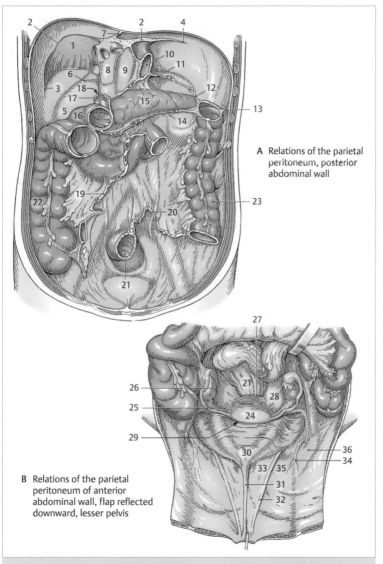

A Relations of the parietal peritoneum, posterior abdominal wall

B Relations of the parietal peritoneum of anterior abdominal wall, flap reflected downward, lesser pelvis

Alimentary System

Fig. 4.24 Relations of the parietal peritoneum.

4.7 Stomach

The **stomach** is a broad, crescent-shaped intraperitoneal hollow organ. It lies in the upper part of the abdomen (A) below the left dome of the diaphragm and above the transverse colon, partially hidden behind the left costal margin in the left hypochondrium. Depending on its shape and amount of contents, it can extend a variable distance into the epigastric region.

Gross Anatomy

The abdominal part of the esophagus (**B1**) opens via the **cardial orifice** (**C2**) into the funnel-shaped entrance to the stomach called the **cardia** (**B3**), which is continuous with the **fundus of the stomach** (**B4**), the highest point of the stomach. The fundus is located below the left dome of the diaphragm, and in an individual standing upright contains swallowed air (*gastric bubble*). The fundus is separated from the heart only by the central tendon of the diaphragm. The junction of the esophagus and fundus of the stomach forms a sharp angle called the **cardial notch** (**B5**). The **body of the stomach** (**B6**) makes up the greater part of the stomach. It is continuous with the **pyloric part** (**BC7**), which may be divided into the *pyloric antrum* (**BC7 a**) and *pyloric canal* (**BC7 b**). The pyloric part opens via the *pyloric orifice* (**C8**), which is surrounded by a ring of muscle known as the *pylorus*, into the duodenum (**BC9**).

The level of the pylorus varies depending on the shape of the stomach. In supine position, it is usually to the right of the midline at the level of the first lumbar vertebra and drops to the fourth lumbar vertebra in erect position, but it is always in front of the inferior vena cava.

In terms of its external features, the stomach may be divided into **anterior and posterior surfaces**. These are separated by the **lesser curvature** (**B10**) and **greater curvature** (**B11**), as well as peritoneal fold attachments. The lesser (concave) curvature of the stomach points upward and toward the right; its lowest point is the *angular incisure* (**B12**), a sharp bend that marks the beginning of the pyloric part and is often visible on radiographs. The greater (convex) curvature of the stomach points downward, and its convex border opposite the angular incisure is referred to as the *angle of the stomach* (**B13**). Arising from the lesser curvature of the stomach is the largest portion of the **lesser omentum**, the *hepatogastric ligament*. The **greater omentum** extends from the greater curvature, forming the *gastrocolic ligament*, which extends between the stomach and transverse colon; *the gastrophrenic ligament* between the fundus of the stomach and diaphragm; and the *gastrosplenic ligament* between the greater curvature of the stomach and the spleen. If the lower border of the liver is lifted up, the lesser omentum can be seen.

Stomach wall and mucosa. The outer surface of the stomach wall is smooth and covered by *visceral peritoneum*. On the interior of the stomach, the gastric mucosa is thrown into large, tortuous, longitudinal **gastric folds** (**C14**), which are visible to the naked eye. The mucosa at the lesser curvature contains a few parallel ridges forming the **gastric canal**. In the rest of the mucosa, the folds are irregularly shaped.

Under a **microscope**, the raised areas and shallow indentations forming the microstructure (**D**) of the gastric mucosa can be seen. The mucosal structure is characterized by raised areas called **gastric areas** (**D15**), into which the evenly spaced **gastric pits** (**D16**) open. The wall of the stomach is only a few millimeters thick. As elsewhere in the intestinal canal, its layers consist of a *mucosa* (**D17**), a *submucosa* (**D18**), a *muscular layer* (**D19**), a thin *subserosa* (**D20**), and a *serosa* (**D20**).

Alimentary System

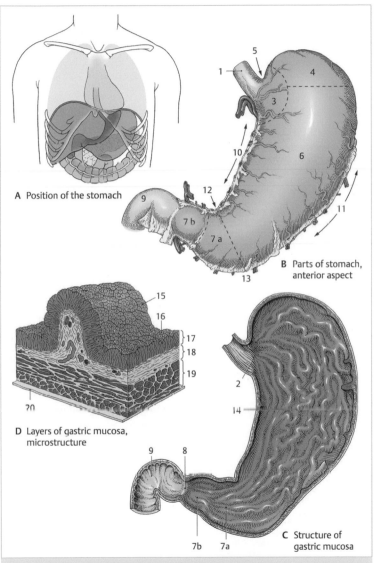

A Position of the stomach

B Parts of stomach, anterior aspect

D Layers of gastric mucosa, microstructure

C Structure of gastric mucosa

Fig. 4.25 Macroscopic structure of the stomach.

Microscopic Anatomy of the Stomach

Given that the structure of the walls of the alimentary canal is largely the same everywhere (see p. 142), only specific features of individual segments will be highlighted.

Mucosa

Throughout the stomach, the surface of the mucosa and gastric pits (**AB1**), with a combined thickness of about 1–2 mm, is lined by a **simple**, **columnar epithelium** (**AB2**), which transitions abruptly at the cardial orifice from the esophageal epithelium. The surface epithelium of the stomach produces a *highly viscous, neutral mucus*, which protects the wall of the stomach from damage. The mucosal connective tissue (*lamina propria*) (**A3**) is occupied by **tubular gastric glands** (**AB4**), which extend to the *muscular layer* (**A5**) and open into the gastric pits.

The glands of the stomach may be divided by region, shape, cellular composition, and function. The *glands in the body and fundus* are known as the **gastric glands proper**; those in the *cardia*, are referred to as the **cardiac glands**; and those in the *pyloric part* of the stomach are called the **pyloric glands**.

Gastric glands proper. The glands in the fundus and body of the stomach (**A**) are closely packed, long, straight glands about 1.5 mm in length. They are composed of three different cell types that occur in different proportions in the different regions of the gland (**B**). The **neck of the gland** contains mainly mucus-producing **mucous neck cells** (**AB6**), which differ morphologically from surface epithelial cells. Frequent division of the neck cells serves to replenish the surface epithelium. The **next portion of the gland** has abundant chief cells and parietal cells. **Chief cells** (**AB7**) are columnar and are highly basophilic. They produce *pepsinogens*, precursors of the digestive enzyme pepsin that breaks down proteins. The **parietal cells** (**AB8**) appear to rest on the tubules. They are large, highly acidophilic, and triangular in shape. The apex of the cell is in contact with the lumen of the gland, and its base projects beyond the borders of the adjacent cells.

Parietal cells produce *hydrochloric acid for the gastric juice* and *intrinsic factor*, which is necessary for absorption of vitamin B_{12} in the ileum. The **base of the gastric glands** contains chief cells and **enteroendocrine cells** (see p. 384).

Cardiac glands. The cardia contains tubular gastric glands with numerous branches and cystic dilatations. The glands secrete mucus and antibacterial lysozyme. They do not contain any chief or parietal cells.

Pyloric glands. In the pyloric part (**C**), the gastric pits are generally deeper than elsewhere in the mucosa. The branches of the glands extend deeply downward, forming coils. They are predominantly lined by **columnar cells** that secrete **neutral to slightly acid mucus**. The pyloric glands also contain gastrin-producing **endocrine cells** (G cells) (see p. 387).

Muscular Layer (D)

The muscular layer of the stomach consists of **three layers**. In addition to those typically found in the intestinal wall, that is, the longitudinal layer (**D9**) and the circular layer (**D10**), the stomach has a third layer consisting of oblique fibers (**D11**). The fibers of the outer **longitudinal layer** are especially thick. They pass along the greater curvature from the cardia to the pylorus and along the lesser curvature to the angular incisure. After the angular incisure, new longitudinal muscle fibers begin and extend beyond the pyloric part of the stomach to continue into the duodenum. The *angular incisure* thus marks the *boundary between two functionally distinct parts of the stomach*: an upper *digestive sac* with digestive functions and a lower *pyloric canal*, with emptying functions. The longitudinal muscle layer acts to regulate longitudinal expansion of the stomach. The well-developed middle **circular layer** is thickened around the pylorus to form the *pyloric sphincter* (**D12**), which projects into the interior of the stomach. The innermost layer of the muscular coat consists of **oblique fibers**, which pass diagonally over the body of the stomach, without covering the lesser curvature, and are continuous with the circular layer.

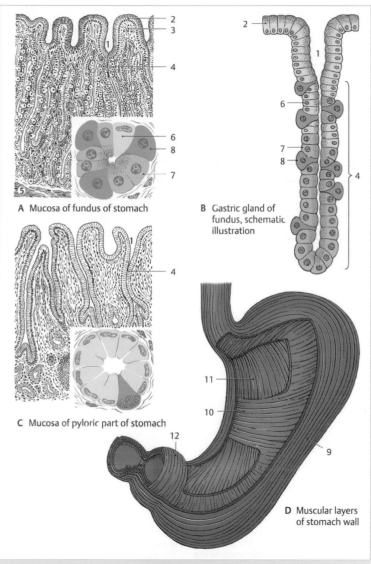

A Mucosa of fundus of stomach

B Gastric gland of fundus, schematic illustration

C Mucosa of pyloric part of stomach

D Muscular layers of stomach wall

Fig. 4.26 Microscopic structure of the stomach wall.

Vessels, Nerves, Lymphatic Drainage

Arteries. The arteries supplying the stomach usually arise from **branches of the celiac trunk (A1)** and join to form **vascular plexuses** along the lesser and greater curvatures. The vascular arch at the **lesser curvature** is formed by the left gastric artery (**A2**) and right gastric artery (**A3**). The **left gastric artery** arises from the *celiac trunk* and initially ascends in a fold of peritoneum known as the upper gastro pancreatic fold, before curving toward the lesser curvature. At the level of the cardia, it distributes small branches to the esophagus and larger branches to the stomach, and anastomoses with the right gastric artery which usually arises from the *hepatic artery proper* (**A4**). During its course, the **right gastric artery** first lies superficially in the hepatoduodenal ligament of the lesser omentum and then proceeds in the hepatogastric ligament to the lesser curvature of the stomach. There it unites with the left gastric artery to form a vascular arch. The vascular arch at the **greater curvature** is formed by the gastro-omental arteries. The **left gastro-omental artery** (**A5**) passes as a branch of the *splenic artery* (**A6**) through the gastrosplenic ligament to the greater curvature, where it runs in the gastrocolic ligament and anastomoses with the **right gastroomental artery** (**A7**), which originates from the *gastroduodenal artery* (**A8**). The fundic region of the stomach receives additional nourishment from the small **short gastric arteries**, branches of the *splenic artery*. **Veins**. The gastric veins run **parallel to the arteries** after which they are named. Blood either drains directly through the *left gastric vein* (**A9**) into the *hepatic portal vein* (**A10**), or flows first to the *splenic vein* and *superior mesenteric vein* and then into the hepatic portal vein.

Nerves. The postganglionic **sympathetic fibers** innervating the stomach arise from the **celiac nerve plexus** (**A11**) and accompany the arteries to the stomach wall. Stimulation of the sympathetic nervous system causes *constriction of the blood vessels of the stomach* and *inhibits gastric motility*. The **parasympathetic fibers** arise from **branches of the vagus nerve**, which form the *anterior vagal trunk* on the anterior surface of the stomach and the *posterior vagal*

trunk on the posterior surface. Stimulation of the parasympathetic system leads to increased *circulation*, increased *secretion of gastric juice and hydrochloric acid*, and an increase in *stomach movements*.

Regional lymph nodes (B). Lymph drains from the mucosal and submucosal and from the muscular and subserous network of the lymphatic vessels of the stomach in three directions: lymph from the cardia and much of the anterior and posterior walls drains along the lesser curvature to reach the **gastric** nodes (**B12**), most of which lie along the *left gastric artery;* lymph from the fundic region of the stomach and the parts of the greater curvature adjacent to the spleen drains into the **splenic nodes** (**B13**); and the remainder of the lymph from the greater curvature drains to the **gastro-omental** nodes (**B14**). Lymph collected by the above-named nodes ultimately drains to the *celiac nodes* (**B15**). Lymph from the pyloric region drains to the **gastro-omental** nodes (**B14**) and usually to the **pyloric nodes** (**B16**) lying behind the pylorus. Most of the lymph is also conveyed to the *celiac nodes*, and a smaller amount flows to the *superior mesenteric nodes* (**B17**). There are numerous connections between these highly complicated lymphatic drainage territories.

> **Clinical note.** Metastasis to the pyloric nodes can result in their fusion with the pancreas (**B18**) behind them, which can present a considerable intraoperative challenge.

Gastric function. Once in the stomach, the food boluses are stacked, chemically broken down, and transformed into chyme. The chyme is surrounded by the wall of the stomach without an increase in wall tension. These tonic contractions of the stomach wall around its contents are referred to as **peristole** and occur only in that part of the stomach forming the digestive sac. The stomach contents are gradually propelled distalward toward the pyloric canal, the inferior region of the stomach, for gastric emptying. Peristaltic waves, or muscular contractions, then propel the stomach contents toward the pylorus, which empties the contents of the stomach in small portions into the duodenum.

> **Clinical note. Gastritis**, characterized by multiple punctate superficial mucosal defects, is the most common acute inflammation of the stomach. The cause is nowadays believed to be colonization with *Helicobacter pylori*, a flagellated Gram-negative, spiral bacterium. **Ulcer disease** is the collective term for various forms of stomach ulcers.

Alimentary System

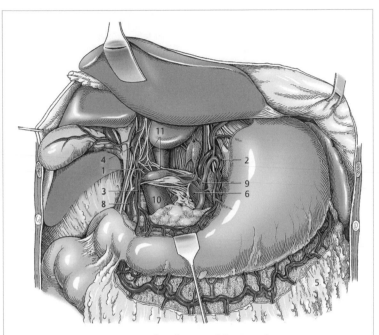

A Vessels and nerves of the stomach

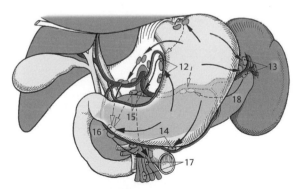

B Lymph nodes and lymphatic drainage of the stomach

Fig. 4.27 Vessels, nerves, and lymphatic drainage of the stomach.

Alimentary System

4.8 Small Intestine

Below the stomach, the alimentary canal is continuous with the **small intestine**. Its segments consist of the **duodenum** (**A1**), **jejunum** (**AC2**), and **ileum** (**AC3**), which opens in the right iliac fossa into the large intestine (**A4**). The average length of the entire small intestine is about 5 m.

Gross Anatomy

Duodenum

The horseshoe-shaped or C-shaped duodenum, 25–30 cm in length, projects toward the *umbilicus*. Lying on the posterior abdominal wall, most of the duodenum lies on the right side of the vertebral column and encloses the head of the pancreas (**B5**).

The duodenum can be divided into **four segments**: the first part, or **superior part** (**B6**), begins at the *pylorus* (**B7**) at the level of L1 to the right of the midline. It ascends slightly from anteroposteriorly and becomes continuous at the *superior duodenal flexure* (**B8**) with the descending part. Because of its dilated appearance on radiographs, the first part of the duodenum is referred to in clinical usage as the *duodenal cap*, or *ampulla*. The superior part is crossed posteriorly by the portal vein and common bile duct. The inferior vena cava is deep to these structures. The **descending part** (**B9**) descends on the right side of the vertebral column to the level of L3. It is continuous at the *inferior duodenal flexure* (**B10**) with the **horizontal part** (**B11**), which travels below the head of the pancreas over the vertebral column. After reaching the left side of the vertebral column it climbs as the **ascending part** (**B12**) to the *duodenojejunal flexure* (**B13**), situated at the level of L2, where it passes into the jejunum.

The *superior part* of the duodenum is situated *intraperitoneally*. Its attachment to the liver by the hepatoduodenal ligament (**B14**) allows for movement. The *descending part and all consecutive segments* are *secondarily retroperitoneal structures*, so only their anterior surfaces are covered by peritoneum. The small intestine becomes *intraperitoneal* again at the duodenojejunal flexure, with nearby peritoneal folds

and recesses. The **superior duodenal fossa** (**B15**) is framed by the **superior duodenal fold** (**B16**) and the **inferior duodenal fossa** (**B17**) by the **inferior duodenal fold** (**B18**). Bundles of smooth muscle fiber cells, forming the **suspensory muscle of the duodenum** (ligament of Treitz), connect the ascending part of the duodenum with the trunk of the superior mesenteric artery.

> **Clinical note.** Incarcerations of small intestinal loops in peritoneal recesses are referred to as internal hernias (**Treitz hernias**). These can potentially lead to life-threatening intestinal necrosis.

Jejunum and Ileum

The small intestine begins looping at the **duodenojejunal flexure** (**B13**). The **jejunum** (**AC2**) forms up to two-fifths of its total length and the **ileum** (**AC3**) up to three-fifths. The loops of the small intestine lie in the infracolic part of the abdominal cavity, framed by the large intestine (**A4**) and covered by the greater omentum. In the right iliac fossa, the ileum opens via the **ileal orifice** into the large intestine. In about 2%, there is a blind pouch located 50–100 cm from the valve, which is known as the ileal diverticulum, or **Meckel diverticulum**, a remnant of the *embryonic vitelline duct*.

The jejunum and ileum are situated *intraperitoneally* and are suspended from the posterior abdominal wall by a **mesentery** (**C19**), which permits their movement. The **root of the mesentery** (**BC20**) is 15–18-cm long and passes along the posterior abdominal wall in a line from the duodenojejunal flexure to the right iliac fossa. The **attachment of the mesentery to the small intestine** is about 4 m long and lies in numerous folds, forming a type of collar around the small intestine. The walls of the jejunum and ileum have a smooth outer surface and peritoneal lining, and cannot be distinguished from each other macroscopically.

> **Clinical note.** Inflammation of the Meckel diverticulum can be mistaken for appendicitis.

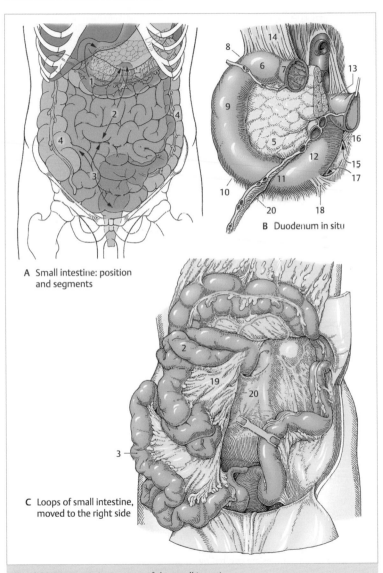

A Small intestine: position and segments

B Duodenum in situ

C Loops of small intestine, moved to the right side

Fig. 4.28 Macroscopic structure of the small intestine.

Structure of the Small Intestinal Wall

Mucosal Landmarks

Duodenum. The mucosal lining of the duodenum contains densely packed, tall **circular folds** (Kerckring valves) (**A1**) that are visible to the naked eye. *Consisting of mucosa and submucosa,* the circular folds enlarge the surface area of the mucosa by 50%. The descending part of the duodenum contains the openings of the excretory passages from the liver and pancreas, that is, the *bile duct* (**A2**) and *pancreatic duct* (**A3**). These produce a longitudinal fold in the mucosa, known as the **longitudinal fold of the duodenum** (**A4**) and normally join to open on a mucosal projection, lying on top of the fold, called the **major duodenal papilla** (**A5**). Located cranial to the major duodenal papilla is the **minor duodenal papilla**, where the *accessory pancreatic duct* usually opens.

Jejunum and ileum. The initial portion of the mucosal lining of the jejunum (**B**) also has tall, densely arranged **circular folds**. Closer to the ileum (**C**), the folds become shorter and are spaced further apart, and in the second half of the ileum they are usually absent. Opposite the mesenteric attachment, the mucosa of the ileum bulges visibly into the lumen, owing to underlying **aggregated lymphoid nodules** (**C6**) (Peyer patches) in the mucosa and submucosa.

Microscopic Anatomy

Mucosa. The microstructure of the mucosa of the small intestine corresponds to the general structure found in the intestine (see p. 142). In addition to circular folds, the surface of all small-intestinal segments is also enlarged by villi and crypts.

Intestinal villi (**D–F7**). Intestinal villi are *leaflike or fingerlike mucosal projections* of the *epithelium* and *lamina propria* that lend a velvety appearance to the mucosa of the small intestine. The epithelium contains various cell types, all derived from the same stem cells. On their surface, the villi are covered by absorptive epithelial cells known as *enterocytes* (**E9**) with scattered goblet cells. The surface area of the luminal side of the enterocytes is vastly enlarged by an arrangement of microvilli which form a *brush border*. Each **villus core** is occupied by *connective tissue* (lamina propria)

containing smooth muscle cells for individual *villus motility*, as well as a *blood vessel* (**E10**) and a *lymph vessel*, along with lymphocytes, plasma cells, and mast cells.

Intestinal glands (**D–F8**) (crypts of Lieberkühn). The short, tubular intestinal glands, which open at the bases of adjacent villi, extend to the muscularis mucosae. The epithelium of the glands has a secretory function and assists in epithelial cell regeneration. It consists mainly of *enterocytes; goblet cells* (**E11**); *Paneth cells* with apical granules containing lysosomal enzymes, and peptidase; and hormone-producing *enteroendocrine cells* (see p. 384). Paneth cells are found mainly at the bottom of the crypts.

Submucosa. The connective tissue of the submucosa contains the **submucosal nerve plexus** (**Meissner plexus**) and loose networks of **blood and lymphatic vessels**. The submucosa of the duodenum (**D**) contains branching tubuloalveolar **duodenal glands** (**D12**), also known as Brunner glands. Their mucilaginous secretions neutralize the substances in the chyme received from the stomach.

Muscular layer. Throughout the small intestine, the muscular layer consists of a well-developed **inner circular layer** and a less prominent **outer longitudinal layer**. The connective tissue between the two layers contains the (autonomic) **myenteric nerve plexus** (**Auerbach plexus**).

The inner circular and outer longitudinal layers of muscle act as **antagonists:** contraction of the longitudinal layer shortens and expands an intestinal, segment, while contraction of the circular layer elongates and narrows it. This produces *pendular* and *rhythmic segmentation contractions* that mix intestinal contents, and *peristaltic contractions* or *waves* that transport them.

Summary

The **duodenum** (**D**) has tall circular folds; tall, leaflike villi; and shallow crypts. Its submucosa contains duodenal glands.

The **jejunum** (**E**) is characterized by tall and densely packed circular folds; tall, fingerlike villi; and crypts that gradually become deeper.

The **ileum** (**F**) contains shorter villi and the crypts become progressively deeper. Its submucosa contains aggregated lymphoid nodules that extend into the lamina propria.

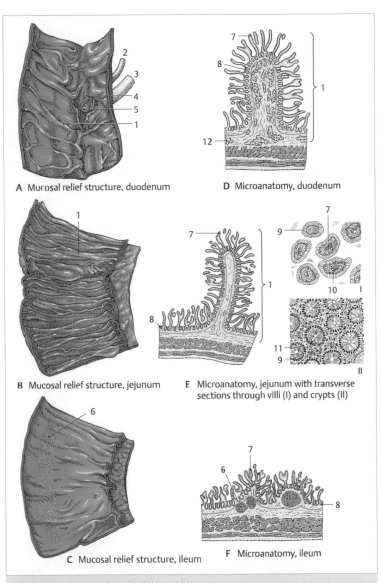

A Mucosal relief structure, duodenum

D Microanatomy, duodenum

B Mucosal relief structure, jejunum

E Microanatomy, jejunum with transverse sections through villi (I) and crypts (II)

C Mucosal relief structure, ileum

F Microanatomy, ileum

Fig. 4.29 Structure of the wall of the small intestine.

Alimentary System

Vessels, Nerves, and Lymphatic Drainage

Duodenum

Arteries. The vessels supplying the duodenum largely correspond to those supplying the head of the pancreas. The **anterior superior pancreaticoduodenal artery** (A1) and **posterior superior pancreaticoduodenal artery** (A2) arise from the *gastroduodenal artery* (A3), a branch of the *common hepatic artery* (A4), which, in turn, is a branch of the *celiac trunk* (A5). They unite with the **inferior** pancreaticoduodenal **artery** (A6), arising from the *superior mesenteric artery* (AB7), to form a vascular loop around the duodenum and the pancreas head, establishing a connection between arterial systems of the celiac trunk and superior mesenteric artery.

Veins. Venous drainage from the duodenum and pancreas is through the **splenic vein** (A8) and **superior mesenteric vein** (AB9) into the *hepatic portal vein* (A10).

Nerves. Extrinsic autonomic innervation of the entire small intestine is provided by nerve plexuses around the mesenteric vessels. The **parasympathetic** fibers arise from the *vagal trunks* and the **sympathetic** fibers from the *celiac ganglia* and *superior mesenteric ganglion*.

Regional lymph nodes. Lymph drains to the small group of **pyloric** nodes (see p. 194) and the pancreaticoduodenal nodes. The *hepatic nodes* serve as the second filtering station, emptying into the *celiac nodes*, which in turn drain into the *intestinal trunks*.

Jejunum and Ileum

Arteries. Jejunum and ileum receive their blood supply from **branches of the superior** mesenteric **artery** (AB7). About **4–5 jejunal arteries** (B11) and about **12 ileal arteries** (B12) course in the mesentery to the jejunum and ileum. Each of these jejunal or ileal arteries initially gives rise to two branches that communicate with the adjacent artery. In their course, there are increasingly numerous interconnections between the vessels, giving rise to progressively smaller **arterial arcades** (B13). The branches passing from the peripheral arcades to the intestinal wall are terminal arteries. Hence, occlusion of these vessels can result in regional intestinal damage.

Veins. Veins accompanying the arteries drain the jejunum and ileum via the *superior mesenteric vein* to the *hepatic portal vein* (A10).

Nerves. The innervation corresponds to that of the duodenum.

Regional lymph nodes. Lymph from the small-intestinal villi and the remainder of the intestinal wall drains via the lymphatic vessels lying along the arteries. Drainage is first to the group of *juxta-intestinal mesenteric nodes* (B14) near the primary arterial arcades, and from there to the *superior mesenteric nodes*, which are adjacent to the *pancreaticoduodenal nodes*, and also via the *celiac nodes* into the *intestinal trunks*.

Function of the Small Intestine

The chief function of the small intestine is digestion and absorption of nutrients. Digestion can be defined as the *enzymatic breakdown of nutrients into absorbable components:* carbohydrates are broken down into monosaccharides; proteins into amino acids; and fats into fatty acids and glycerin. Pancreatic secretions released into the duodenum provide an important *source of protein*. Digestion of fat requires bile acids, which are also secreted, into the duodenum. The intestinal mucosa contains *absorptive* and *mucus-producing epithelial cells* as well as *endocrine cells*. The latter secrete hormones that regulate pancreatic and gallbladder secretion, as well as intestinal motility. The chyme is moved through the small intestine by *mixing and propulsive movements*.

Clinical note. Proliferation of duodenal epithelial cells in month 2–3 of embryo development causes complete temporary occlusion of the lumen. Failure to become recanalized later in pregnancy results in **duodenal stenosis**, in which the lumen is narrowed, or **atresia**, in which it is completely occluded. **The small** intestine is crucial for the absorption of nearly all components of the diet. It absorbs between 7 L and 12 L of fluid daily. Inflammatory diseases of the small intestine inevitably lead to disturbance of intestinal fluid and electrolyte balance, usually manifested clinically as diarrhea.

Ulcers are the most common disease in the duodenum. They generally occur in the duodenal bulb, with a peak incidence between the ages of 30 and 50 years. Men are affected four times more often than women. Typical symptoms include epigastric pain at night or when fasting, along with bloating, belching, meteorism, and vomiting.

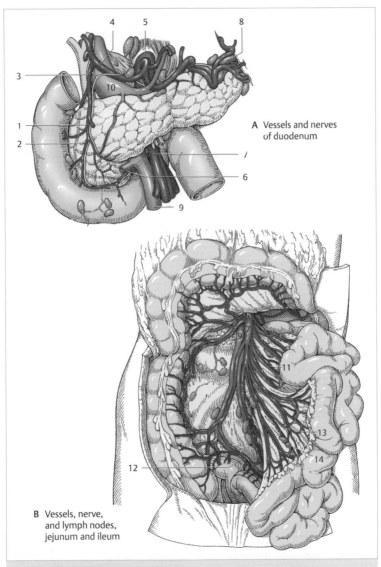

A Vessels and nerves of duodenum

B Vessels, nerve, and lymph nodes, jejunum and ileum

Fig. 4.30 Vessels, nerves, and lymphatic drainage of the small intestine.

4.9 Large Intestine

Segments of the Large Intestine: Overview

The **large intestine** is 1.5–1.8-m long. It lies in the infracolic part of the abdominal cavity, framing the loops of the small intestine. The large intestine may be subdivided into four parts: the **cecum (A1)** and *vermiform appendix* (**AC2**); the **colon**, consisting of the *ascending colon* (**A3**), *transverse colon* (**A4**), *descending colon* (**A5**), and *sigmoid colon* (**A6**); the **rectum (A7)**; and the **anal canal (A8)**. With the exception of the anal canal, which originates from the ectoderm, the entire large intestine originates from the endoderm.

Typical Features

The cecum and colon are characterized by typical features on their outer surfaces that make them readily distinguishable from the small intestine. The **teniae coli (B9)** are *thickened bands of the outer longitudinal layer of muscle*, about 1-cm wide. They are referred to by their location on the transverse colon as *mesocolic tenia, omental tenia*, and *free tenia* (**B10**). Projecting into the intestinal lumen are the **semilunar folds of the colon (B11)**. Consisting of all wall layers, they are produced by muscular contractions and thus vary in number and location. Around the outside of the wall of the large intestine, they create transverse constricting furrows. Between neighboring furrows, the colon wall bulges outward, forming sacculations knows as the **haustra of the colon (B12)**. Also on the outer surface are subserosal fatty tags called **omental (or epiploic) appendices (B13)**.

Cecum and Vermiform Appendix

Cecum. The initial segment of the large intestine is 6–8 cm long, saccular, and located in the *right iliac fossa*, and contains the opening of the ileum (**C14**) in its medial wall. The **mesocolic tenia** faces posteromedially; the **omental tenia** posterolaterally; and the **free tenia (B10)** lies between them and is visible from the anterior.

Vermiform appendix (AC2). The vermiform appendix is continuous with the *posteromedial end of the cecum*. Its position depends on that of the cecum and is therefore highly variable (**D**): in about 65%, the vermiform appendix lies posterior to the cecum in the (ascending) *retrocecal position;* in 31% it extends beyond the linea terminalis into the lesser pelvis, lying in the (descending) *subcecal position;* in more than 2% it lies posterior to the cecum in the (transverse) *retrocecal position;* in 1% it lies anterior to the ileum in the (ascending) *paracecal, preileal position;* in about 0.5% it lies posterior to the ileum in the (ascending) *paracecal, retroileal position.* In the **ascending, retrocecal position**, which is the most common, the base of the vermiform appendix projects toward the **McBurney point** on the anterior abdominal wall (**E**). This point lies about one-third of the distance from the beginning of an imaginary line drawn from the anterior superior iliac spine to the umbilicus. The vermiform appendix is, on average, 10-cm long and 6-mm thick. The three teniae of the cecum (**C**) converge at the opening to the vermiform appendix, and do not form bands in the *longitudinal muscle layer* of the vermiform appendix, which has no tenia.

Peritoneal relations. The peritoneal relations of the large intestine vary. The cecum may be almost completely covered on all sides by peritoneum, in which case it is referred to as a **free cecum**, sometimes with its own mesocolon. A **fixed cecum** is a secondarily retroperitoneal cecum that is affixed to the fascia of the iliacus muscle. Located above and below the ileocecal junction, and hidden behind the two peritoneal folds, that is, the **vascular fold of the cecum** and the **ileocecal fold**, are the **superior ileocecal recess** and **inferior ileocecal recess (C15)**. Behind the right side of the cecum, there is often a **retrocecal recess (C16)**.

The vermiform appendix lies in an intraperitoneal position and has its own **mesoappendix (C17)**.

Clinical note. The course of the teniae can help the surgeon to quickly locate the vermiform appendix.

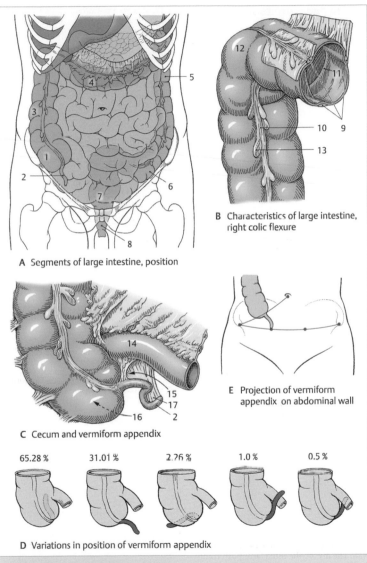

A Segments of large intestine, position

B Characteristics of large intestine, right colic flexure

C Cecum and vermiform appendix

E Projection of vermiform appendix on abdominal wall

65.28 %   31.01 %   2.26 %   1.0 %   0.5 %

D Variations in position of vermiform appendix

Fig. 4.31 Segments of the large intestine, cecum.

Alimentary System

Alimentary System

Cecum and Vermiform Appendix, cont.

Mucosal Landmarks

The **semilunar folds of the colon** (**A1**) are visible in the interior of the cecum. Opening into its wall is the ileum (**AB2**), with its two mucosa-covered valve lips known as the ileocecal lip (**AB3**) and **ileocolic lip** (**AB4**), projecting into the cecal lumen. These form the ileocecal valve that surrounds the **ileal orifice** (**AB5**). In the cadaver, the ileal orifice is a transverse opening; in the living body, the pair of lips bulges far into the cecum, forming the ileal papilla (**B6**) and giving the opening a rather star-shaped appearance. The mucosa-covered lips unite at their outer ends to produce a fold called the **frenulum of the ileal orifice** (**A7**). The mucosa-covered lips and folds, produced for the most part by the invaginated muscular layer of the terminal ileum, act to prevent backflow of the contents of the large intestine into the small intestine.

At a short distance distal to the ileum, the vermiform appendix opens via the orifice of **the vermiform appendix** (**AB8**) into the cecum.

Microscopic Anatomy

Cecum (**C**). The colonic mucosa, which is the same in all segments, begins directly after the ileocecal valve. The mucosa of the cecum *does not contain villi;* it possesses only crypts, or *intestinal glands* (**C9**), which are especially deep and packed close together in this part of the large intestine. The surface epithelium is composed of *enterocytes* (**C10**) with a tall *brush border*, as well as *goblet cells* (**C11**). The submucosa contains areas of *lymphatic follicles*. The *circular layer* of the muscular layer forms a continuous layer, while the *longitudinal layer* is mostly limited to the three teniae.

Vermiform appendix (**D**). The histologic appearance of the vermiform appendix is also similar to that of the rest of the large intestine, but its irregular crypts are shallow. A typical feature is the massive collection of lymphatic follicles, or **aggregated lymphoid nodules** (**D12**), extending from the lamina propria through the muscularis mucosae to the submucosa. The vermiform appendix is an **important component of the immune system** (see p. 384). Its muscular layer is continuous, consisting of a *circular layer* and a *longitudinal layer*.

C17 Muscularis mucosae, **C18** Submucosa, **C19** Circular muscle layer, **C20** Longitudinal muscle layer, **C21** Serosa, **D22** Mesoappendix

Vessels, Nerves, and Lymphatic Drainage

Arteries (**E**). The cecum and appendix are both supplied by the **ileocolic artery** (**E13**), which arises as the last branch from the *superior mesenteric artery*. It gives rise to the following branches:

the *appendicular artery* (**E14**), which runs in the mesoappendix to the vermiform appendix;

the *anterior cecal artery* (**E15**), which runs in the *vascular fold of the cecum* to the anterior wall of the cecum;

the *posterior cecal artery* (**E16**) to the posterior wall of the cecum;

the *ileal branches* to the terminal ileum (**E17**).

Veins. Venous drainage is via the veins of the same name, which empty via the superior *mesenteric vein* into the *hepatic portal vein*.

Nerves. Autonomic innervation is identical to that of the small intestine.

Regional lymph nodes. Lying in the angle between the ileum and cecum, the ileocolic *nodes, prececal nodes, retrocecal nodes,* and *appendicular nodes* collect lymph from the cecum and vermiform appendix and drain via the *mesenteric nodes* into the *intestinal trunks*.

Function. The main function of the **cecum** and **colon** is **reabsorption of water and electrolytes**, which enter the intestinal lumen along with digestive juices. After the digestive processes are completed in the ileum, the large intestine receives indigestible residues, which are broken down by bacteria. Intestinal contents are transported through the large intestine and converted to solid waste by means of slow peristalsis and antiperistalsis. A few propulsive movements are sufficient to propel the intestinal contents distalward into the colon.

The **vermiform appendix** is an important site serving the **immune system of the digestive tract** (see p. 418).

Clinical note. In its function as part of the immune system, the vermiform appendix can overreact to infection. Inflammation, or **appendicitis**, can result in perforation, with a resultant spread of inflammation to the abdominal cavity (**peritonitis**). Terminal ileitis (Crohn disease) can present like appendicitis because of the proximity to the vermiform appendix.

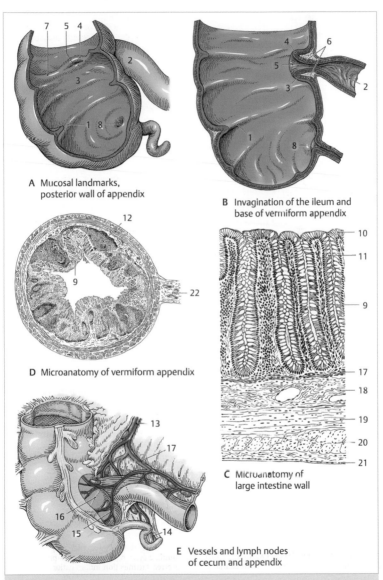

A Mucosal landmarks,
posterior wall of appendix

B Invagination of the ileum and
base of vermiform appendix

D Microanatomy of vermiform appendix

C Microanatomy of
large intestine wall

E Vessels and lymph nodes
of cecum and appendix

Fig. 4.32 Cecum and vermiform appendix, continued.

Alimentary System

Colon Segments

Ascending colon. Above the ileal orifice, the cecum (**A1**) is continuous with the ascending colon (**A2**). The ascending colon lies in the lower right part of the abdomen and extends to the **right colic flexure** (**A3**), which is usually situated between the right inferior pole of the kidney and the right lobe of the liver, where it produces the *colic impression*. The ascending colon is a **secondarily retroperitoneal** organ.

Transverse colon (**A4**). The transverse colon begins at the right colic flexure. It is an **intraperitoneal** organ and its position may vary considerably, sometimes lying as high as the level of the navel or, in extreme cases, as low as the lesser pelvis. It is attached to the posterior abdominal wall but mobile (see p. 188 **A**), by the **transverse mesocolon** (**B5**), to the liver by the **hepatocolic ligament**, and to the stomach by the **gastrocolic ligament**.

Descending colon. The transverse colon turns sharply at the **left colic flexure** (**A6**), below the left dome of the diaphragm and joins the descending colon (**A7**). The sharp bend in the colon is fixed in position by the **phrenicocolic ligament**. Its fixed position can obstruct the passage of intestinal contents. The descending colon lies on the left side of the lower abdomen and, as a **secondarily retroperitoneal** organ, is affixed to the posterior abdominal wall.

Sigmoid colon. The descending colon becomes continuous with the sigmoid colon (**AB8**) in the left iliac fossa. The sigmoid portion of the colon is again **intraperitoneal**. It is attached to the posterior abdominal wall by the **sigmoid mesocolon** (**A9**), the root of which may contain the **intersigmoid recess**. The sigmoid colon follows an S-shaped course toward the midline of the body, where it becomes continuous with the rectum at the level of L2 or L3.

All segments of the colon bear the **characteristic features of the large intestine**; each has three teniae, of which only the *free tenia* (**A10**) *is readily visible*. On all secondarily retroperitoneal parts, the mesocolic and omental teniae face the posterior abdominal wall; on the transverse colon, the mesocolic tenia is located at the attachment of the transverse mesocolon, and the omental tenia is at the attachment of the greater omentum (**A11**).

Mucosal landmarks and microanatomy. The surface structure of the mucosa is formed by the **semilunar folds** of the **colon**, and is similar to that of the cecum (see p. 204). The crypts become progressively shallower toward the anus.

Vessels, Nerves, and Lymphatic Drainage

Arteries (**B**). The ascending colon and about two-thirds of the transverse colon receive their blood supply from the **right colic artery** and **middle colic artery** (**B12**), arising from the *superior mesenteric artery* (see p. 200 **B**). The right colic artery usually anastomoses with both the *ileocolic artery* and the *middle colic artery*. The left one-third of the transverse colon is nourished, as is the descending colon, by the **left colic artery** (**B13**), arising from the *inferior mesenteric artery* (**B14**). The middle colic artery anastomoses with the left colic artery; hence, there is communication between the superior and inferior mesenteric arterial systems. The **sigmoid artery** (**B15**) joins the left colic artery and anastomoses with this vessel and with the superior rectal artery.

Veins. Veins of the same name follow the course of the respective arteries and drain via the *superior mesenteric vein* or *inferior mesenteric vein* (**B16**) to the *hepatic portal vein*.

Nerves. Fibers arising from the *vagus nerve* provide **parasympathetic** innervation of the colon as far as a point between the middle and left thirds of the transverse colon (**Cannon-Boehm point**); beyond this point, the parasympathetic fibers to the colon originate in the *sacral spinal cord* at the level of S2–S5 and pass cephalad via the *sacral splanchnic nerves* to the autonomic plexuses lying along the blood vessels. **Sympathetic** fibers arise from the superior *mesenteric plexus* or *inferior mesenteric plexus* (**B17**).

Regional lymph nodes. The lymphatic vessels follow the course of the colic arteries and veins. The **paracolic nodes** lie directly on the colon. The **colic nodes** (**B18**) are located along the nourishing vessels. They drain to the *mesocolic nodes*, which in turn drain to the *celiac nodes*.

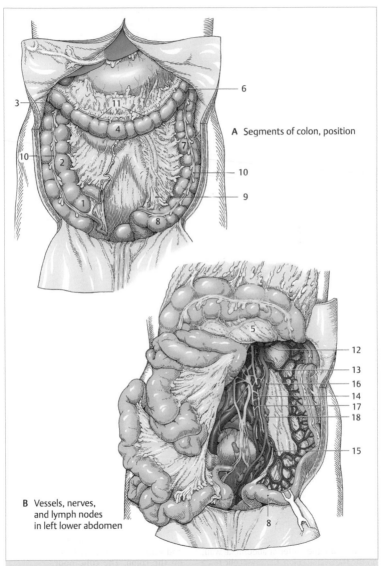

A Segments of colon, position

B Vessels, nerves, and lymph nodes in left lower abdomen

Fig. 4.33 Segments of the colon.

Alimentary System

Rectum and Anal Canal

At the level of S2 or S3, the sigmoid colon (**A1**) becomes continuous with the **rectum** (**A2**). The rectum is about 15 cm long. The portion of the rectum in the lesser pelvis, namely the **sacral flexure of the rectum** (**A3**), follows the anterior concavity of the sacrococcygeal curve. At the **anorectal flexure of the rectum** (**A4**), an anterior convexity of the rectum, it bends to pass posteriorly through the *pelvic diaphragm* and become continuous with the anal canal. In addition to the *curvatures in the sagittal plane*, the rectum also *bends in the frontal plane* (**lateral flexures**). The rectum does not share the characteristics typical of the large intestine-haustra, omental appendices, and teniae, and its *longitudinal muscle layer is a continuous layer* rather than gathered in bands.

The **anal canal** (**A5**), about 4-cm long, is the final portion of the intestinal canal. It is surrounded by a complex sphincter apparatus and opens at the **anus** (**A6**).

The upper part of the rectum is covered on its anterior aspect and laterally by peritoneum. In the male pelvis, the peritoneum reflects onto the urinary bladder, forming the **rectovesical pouch**. In the female pelvis, it reflects onto the uterus, forming the **rectouterine pouch** (**A7**). The *upper portion of the rectum is therefore retroperitoneal*. Like the anal canal, the distal portion of the rectum has *no peritoneal covering*.

Mucosal landmarks and microanatomy

Above the anal canal in the region of the sacral flexure, the rectum can form a dilatation known as the **rectal ampulla**. There are usually three constant transverse folds projecting into the interior of the rectum, known as the **transverse folds of the rectum**. The upper and lower folds project from the left, while the middle and largest of the three, the **Kohlrausch fold** (**A8**), projects from the right. It is located about 6 cm from the anus. In the female pelvis, the Kohlrausch fold lies at the height of the

rectouterine pouch, the lowest point in the peritoneal cavity.

The **structure of the walls** of the rectum resembles that found elsewhere in the large intestine.

Sphincter Apparatus

Surrounding the anal canal is a complex sphincter apparatus. Its components consist of an inner layer of the smooth muscle forming the **internal anal sphincter** (**B–D9**), and an outer layer of striated muscle forming the **external anal sphincter** (**B–D10**), the fibers of which pass caudal to the pelvic floor musculature to blend with the *levator ani* muscle.

Internal anal sphincter. This is a *thickened continuation of the circular muscle layer* of the large intestine, about 2-cm long. It extends as far as the **anocutaneous line** and can be palpated there as a muscular ring surrounding the anal canal.

External anal sphincter. This surrounds the outer surface of the smooth muscle of the internal anal sphincter. It is divided into three components: a *subcutaneous part* (**B10 a**), a *superficial part* (**B10 b**), and a *deep part* (**B10 c**). The external anal sphincter is connected by the *anococcygeal body* (**AD11**) to the coccyx. Its inferior portion blends with the **puborectalis** (**B12**) part of the *levator ani* muscle.

The external and internal anal sphincters are separated by a thin layer of longitudinal smooth muscle cells (**B–D13**). These longitudinal bundles are the continuation of the *longitudinal muscle layer* of the intestinal wall and fan out as the **corrugator cutis muscle of the anus**, into the perianal skin. During their course, they permeate the subcutaneous part of the striated sphincter muscle.

The **internal anal sphincter** is normally *in a state of contraction*, which is mostly influenced by sympathetic innervation. Although the **external anal** sphincter is also in a state of *involuntary tonic contraction*, the pudendal nerve also mediates *voluntary contraction*.

CD14 Perineal body, **CD15** Ischioanal fossa, **D16** Bulb of penis

Alimentary System

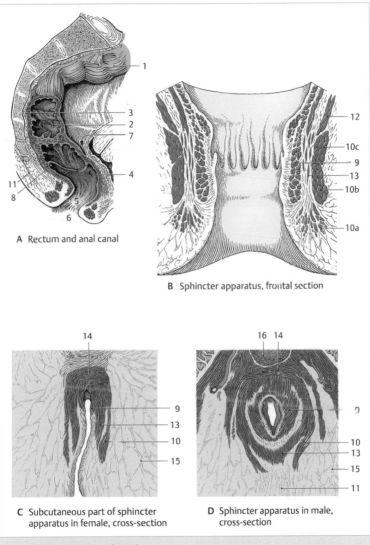

A Rectum and anal canal

B Sphincter apparatus, frontal section

C Subcutaneous part of sphincter apparatus in female, cross-section

D Sphincter apparatus in male, cross-section

Fig. 4.34 Rectum and anal canal.

Rectum and Anal Canal, cont.

Mucosal Landmarks and Microscopic Anatomy of the Anal Canal

Mucosal landmarks. Lying at the upper end of the **anal columns** (**A1**), the **anorectal junction** (**A2**) marks the junction between the rectum and the anal canal and the transition from rectal mucosa to the irregular mucosa of the anal canal. The anal columns are *six to ten longitudinal mucosal folds* between which lie depressions called **anal sinuses** (**A3**). At their lower ends, the anal columns are connected by transverse folds known as the **anal val**ves (**A4**), demarcating the slightly jagged pectinate line. The anal columns overlie the arteriovenous plexuses surrounding the **rectum** (**A5**), which are fed by the *superior rectal artery*.

Histology. The mucosal composition of the anal canal alternates at the anal columns between *columnar epithelium* and *stratified, nonkeratinized squamous epithelium*. Distal to the anal columns is the anal transition zone (**A6**), a strip of mucosa that appears white to the naked eye and consists entirely of *stratified, nonkeratinized squamous epithelium*. The mucosa of the anal transitional zone is highly sensitive to pain and is firmly attached to the underlying layers. It ends at the anocutaneous line (**A7**), where the stratified, nonkeratinized squamous epithelium of the mucosa transitions into the *stratified, keratinized squamous epithelium* of the skin.

> **Clinical note.** Internal hemorrhoids result from prolapse of the arteriovenous plexuses underlying the anal columns, with loss of blood that is bright red in color, indicating its arterial source.

Vessels, Nerves, and Lymphatic Drainage

Arteries. Most of the rectum is nourished by the **superior rectal artery** (**B8**), which arises from the *inferior mesenteric artery*. The inconstant **middle rectal artery** (**B9**) (from the *internal iliac artery*) passes to the wall of the rectum at the level of the pelvic floor. The **inferior rectal artery** (**B10**) originates from the *internal pudendal artery* and supplies the anal canal and external anal sphincter.

Veins. The veins draining the rectum anastomose to form the **rectal venous plexus** that surrounds it. Venous drainage corresponds to arterial supply: drainage is **via the superior rectal vein** to the *inferior mesenteric vein* and then to the *hepatic portal vein* (portal circulation), or via the middle and inferior rectal veins to the *internal iliac vein* and then *inferior vena cava* (systemic circulation).

Nerves. Autonomic nerve supply to the rectum and anal canal is from the sacral portion *of the parasympathetic nervous system* and the *lumbar sympathetic trunk*. The nerve fibers pass to the intestine via the **inferior hypogastric plexus** (**B11**). Sensory innervation of the anal skin is by the **inferior rectal nerves**, which are branches of the **pudendal nerve**.

Regional lymph nodes. Lymph from the rectum drains via the superior rectal nodes lying along the *superior rectal artery* to the *inferior mesenteric nodes*. Lymph from the anal canal drains to the **superficial inguinal nodes**.

Function

The functions of the rectum and anal canal may be summed up in two words: **continence** and **defecation**.

Continence. The **sustained tonic contraction of the sphincter** normally keeps the anus closed. The **puborectalis** forms a muscular sling around the anorectal flexure, drawing it forward and also closing the anal canal. The blood-filled **arteriovenous plexuses surrounding the body of the rectum** also help ensure complete closure of the anal canal.

Defecation. Defecation is preceded by movement of the contents of the colon into the rectum. Accumulation of feces in the rectum increases wall tension, stimulating defecation, which in turn leads to **reflexive relaxation** of the internal anal sphincter. **Voluntarily** relaxing the puborectalis and internal anal sphincter, and using intra-abdominal pressure, leads to voluntary defecation.

> **Clinical note.** In clinical practice, the sphincter apparatus is viewed as only one component in the entire **organ of continence** (consisting of the *rectum, anal canal, sphincter apparatus, puborectalis, arteriovenous plexuses of the rectum*, and *autonomic nerves*) which works as a unit to achieve proper closure of the rectum and ensure continence.

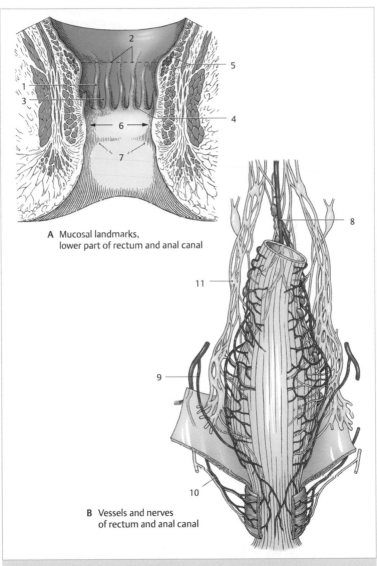

A Mucosal landmarks,
lower part of rectum and anal canal

B Vessels and nerves
of rectum and anal canal

Fig. 4.35 Rectum and anal canal, continued.

4.10 Liver

Gross Anatomy

The **liver** (**A1**) lies mostly below the right dome of the diaphragm. The inferior border of this reddish-brown organ is nearly flush with that of the right costal margin. The border of the liver runs diagonally to the left and passes through the epigastric region as it intersects the midclavicular line. The liver is an **intraperitoneal** organ and, except for the triangular bare area (**C7**), is completely covered by visceral peritoneum. It is attached by the *falciform ligament* to the parietal peritoneum of the anterior abdominal wall, by the *lesser omentum* or *hepatoduodenal ligament* to the duodenum, and by the *hepatogastric ligament* to the lesser curvature of the stomach. The peritoneum surrounding the liver gives it a smooth, glistening appearance. With the naked eye, a convex **diaphragmatic surface** and a **visceral surface** with a complex arrangement of structures can be seen.

Diaphragmatic Surface

The diaphragmatic surface consists of various parts, the largest being the **anterior part** (**B**), which faces anteriorly. The anterior part is divided on the surface by the sagittally oriented **falciform ligament** (**BC2**) into a **right lobe of the liver** (**BC3**) and a **left lobe of the liver** (**BC4**). The anterior surface converges with the visceral surface, which ascends backward, at the distinct **inferior border** (**B5**). The fundus of the gallbladder projects over the inferior border to the right of the falciform ligament. The **superior part** (**C**) of the liver faces cephalad. Near the inferior vena cava (**CD6**), the liver is attached to the diaphragm in the **bare area** (**C7**), which is not covered by visceral peritoneum. Once the liver is freed from its attachments, the bare area is framed by reflections of the visceral peritoneum onto the parietal peritoneum: the **coronary ligament** (**C8**) continues on the right side as the *right triangular ligament* (**C9**) and on the left side as the *left triangular ligament* (**C10**). The latter terminates in a fibrous band called the *fibrous appendix of the liver* (**C11**). The coronary ligament from either side passes anteriorly to become continuous with the falciform ligament (**BC2**). On the left side, in front of the inferior vena cava, the heart lies adjacent to the superior part of the liver, separated from the *cardiac impression* by the diaphragm. The **right part** refers to the right, lateral portion of the diaphragmatic surface and the **posterior part** to the small, posteriorly directed portion.

Visceral Surface

The slightly concave visceral surface of the liver extends diagonally from posterosuperior to anteroinferior. It lies in close proximity to the adjacent organs. It is subdivided by a set of **H-shaped grooves**. The **porta hepatis** (**D12**) forms the (horizontal) crossbar of the H. Entering the liver at the porta hepatis are the *portal veins* (**D13**), *two branches of the hepatic artery proper* (**D14**), and *nerves;* the *right hepatic duct* (**D15**), *left hepatic duct* (**D16**), and *lymphatic vessels* leave through the porta hepatis. The **left** (sagittal) limb of the H is formed by the **fissure for the round ligament** (**D17**), containing the *round ligament of the liver* (**D18**), a vestige of the *umbilical vein;* and the **fissure for the ligamentum venosum** (**D19**) housing the *ligamentum venosum* (**D20**), a remnant of the *ductus venosus* (duct of Arantius). The **right** (sagittal) limb of the H is formed by a groove called the **fossa for the gallbladder**, which houses the *gallbladder* (**D21**) and the **groove for the vena cava** (**D22**), which contains the *inferior vena cava* (**CD6**). The left limb of the H divides the right and left lobes of the liver, while the right limb divides the right lobe of the liver from the **quadrate lobe** (**D23**) in front and the **caudate lobe** (**CD24**) behind. The *papillary process* projects inferiorly from the caudate lobe; the *caudate process* projects into the right lobe of the liver.

The visceral surface of the liver is marked by visible impressions from adjacent organs attached to it: its **left side** is marked by an elevation known as the *omental tuberosity* (**D25**) as well as the *esophageal impression* (**D26**) and *gastric impression* (**D27**). Indenting the **right side** of the liver are the *duodenal impression* (**D28**), *colic impression* (**D29**), *renal impression* (**D30**), and *suprarenal impression* (**D31**).

CD32 Ligament of vena cava

Note to D: The liver is oriented as it appears when the patient is supine, according to the internationally accepted computed tomography view (posterior below and anterior above).

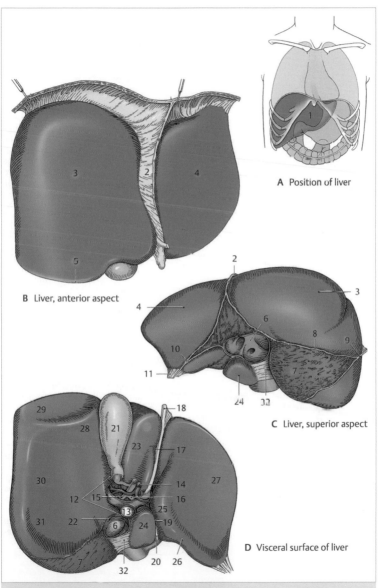

A Position of liver

B Liver, anterior aspect

C Liver, superior aspect

D Visceral surface of liver

Fig. 4.36 Macroscopic structure of the liver.

Liver Segments

The liver may be divided either into lobes based on macroscopic features, or into **liver segments** based on the **distribution of intrahepatic vessels**, that is, the *hepatic portal vein, hepatic artery proper*, and *bile ducts*. These segments are variable and are also described differently in the literature, but are generally seen as consisting of a **right part of the liver** and a **left part of the liver**. The left part of the liver can be further subdivided into *medial* and *lateral* parts (see Fig. **BC**, p. 216 A). The boundaries between these segments, or functional units, differ from the boundaries between the right and left lobes.

Microscopic Anatomy

The liver is enclosed in the visceral peritoneum and a **fibrous capsule** that accompanies the hepatic vessels as they pass into the interior of the organ, forming a supporting framework of connective tissue also known as the *perivascular fibrous capsule (Glisson capsule)*. Lying in the spaces within the connective tissue framework are **hepatocytes** (**A1**), the epithelial cells of the liver. Together, the connective tissue, hepatocytes, and vessels form the architectonic structural units of the liver known as the **lobules of the liver** (**AB2**).

Lobules of the Liver

Classical lobule model. Located at the center of each functional unit is a **central vein** (**AB3**). Each polygonal lobule is surrounded by a small amount of connective tissue that becomes denser at the corners between adjacent lobules, forming triangular regions called **portal areas** (**B4**). Each portal area contains three main structures—a branch of the hepatic portal vein, that is, an *interlobular vein* (**A5**); a branch of the hepatic artery proper, that is, an *interlobular artery* (**A6**); and a bile duct, that is, an *interlobar duct* (**A7**)—encased in the connective tissue of the Glisson capsule and collectively known as a **portal or Glisson triad**. The hepatocytes radiate toward the periphery of the lobule. They are composed of cell plates between which long, **sinusoidal capillaries** (**A8**) also radiate outward. The sinusoidal capillaries receive blood from both the *hepatic*

artery proper and the *hepatic portal vein;* in other words, they receive oxygenated, nutrient-rich blood. After transfer of substances within the sinusoids between the blood and hepatocytes, the blood drains via the *central vein* into the *collecting veins* and then into the *hepatic veins*. Between the vessel walls of the hepatic sinusoids and the surfaces of the hepatocytes is a space called the **perisinusoidal space** (**CD9**) (Disse space). The *microvilli* (**D10**) of the hepatocytes project into this space, which also contains fat-storing cells called *Ito cells*. The endothelial cells of the sinusoids are flat, with large transcellular pores (width about 100 nm) not closed by a diaphragm, that is, **discontinuous endothelium** (**D11**). There is no basement membrane. Hepatic macrophages known as Kupffer cells, which are part of the mononuclear phagocyte system (MPS), are found on the luminal surface of the endothelium. The microvilli projecting into the perisinusoidal space have direct contact with blood that percolates through the endothelial pores to reach them.

Portal lobule model (**B**). This model places the **portal area** at the center of the lobule, emphasizing the **flow direction of the bile**. Bile is produced by the hepatocytes and secreted into the **bile canaliculi** (**C12**). Bile canaliculi resemble channels whose sides are formed by cell contacts in the *spaces between the hepatocytes* (**D13**). Bile flows from the region around the central veins to the interlobular ducts, which in turn form **biliary ductules** that empty into the **right hepatic duct** and **left hepatic duct**. The portal lobule is *triangular* in shape and contains the central veins at its corners.

The axis of the **rhombic hepatic acinus** (**B**) contains a branch of the hepatic artery proper. In the **outer zone** (zone 1), the adjacent hepatocytes have a high *metabolic rate*. Cells of the outer zone receive highly oxygenated blood because of their proximity to distributing arteries. In the **inner zone** (zone 3), the *metabolic rate* of the hepatocytes, as well as their *oxygen supply*, is diminished.

Liver functions. As the **largest metabolic organ** in the body, the liver fulfills important functions, such as assisting in the metabolism of carbohydrates, proteins, and fats, as well as detoxification processes. In its function as an **exocrine gland**, it produces *bile*, which is secreted as needed into the duodenum via a duct system. During *fetal life*, it is involved in *hematopoiesis*.

Alimentary System

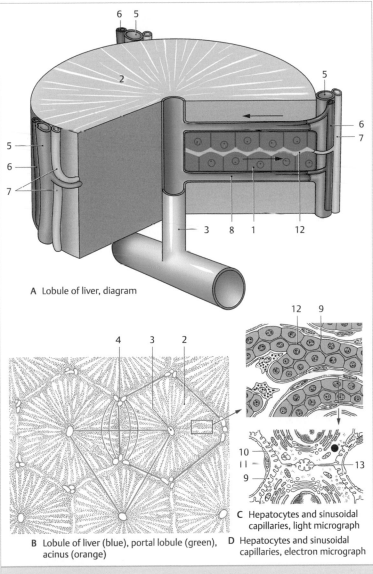

A Lobule of liver, diagram

B Lobule of liver (blue), portal lobule (green), acinus (orange)

C Hepatocytes and sinusoidal capillaries, light micrograph

D Hepatocytes and sinusoidal capillaries, electron micrograph

Fig. 4.37 Segmental and microscopic structure of the liver.

Vessels, Nerves, and Lymphatic Drainage

Arteries (B). The liver receives oxygenated blood from the **hepatic artery proper (B1)** (from the *common hepatic artery* from the *celiac trunk*), which passes in the hepatoduodenal ligament to the porta hepatis and divides into two branches, a *right branch* (**B2**) and a *left branch* (**B3**).

Veins. Venous blood drains from the liver through several short **hepatic veins** to the *inferior vena cava*. Nutrient-rich blood from the gastrointestinal tract flows via the **portal veins** to the liver (see below).

Nerves. Nerve supply to the liver is provided by autonomic nerves, the hepatic plexus, a continuation of the **celiac nerve plexus**.

Regional lymph nodes. Lymph is drained via the **hepatic nodes** lying along the porta hepatis, to the *superior diaphragmatic nodes* and *parasternal nodes*.

Hepatic Portal Vein System (C)

Hepatic portal vein (BC4). The hepatic portal vein receives *blood from* **three major tributaries** (see below) that *drain the unpaired abdominal organs*. This enables the nutrients absorbed in the intestine to reach the liver via the shortest pathway. After entering the liver, the hepatic portal vein divides into a **right branch** to the right lobe of the liver and a **left branch** to the left lobe of the liver. These large hepatic portal branches each ramify into the *interlobular veins*.

Tributaries. The **splenic vein (BC5)** accompanies the splenic artery along the upper border of the pancreas. It receives the *pancreatic veins*, *short gastric veins*, and *left gastro-omental vein*. The **inferior mesenteric vein (BC6)**, which opens into the splenic vein behind the body of the pancreas, receives the *left colic vein* (**C7**), *sigmoid veins*, and *superior rectal vein*. It courses in a fold of peritoneum known as the superior duodenal fold over the duodenojejunal flexure to behind the pancreas. Behind the head of the pancreas, the splenic vein unites with the superior mesenteric vein to form the portal vein, which is 5–8-cm long. The **superior mesenteric vein (BC8)** receives the *jejunal* and *ileal veins* (**C9**), *right*

gastro-omental vein, pancreatic veins, pancreaticoduodenal veins, ileocolic vein (**C10**), *right colic vein* (**C11**), and *middle colic vein* (**C12**). The superior mesenteric vein and its tributaries accompany the corresponding arteries of the same name. A few smaller, surrounding veins empty directly into the trunk of the hepatic portal vein. These are the *cystic vein, right* and *left gastric veins, prepyloric vein,* and *paraumbilical veins.* The *paraumbilical veins* accompany the round ligament of the liver and communicate with the subcutaneous veins of the abdominal wall and hepatic portal vein.

Portal-caval Anastomoses

In specific regions of the body, the drainage area of the hepatic portal vein communicates with that of the superior and inferior venae cavae. The hepatic portal drainage area meets the caval system in the following locations:

1. Esophagus. The **gastric veins** connect with **esophageal veins,** which drain via the *azygos vein* and *hemiazygos vein* into the *superior vena cava* (I). In hepatic portal vein occlusion, increased drainage to the esophageal veins can result in dilated blood vessels, known as **esophageal varices.**

2. Abdominal wall. The hepatic portal vein is connected via the **paraumbilical veins (II)** with superficial veins of the abdomen that empty via the *thoracoepigastric veins* into the *superior vena cava.* An increased volume of blood in the abdominal region can cause dilation of superficial abdominal vessels and may result in a condition called **caput medusae.**

3. Rectum. The **superior rectal vein,** which empties via the *inferior mesenteric vein* into the *hepatic portal vein,* connects with the **middle** and **inferior rectal veins (III),** which drain via the *internal iliac vein* into the *inferior vena cava.* A backup of portal blood in this region can result in **hemorrhoids.**

> **Clinical note.** When portal vein flow through the liver to the heart is impeded, blood pressure in the portal vein rises, resulting in *portal hypertension.* The main hazard of portal hypertension is bleeding from esophageal varices, which is difficult to control and is fatal in about 60% of cases.

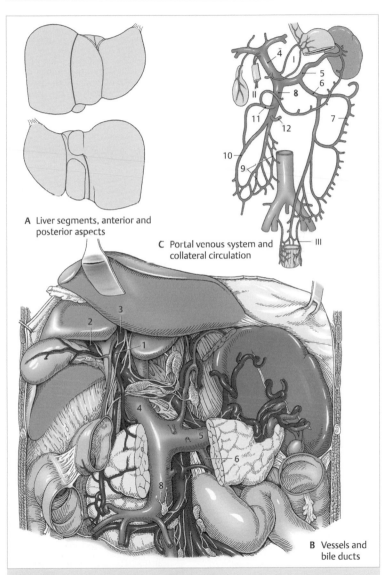

A Liver segments, anterior and posterior aspects

C Portal venous system and collateral circulation

B Vessels and bile ducts

Fig. 4.38 Portal venous system.

Alimentary System

Bile Ducts

For clinical purposes, the bile ducts may be divided into an **intrahepatic** and **extrahepatic** part.

Intrahepatic bile ducts. The intrahepatic bile ducts begin at the **bile canaliculi** between the hepatocytes (see p. 214). These tiny channels open through the short *canals of Hering* into the **interlobular bile ducts**, which unite to form **larger bile ducts**. The larger bile ducts accompany the hepatic vessels and empty into the **right hepatic duct** and **left hepatic duct**, which arise from the right and left lobes of the liver and receive a *right duct of the* caudate lobe and a left duct of the caudate *lobe* respectively.

Extrahepatic bile ducts. Near the porta **hepatis, the** right hepatic duct (**AB1**) **and** left *hepatic duct* (**AB2**) unite to form the **common hepatic duct** (**AB3**). The common hepatic duct is the initial part of the extrahepatic duct system. It is 4–6-cm long and contained within the hepatoduodenal ligament, anterior to and to the right of the portal vein. After receiving the **cystic duct** (**AB4**), which joins it at a sharp angle, it continues as the 6–8-cm long **bile duct** (**AB5**). The bile duct initially lies in the free border of the hepatoduodenal ligament, before traveling behind the superior part of the duodenum to the medial side of the descending part of the duodenum. There it usually joins the *pancreatic duct* (B6), with which it opens on the **major duodenal papilla** (**B7**) (see p. 198). Before its junction with the pancreatic duct, the bile duct is surrounded by a sphincter **called the** sphincter of the bile duct. **The junction** of the two ducts is often expanded to form the **hepatopancreatic ampulla** (**B8**), **which has its own** sphincter of the ampulla. The mucosa of the extrahepatic bile ducts has almost no folds, with the exception of the cystic duct, which has a complex *spiral fold*.

Microanatomy. The extrahepatic bile ducts are lined by **columnar epithelium** overlying a thin layer of connective tissue (**lamina propria**). Beneath this, the **muscular layer** consists of a thin layer of smooth muscle cells. The connective tissue **adventitia** contains the *glands of the bile duct*.

Gallbladder

The **gallbladder** (**C9**) is a thin-walled, pear-shaped sac 8–12-cm long and 4–5-cm wide, which can hold 30–50 mL of fluid. It can be divided into the **fundus of the gallbladder** (**C10**), **body of the gallbladder** (**C11**), and **neck of the gallbladder** (**C12**). The gallbladder rests on the gallbladder fossa of the liver and is attached to it by connective tissue. The fundus of the gallbladder extends past the inferior border of the liver. The neck, which lies above the superior part of the duodenum, faces backward and upward. The gallbladder is covered by peritoneum only on the surface that faces the intestine.

The mucosa forms *ridgelike and interconnected mucosal folds that allow expansion of the gallbladder*, producing a *pattern of polygonal areas* that are visible to the naked eye.

Microanatomy. The **mucosa** is composed of *columnar epithelium* with *goblet cells* and *subepithelial, highly vascular connective tissue*. The **muscular layer** contains a *spiral arrangement of smooth muscle cells* and is covered on its outer aspect by a thick subserosa and a **serous coat**.

Vessels, Nerves, and Lymphatic Drainage

Arteries. The gallbladder is supplied by the cystic artery (from the *right branch of the hepatic artery proper*).

Veins. The **cystic veins** empty directly into **the** hepatic portal vein.

Nerves. The autonomic nerve fibers to the bile ducts and gallbladder arise from the **celiac nerve plexus**. The peritoneal covering surrounding the gallbladder and liver is innervated by sensory fibers from the **right phrenic nerve**.

Regional lymph nodes. Lymph from the gallbladder walls drains to the **hepatic nodes** at the porta hepatis.

Function. The gallbladder stores and concentrates bile, and the bile ducts transport it.

Clinical note. The gallbladder and bile ducts can be visualized using contrast radiography or ultrasonography, another excellent means of viewing these structures.

Alimentary System

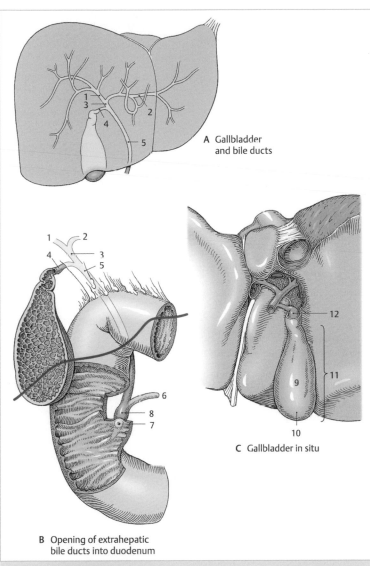

A Gallbladder and bile ducts

B Opening of extrahepatic bile ducts into duodenum

C Gallbladder in situ

Fig. 4.39 Bile ducts and gallbladder.

4.11 Pancreas

Gross and Microscopic Anatomy

The **pancreas** (**A1**) is a wedge-shaped organ, 13–15-cm long, that lies on the posterior abdominal wall at the level of L1–L2. It extends almost horizontally from the C-shaped duodenum to the splenic hilum and may be divided by its macroscopic features into **three parts:**

Head of the pancreas (**B2**). The head of the pancreas, which lies in the C-shaped duodenal loop, is the thickest part of the organ. The hook-shaped **uncinate process** (**B3**) projects posteriorly and inferiorly from the head of the pancreas surrounding the *mesenteric vessels* (**B4**). Between the head of the pancreas and the uncinate process is a groove called the *pancreatic notch* (**B5**).

Body of the pancreas (**B6**). Most of the thinner and horizontal body of the pancreas lies in front of the vertebral column and abdominal aorta. The body has an eminence, near the neck, called the **omental tuberosity** (**B7**), which projects into the omental bursa (see p. 222).

Tail of the pancreas (**B8**). The tail of the pancreas extends to the splenorenal ligament of the spleen.

The **retroperitoneal** pancreas is covered on all sides by connective tissue. The *transverse mesocolon* (**B9**) passes horizontally along the diaphragmatic anterior surface of its head and body. The anterior surface is divided by the *root of the mesocolon* into an **anterosuperior surface** (**B10**), which faces upward, and an **anteroinferior surface** (**B11**), facing downward.

The 2-mm thick **pancreatic duct** (**B12**) runs along the long axis of the gland near its **posterior surface**. It usually opens with the bile duct onto the *major duodenal papilla* (**B13**). In rare instances, the ducts may open independently into the duodenum. A patent **accessory pancreatic duct** (**B14**) is not uncommon. It drains above the main excretory duct into the *minor duodenal papilla*. **Microanatomy**. The pancreas is a **predominantly exocrine gland**. The endocrine part consists of the pancreatic islets (see p. 344). The exocrine part (**C**) is **purely serous**, and its secretory units, or **acini** (**C15**), contain polarized *epithelial cells*. Draining the secretory units are **long intercalated ducts** (**C16**)

that begin within the acini and form the first part of the excretory duct system. In cross section, the invaginated intercalated ducts appear as *centroacinar cells* (**CD17**). Several intercalated ducts combine to form intralobular ducts, which drain into **interlobar excretory ducts**. These ultimately unite to form the **pancreatic duct** through which secretion drains into the duodenum. The fibrous capsule surrounding the pancreas sends delicate fibrous septa into the interior of the organ, dividing the parenchyma into lobes and lobules.

Vessels, Nerves, and Lymphatic Drainage

Arteries. Arterial supply to the head of the pancreas, like that of the duodenum (see p. 200), is provided by **branches of the gastroduodenal artery** (from the *common hepatic artery*): the *posterior superior pancreaticoduodenal artery* and the *anterior superior pancreaticoduodenal artery*. Both vessels anastomose with the *inferior pancreaticoduodenal artery* from the superior mesenteric artery. The body and tail of the pancreas receive their blood supply from the pancreatic branches, which are **branches of the splenic artery**.

Veins. Venous drainage is via short veins named after the corresponding arteries. They empty via the *splenic vein* and *superior mesenteric vein* into the *hepatic portal vein*. **Nerves**. Sympathetic fibers to the pancreas arise from the *celiac plexus*; parasympathetic fibers arise from the **vagus nerve**. **Regional lymph nodes**. Lymph from the head of the pancreas drains into the **pancreaticoduodenal nodes** and from there usually to the *hepatic nodes*. Lymph from the body and tail of the pancreas drains to the **pancreatic nodes** lying along the superior and inferior borders of the pancreas. The pancreatic nodes drain into the *celiac nodes*.

Function. The exocrine pancreas produces a secretion containing *lipase*, which breaks down fat, *amylase*, which breaks down carbohydrates, and precursors of *protease*, which breaks down protein.

> **Clinical note.** Acute **pancreatitis**, is a life-threatening disease that arises as a result of activation of pancreatic enzymes within the gland itself, thereby destroying the parenchyma ("autodigestion").

Alimentary System

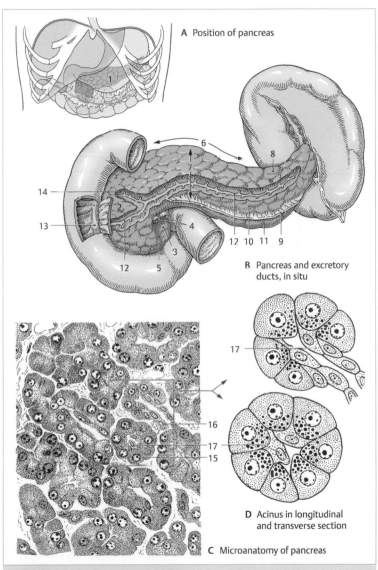

A Position of pancreas

B Pancreas and excretory ducts, in situ

C Microanatomy of pancreas

D Acinus in longitudinal and transverse section

Fig. 4.40 Macroscopic structure and microscopic structure.

Topography of the Omental Bursa and Pancreas

Omental Bursa

The omental bursa is a nearly completely closed **peritoneal cavity containing a capillary film** that lies *behind* the stomach (**A1**) and lesser omentum, and *in front of* the parietal peritoneum-covered pancreas (**A2**). The **omental foramen** (arrow) is the only natural entrance to the omental bursa. The peritoneal relations in and around the omental bursa have already been discussed in greater detail (see p. 188).

The omental bursa is visible in its entirety only after it has been freed by one of various surgical routes (dividing the lesser omentum, gastrocolic ligament, or transverse mesocolon).

Omental foramen. The anterior boundary of the omental foramen is formed by the **hepatoduodenal ligament**, a part of the lesser omentum. Lying in the hepatoduodenal ligament are the *hepatic artery proper* (B7), the *bile duct* (B8), and the *hepatic portal vein* (B9). On inserting a finger into the omental foramen, the hepatic portal vein, lying furthest posteriorly in the hepatoduodenal ligament, can be felt at the anterior boundary of the omental foramen; behind the hepatic portal vein the inferior vena cava can be palpated. The pulse of the left gastric artery (**B10**) can be palpated in the gastropancreatic fold (**A4**). The *caudate lobe of the liver* is above and the *superior part of the duodenum* is below.

Vestibule of the omental bursa. The omental foramen leads to the vestibule of the omental bursa, which is bounded anteriorly by the *lesser omentum* and posteriorly by the *parietal peritoneum*. Projecting into the vestibule is the **papillary process** of the caudate lobe of the liver (**AB3**). To the left of the papillary process is the prominent **gastropancreatic fold** (**A4**), which divides the vestibule from the main part of the cavity.

Main cavity. The greater part of the omental bursa consists of the **superior recess of the omental bursa**, extending upward between the *esophagus* and *inferior vena cava* as far as the gastric fundus; the **splenic recess of the omental bursa** (**A5**), extending to the left between the *splenic ligaments*

and *stomach;* and the **inferior recess of the omental bursa** (**A6**), extending downward between the *greater curvature of the stomach* and the *transverse colon*.

Pancreas

The **pancreas** forms the **posterior wall of the omental bursa**. Its **anterior surface** is covered by parietal peritoneum, and its head is surrounded by the duodenum. The pancreas lies in close proximity to the **large trunks in the upper abdomen**. Running along its *superior border* (**B11**) is the *splenic artery* (**B12**), which is accompanied by the *splenic vein* (**B13**), passing deep to it. Behind the body of the pancreas, the splenic vein receives the *inferior mesenteric vein*, which unites behind the head of the pancreas with the *superior mesenteric vein* (**B14**), to form the *hepatic portal vein* (B9). The *superior mesenteric artery* (**B15**), which originates from the aorta, passes behind the pancreas, and descends along the duodenojejunal flexure (**B16**) before proceeding through the pancreatic notch to the uncinate process, over the superior border of the horizontal part of the duodenum and into the root of the mesenteries.

Additional structures lying **posterior** to the pancreas are (from right to left): the *bile duct, inferior vena cava, aorta, left adrenal gland, left kidney,* and *vessels of the left kidney*. The tail of the pancreas projects into the splenic hilum and thus also has a topographical relationship to the *left colic flexure* and *descending colon* (**B17**).

Clinical note. Disorders of the pancreas (inflammation, cancer of the pancreatic head) can spread to the adjacent duodenum or cause obstruction of the hepatic, bile, and pancreatic ducts, with resultant **obstructive jaundice.** Pancreatic disease can also cause a backup in the hepatic portal vein or inferior vena cava, leading to ascites and edema of the lower limbs.

Diagnosis of pancreatic disease has been greatly improved by the use of modern imaging techniques such as computed tomography (CT) and ultrasonography.

AB18 Right lobe of liver, **AB19** Gallbladder, **A20** Round ligament of liver, **AB21** Left lobe of liver, **AB22** Spleen

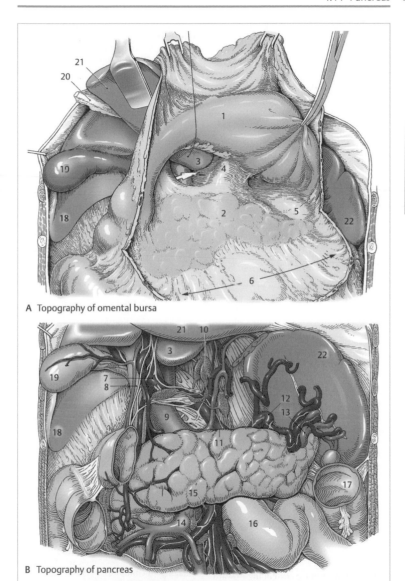

A Topography of omental bursa

B Topography of pancreas

Fig. 4.41 Topography of the omental bursa and pancreas.

4.12 Topographical Anatomy II

Cross-Sectional Anatomy of the Upper Abdomen

Modern imaging techniques are frequently used to diagnose abdominal disorders, particularly those involving the upper abdominal region. The **standard imaging plane** is the **transverse plane**. The following thus describes three transverse sections through the upper abdomen and one through the lower abdomen.

Transverse Section through the Body at T11/T12

The first section is at the level of the intervertebral disc between T11 and T12. In the posterolateral part of the abdomen, the section cuts through the *costodiaphragmatic recess* (**A1**). The section through the *diaphragm* (**A2**) is between the *esophageal hiatus* and *aortic hiatus*. The *aorta* (**A3**) is thus depicted at the level of the thoracic part, that is, before it passes through the diaphragm. The section cuts through the liver above the porta hepatis. The *right* (**A4**) and *left lobes of the liver* (**A5**), as well as the *caudate lobe* (**A6**), surrounding the *inferior vena cava* (**A7**) can be identified. In the connective tissue within the liver parenchyma, the division of the hepatic portal vein into a *right branch* (**A8**) and *left branch* (**A9**) can be identified. The section is through the *stomach* just below the opening of the *esophagus* (**A10**), that is, near the *cardia* (**A11**). Behind the stomach, the section cuts through the upper pole of the *spleen* (**A12**). Between the stomach and spleen, the *gastrophrenic ligament* (**A13**) can be identified.

Transverse Section through the Body at T12

The second transverse section is at the inferior border of T12. It cuts through the inferior portion of the *costodiaphragmatic recess* (**B1**) and is at the level of the passage of the *aorta* (**B3**) through the diaphragm. In this section, the superior part of the *retroperitoneal space* on the right side of the body is occupied by the *adrenal gland* and on the left side it is occupied by the *adrenal gland* (**B14**) and *kidney* (**B15**).

The section cuts through the liver just above the *porta hepatis*, and through the *gallbladder* at the level of the *neck of the gallbladder* (**B16**). Adjacent to this, the section cuts through the *hepatic portal vein* (**B17**) and the *common hepatic artery* (**B18**) on the other side of it. The origins of the common hepatic artery, as well as the *splenic artery* (**B19**), arising from the *celiac trunk* (**B20**), can also be visualized. Owing to the tortuous course of the *splenic artery*, it appears several times in this section. Near the *celiac trunk* are large *lymph nodes* (**B21**). The section cuts through the *stomach* near the *body of the stomach* (**B22**). The mucosal structure exhibits the typical longitudinal folds. Behind the stomach and to its left, the *spleen* (**B12**) can be identified. The section cuts through the *left colic flexure* (**B23**) lying behind and between the stomach and spleen. This is not a typical position for the left colic flexure and is possibly an anatomical variation.

> **Clinical note.** Diseases of the solid upper abdominal organs (liver, biliary tract, pancreas, spleen, and lymph nodes) can be diagnosed with roughly equal sensitivity and specificity with all imaging methods. In the lower abdomen, **ultrasonography** is used to diagnose disease of solid organs while computed tomography (**CT**) or magnetic resonance imaging (**MRI**) is more useful for imaging disease of the small and large intestine. An exception is chronic inflammatory bowel disease or diverticulitis, as the thickened intestinal wall can often be detected readily by ultrasonography.

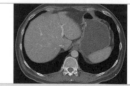

Fig. 4.42C Corresponding plane to Fig. 4.42A on CT.

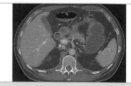

Fig. 4.42D Corresponding plane to Fig. 4.42B on CT.

Alimentary System

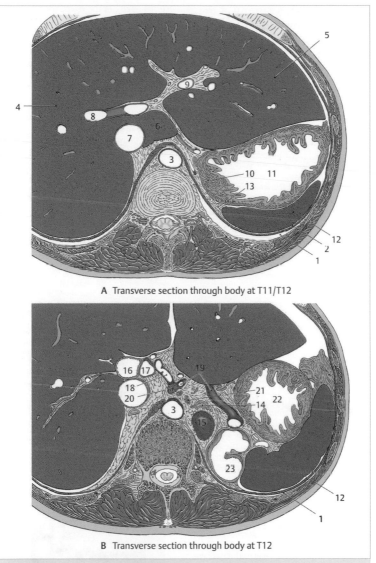

A Transverse section through body at T11/T12

B Transverse section through body at T12

Fig. 4.42 Cross-sectional anatomy of the upper abdomen.

Cross-Sectional Anatomy of the Upper and Lower Abdomen

Transverse Section through the Body at L1

The section cuts through L1 at the level of the *costal process* (**A1**). Only the lateral part of the pleural cavity is visible at the narrow *costodiaphragmatic recess* (**A2**). In the *retroperitoneal space* on the right side of the body, the *adrenal gland* (**A3**) can be seen adjacent to the *superior pole of the kidney* (**A4**). On the left side of the body, only the *kidney* (**A4**) is visible. Immediately adjacent to the right adrenal gland is the *inferior vena cava* (**A5**), and directly in front of the vertebral column is the *aorta* (**A6**). Of the *liver* (**A7**), only the *right lobe* is visible. Nestled in the *fossa of the gallbladder* on the right lobe is the *gallbladder* (**A8**). Directly adjacent to the gallbladder is the *descending part of the duodenum* (**A9**). A section of the *superior part* (**A10**) is also visible, into which the stomach opens via the *pyloric sphincter* (**A11**). The anterior (**A12**) *and posterior walls* (**A13**) of the *stomach* are both visible. Behind the stomach, the cavity constituting the *omental bursa* (**A14**) is easily identified. Lying on the posterior wall of the omental bursa is the *pancreas* (**A15**), with the *uncinate process* (**A16**) projecting from it and surrounding the *superior mesenteric artery* (**A17**) and superior *mesenteric vein* (**A18**). Adjacent to these vessels, part of the course of the *splenic vein* (**A19**) can be traced. In this individual, the *tail of the pancreas* (**A20**) does not reach the *splenic hilum* (**A21**). Between the two organs, the *left colic flexure* (**A22**) can be observed. Anterior to the liver and stomach, the section is through the dilated *transverse colon* (**A23**), which is connected with the stomach by the *gastrocolic ligament* (**A24**).

Transverse Section through the Body at L3

The transverse section is at the level of L3 and shows the lower abdominal organs.

On the right and left sides of the posterior abdominal wall, the section cuts through the *psoas major* (**B25**) *and iliacus muscles* (**B26**). Lying immediately in front of the vertebral column, it cuts through the *common iliac veins* (**B27**) and *common iliac arteries* (**B28**). In the retroperitoneal space on the left side of the body, the section cuts through the *descending colon* (**B29**). The peritoneal cavity is mostly filled by *loops of small intestine* (**B30**) and *mesenteries* (**B31**). On the right side, the section is through the distended *cecum* (**B32**).

The layers of the anterior abdominal wall can be easily distinguished. On its lateral aspect are the *external oblique muscle of the abdomen* (**B33**), the *internal oblique muscle of the abdomen* (**B34**), and the *transverse abdominal muscle* (**B35**). Adjacent to the midline is the *rectus abdominis* (**B36**), and exactly in the center of the anterior abdominal wall is the inferior border of the umbilicus (**B37**).

Clinical note. In the lower abdomen, *ultrasonography* is used primarily in the diagnosis of diseases of the kidneys and urinary tract, bladder, and prostate. By contrast, pathological processes of the intestine are not always imaged successfully. **Virtual colonoscopy** can then be employed: this consists of computer-assisted 3D reconstruction of serial computed tomography (CT) or magnetic resonance imaging (MRI) scans of the abdominal cavity.

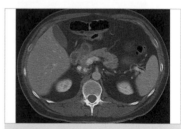

Fig. 4.43C Corresponding plane to Fig. 4.43A on CT.

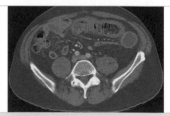

Fig. 4.43D Corresponding plane to Fig. 4.43B on CT.

Alimentary System

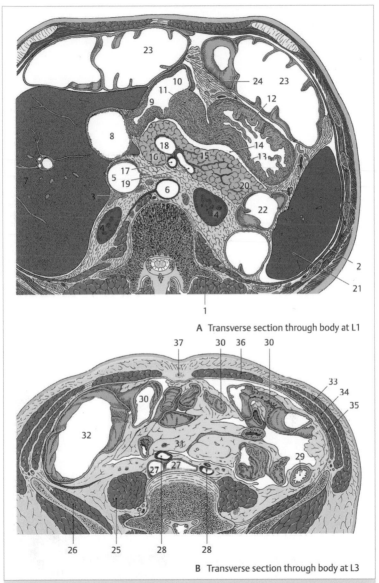

A Transverse section through body at L1

B Transverse section through body at L3

Fig. 4.43 Cross-sectional anatomy of the upper and lower abdomen.

5 Urinary System

5.1 Overview

The organs of the urinary and genital systems have traditionally been grouped together as the "urogenital system," a term that reflects their common embryological origin (see p. 332 ff) but is less suitable for describing morphological and functional aspects of mature organ systems. This book therefore presents the organs of the urinary system and of the male and female genital systems in separate consecutive chapters, followed by a section comparing the topographical anatomy of the male and female pelves, which house most of the organs of the urinary and genital systems.

Organization and Position of the Urinary Organs

The organs of the **urinary system** consist of the paired **kidneys** (A–C1), the paired **renal pelves** (BC2), the paired **ureters** (A–C3), the unpaired **urinary bladder** (AB4), and the **urethra** (A5).

Functional arrangement. The organs of the urinary system are divided into those that are involved in **urine formation** and those involved in its **excretion**. Urine is produced and concentrated in the kidney from an ultrafiltrate of blood plasma. It is collected by the renal pelvis and transported into the ureter, which empties into the urinary bladder. There it is briefly stored before being excreted via the urethra.

Regional arrangement. The organs of the urinary system lie outside of the peritoneum lining the abdominal cavity. They are situated either in the retroperitoneal space or in the connective tissue of the lesser pelvis, known as the subperitoneal space (see p. 2). The *kidneys* and the *larger, proximal part of the ureter* are situated in the **retroperitoneal space,** while the *distal part of the ureter,* the *urinary bladder,* and the *female urethra* are located in the **subperitoneal space**. The *male urethra* leaves the lesser pelvis after a short distance and then continues in the male sex organ, the **penis**.

Retroperitoneal Space

The retroperitoneal space (**C**) lies **in front of** the vertebral column and **behind** the peritoneal cavity. On either side of the vertebral column are **muscles underlying each kidney,** that is, the *quadratus lumborum* (**C6**) and *psoas major* (**C7**). Near these muscles is an indentation alongside either side of the vertebral column, referred to as the lumbar gutter. The lumbar gutters extend from the 12th rib to the iliac crest and are bounded laterally by the lateral edge of the quadratus lumborum. The retroperitoneal space extends **superiorly** to the diaphragm and is continuous **inferiorly** with the subperitoneal space of the lesser pelvis.

> **Clinical Note.** Inflammation involving the retroperitoneal space can spread via the *muscular space* along the psoas major to the lesser trochanter of the femur. The kidneys move with respiration and their position is also affected by posture. During inspiration and when erect, the lower pole of the kidney is 3 cm lower than in expiration and when lying down.

Organs in the retroperitoneal space. In addition to the **organs of the urinary system,** the retroperitoneal space also contains the **adrenal glands** (**C8**), the great vessels, that is, the **aorta** (**C9**) and **inferior vena cava** (**C10**), and the **sympathetic trunk** (**C11**). Retroperitoneal organs are surrounded by *loose connective tissue* and *adipose tissue*.

For topographical anatomy of the retroperitoneal space, (see p. 240).

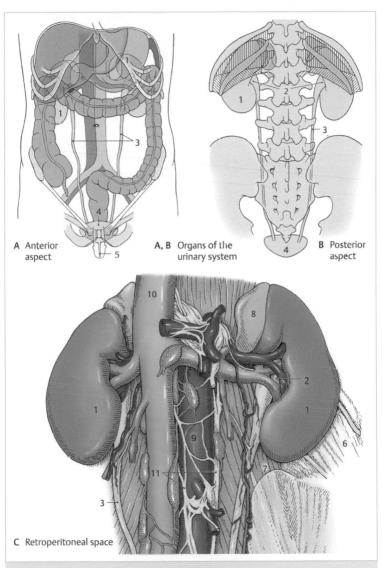

A Anterior aspect

A, B Organs of the urinary system

B Posterior aspect

C Retroperitoneal space

Fig. 5.1 Organization and position of the urinary organs.

5.2 Kidney

Gross Anatomy
External Features

The **kidney** may be divided into two surfaces, an **anterior surface** (**A**) and a **posterior surface** (**B**), as well as a wide **superior pole** (**AB1**) and conical **inferior pole** (**AB2**). The anterior and posterior surfaces are bounded by the convex **lateral border** (**AB3**), which is continuous with the superior and inferior poles, and a concave **medial border** (**A4**). On the medial border is a depression called the **hilum of the kidney** (**A5**) which allows passage of vessels into and out of the organ and also houses the renal pelvis. The hilum of the kidney (**C**) leads to the **renal sinus** (**C6**), a cavity surrounded on all sides by the parenchyma.

An adult kidney is 10–12-cm long, 5–6-cm wide, and 4-cm thick. Each kidney weighs 120–300 g, and the right kidney is usually smaller than the left.

Renal sinus. The renal sinus is a cavity enclosed by renal parenchyma. It can be visualized after removing the vessels, nerves, fat, and renal pelvis. The boundary around its entrance is formed by a liplike indentation on the medial border. Projecting into the renal sinus are pyramidal elevations called **renal papillae** (**C7**). The human kidney has more than one papilla (7–14); these are multiple because the kidney is developed from multiple kidney lobes that later merge. Traces of the structure of the multiple kidney lobes can still be identified (*lobulated kidney*) on the kidney of a neonate.

Surface. In the adult, the surface of the kidneys is usually smooth. It is covered by a tough **fibrous capsule** (**D8**) that contains collagen fibers and is attached to the renal parenchyma by loose connective tissue. The fibrous capsule can be removed easily from a healthy kidney.

Internal Structure

A cross section or longitudinal section of the kidney reveals two distinct regions forming its internal structure: the **renal medulla** (**D9**) and the outer **renal cortex** (**D10**). The macroscopic appearance of the sectioned kidney is produced by the organization of uriniferous tubules and vessels (see pp. 234–236).

Renal medulla. The renal medulla is composed of conical **renal pyramids** (**D11**) that appear pale and striated in cross section because of the straight segments of the renal tubules. The *bases of the renal pyramids* (**D12**) are directed toward the cortex of the kidney. The rounded and wartlike apices form the *renal papillae* (**D13**), which project toward the hilum and into the renal calices of the renal pelvis. On its surface, each renal papilla bears a *cribriform area* of numerous perforations produced by the *openings of papillary ducts*, the openings of the uriniferous tubules. On closer inspection, a renal pyramid can be further subdivided into a reddish **outer zone** and a lighter **inner zone**.

Renal cortex. The renal cortex lies immediately beneath the fibrous capsule. It is about 1-cm thick and in the unmounted specimen has a reddish-brown color. It overlies the pyramids of the renal medulla like an upturned beaker between the lateral aspects of the renal pyramids, sending extensions called **renal columns** (**D14**) into the interior of the organ. The renal cortex is permeated by longitudinal striations known as **medullary rays** (**D15**), which are continuations of the medullary substance radiating from the bases of the pyramids toward the capsule. The cortical part containing the medullary rays is known as the **cortex corticis**, and the cortical substance between the medullary rays is the **cortical labyrinth**.

Kidney lobes. Each kidney lobe consists of a **renal pyramid** and its **surrounding cortex** (see above). Individual kidney lobes are bounded by the renal columns.

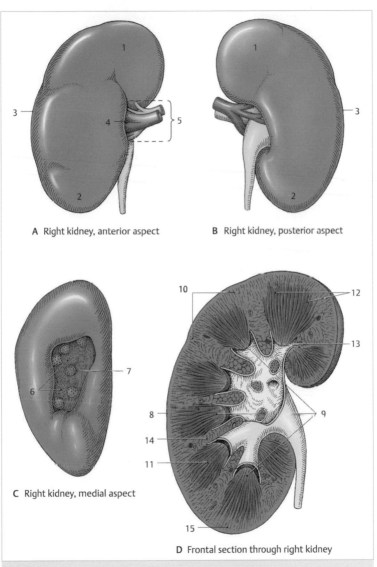

A Right kidney, anterior aspect

B Right kidney, posterior aspect

C Right kidney, medial aspect

D Frontal section through right kidney

Fig. 5.2 Macroscopic structure of the kidney.

Urinary System

Microscopic Anatomy

The macroscopically distinct portions of the parenchyma of the kidney (see p. 232) are produced by a characteristic pattern of distribution of different structural units of the organ. These structural units include the numerous, densely packed **uriniferous tubules**, as well as **blood vessels** and **connective tissue** containing **nerves** and **lymphatic vessels**.

Uriniferous Tubules

The uriniferous tubules consist of two components, a nephron and collecting ducts, which have different embryological origins.

Each **nephron**, or basic functional unit of the kidney, consists of a renal corpuscle and an associated renal tubule, which is a segment of the uriniferous tubules.

Renal corpuscle (**A1**). Each renal corpuscle consists of a cluster of capillaries called a **glomerulus** (**A2**) and a surrounding **glomerular capsule** (**A3**).

Renal tubule. Connected to the renal corpuscle is a continuous system of renal tubules that may be divided into various segments. They are either convoluted or straight. The renal tubules begin with a **proximal tubule**, which has a twisted part known as the *proximal convoluted tubule* (**A4**), and a straight part called the *proximal straight tubule* (**A5**). Following the proximal tubule is the **intermediate tubule**, or thin tubule (**A6**), which can be divided into the *descending thin limb* (**A6 a**) and *ascending thin limb* (**A6 b**). The intermediate tubule is continuous with the **distal tubule**, consisting of a *distal straight tubule* (**A7**) followed by the *distal convoluted tubule* (**A8**).

The tortuous segment of the distal tubule is connected by a **junctional tubule** (**A9**) with a **collecting duct** (**A10**). Each collecting duct receives fluid from approximately 10 nephrons and empties into a **papillary duct** (**A11**), which opens on the tip of the papilla.

Intrarenal Blood Vessels

The functions of the kidney rely closely on the interaction between nephrons, collecting ducts, and intrarenal blood vessels.

The **renal artery** carries waste-laden blood to the kidneys. Its principal branches divide and give off the **interlobar arteries of kidney** (**A12**), which pass between adjacent renal pyramids into the parenchyma and toward the cortex, becoming continuous with the **arcuate arteries of the kidney** (**A13**) at the corticomedullary border. Springing from the arcuate arteries are numerous **interlobular arteries of the kidney** (**A14**). These radiate toward the fibrous capsule and give off **afferent glomerular arterioles** (**A15**) that feed the capillary tufts (**glomeruli**) (**A2**) of the renal corpuscles. Blood flows from the glomeruli via the **efferent glomerular arterioles** (**A16**) into the capillary network of the renal cortex and via the **interlobular veins** (**A17**), **arcuate veins** (**A18**), and **interlobar veins** (**A19**) to the **renal vein**. The **straight arterioles** (**A20**) are branches of the efferent arterioles that radiate from the glomeruli near the renal cortex down into the renal medulla. Ascending parallel to these are the **straight venules** (**A21**), which transport blood via the *arcuate veins* to the *interlobar veins*.

Note: The kidneys receive about 1,500 L of blood daily (roughly 20% of cardiac output). The same vessels supply the parenchyma, where the blood is filtered to produce urine, so they are both nutrient and functional arteries.

The glomerular capillaries are in the arterial limb of the local circulation and constitute an arterial "rete mirabile."

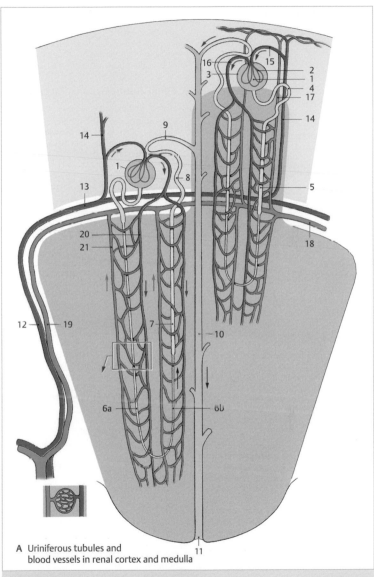

A Uriniferous tubules and
blood vessels in renal cortex and medulla

Fig. 5.3 Microscopic structure of the kidney.

Microscopic Anatomy of the Kidney, cont.

Renal Corpuscles

Glomerulus (**A1**). The glomerulus forming the renal corpuscle consists of **30–40 capillary loops** and is situated between an *afferent glomerular arteriole* (**A2**), leading to it, and an *efferent glomerular arteriole* (**A3**) draining it. The afferent and efferent arterioles anastomose with and lie in close proximity to one another, forming the **vascular pole** (**A4**) of the renal corpuscle. Each glomerulus is surrounded by a dual-layered **glomerular capsule** (Bowman capsule). The *internal part* (**A5**) lies adjacent to the capillary loops as a "visceral layer," and the *external part* acts as a "parietal layer" (**A6**), to separate the glomerulus from its surroundings. The space between the two layers, the capsular space, collects glomerular filtrate and conveys it via the **urinary pole** (**AB18**) into the tubule system.

Glomerular capillaries (**B**). The glomerular capillaries are composed of an **endothelium** (**B7**), with open **fenestrations** (diameter 50–100 μm) between the endothelial cells, and a **continuous, triple-layer basement membrane**, the middle layer of which acts as a mechanical filter. The outer layer, facing the capsular space, is covered by **podocytes** (**A8**), branching cells with numerous processes. The long *primary processes* (**A9**) of the podocytes give rise to *secondary* or *foot processes* that interdigitate like fingers with those of adjacent podocytes, leaving narrow gaps, or *filtration slits*, between them.

Special connective tissue cells known as mesangial cells (**intraglomerular mesangial cells**) (**B10**) lie between the adjacent capillaries of a glomerulus. Mesangial cells also lie at the vascular pole between the afferent arteriole and efferent arteriole (**extraglomerular mesangial cells**) (**AB11**). The mesangial cells are part of the **juxtaglomerular apparatus** of the kidney, which also includes the macula densa (**AB12**) and polar cushion (**AB13**). The **macula densa** refers to specialized epithelial cells lying along the distal convoluted tubule in places of contact with the vascular pole. The **polar cushion** refers to the (granular) myoepithelial cells of the juxtaglomerular apparatus in the preglomerular part of the afferent arteriole. Renin and angiotensinase A have been detected in cells of the polar cushion.

Renal Tubules and Collecting Ducts (C)

The walls of the renal tubules are lined by **simple epithelium**, which varies by region but always has the typical features of transport epithelia.

The **proximal tubule** (**C14**) is lined by cuboidal epithelial cells with a high brush border, as well as infoldings of the cell membrane at the base of the cell and abundant mitochondria.

The **intermediate tubule** (**C15**) is lined by flattened epithelial cells with short microvilli.

The **distal tubule** (**C16**) has tall low cuboidal cells with basal striations (basolateral interdigitations). The cells are somewhat flatter than those of the proximal tubule and have only short microvilli projecting from them.

Part of the area of connecting tubules has tall epithelial cells with many mitochondria and part has cuboidal epithelium with basal folds instead of interdigitations.

The **collecting ducts** (**C17**) are composed of about two-thirds pale-staining epithelial cells with distinct cell borders, and one-third is composed of dark-staining intercalated cells. The epithelial cells lining the collecting ducts become progressively flatter as the duct progresses toward the papillae.

Function of the kidneys. The renal corpuscles form the **filter** that "squeezes" 180 L of **ultrafiltrate** (**primary urine**) out of the blood daily. Of these, 178 L are reabsorbed in the tubule system, and 1.5–2 L of **final urine** (secondary urine) are formed per day. Urine is excreted by the excretory organs. The juxtaglomerular apparatus functions as part of the renin–angiotensin system involved in **blood pressure regulation** and control of **filtrate production**.

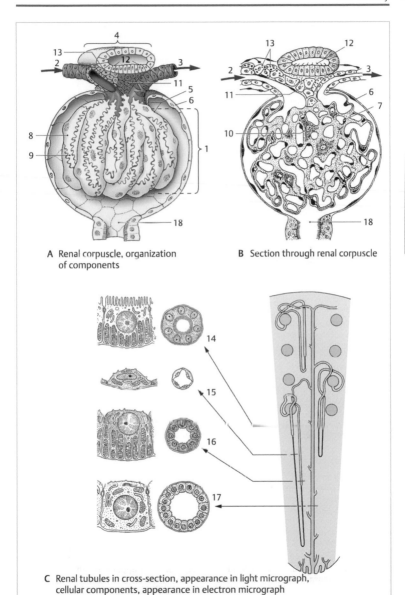

A Renal corpuscle, organization of components

B Section through renal corpuscle

C Renal tubules in cross-section, appearance in light micrograph, cellular components, appearance in electron micrograph

Fig. 5.4 Microscopic structure of the kidney, continued.

Urinary System

Vessels, Nerves, and Lymphatic Drainage

Arteries. Waste substances are carried to the kidneys by the **renal artery** (**A1**). The *right renal artery* springs from the abdominal aorta (**A2**) at the level of L1. In most people, the *left renal artery* arises at a short distance above it. The left renal artery is usually shorter than the right renal artery. The primary intrarenal branches of the two main arteries are **end arteries** and supply specific regions of the parenchyma. These regions may be classified as **renal segments**: the *superior segment, anterior superior segment, anterior inferior segment, inferior segment,* and *posterior segment*. Given the complex nature of kidney development, these segments may vary considerably; anomalies in the course of the renal artery also occur.

Veins. Venous drainage from the kidney is via the **renal vein** (**AC3**). The right renal vein is short and has a straight course while the path of the left renal vein is longer and curving. During its course it receives the *left suprarenal vein* and the *left testicular vein* or *left ovarian vein*.

Nerves. Sympathetic fibers to the kidneys arise from the **renal nerve plexus**, which accompanies the renal artery and is mainly formed by fibers from the adjacent *celiac plexus*. Intrarenal vessels are accompanied and innervated by sympathetic fibers as far as the glomerular vascular pool.

Regional lymph nodes. Lymph from the kidneys drains to the **lateral aortic nodes** through lymphatic capillaries in perivascular connective tissue.

Topography of the Kidneys

Position. The kidneys lie on either side of the vertebral column in the **lumbar groove**. Their long axes are directed upward and backward, so that if an imaginary line is drawn as a continuation from each axis, these lines would intersect. The **superior pole** lies at the level of *T12*, and the **inferior pole** at the level of *L3*. The **hilum of the kidney** is located at the level of *L1*. The right kidney usually lies about half a vertebra lower than the left kidney. The position of the kidneys varies with respiration and posture. **Posterior** to the kidney, the *12th rib* (**A4**) passes diagonally over the boundary between the upper and middle thirds of

the organ. Crossing between the kidney and posterior abdominal wall, nearly parallel to the 12th rib in a craniocaudolateral direction, are the *subcostal nerve* (**A5**), *iliohypogastric nerve* (**A6**), and *ilio-inguinal nerve*.

The costodiaphragmatic recess of the pleura is between the 12th rib and the kidney, so that there is no contact between the rib and the posterior surface of the kidney.

Adjacent organs and vessels. Lying anteriorly on the superior poles of the kidneys are the *suprarenal/adrenal glands* (**A7**). The anterior surface of the right kidney is in contact with the *liver* and *right colic flexure*; near the hilum of the right kidney are the *inferior vena cava* (**A8**) and *duodenum*. The anterior surface of the left kidney is in contact with the *stomach, pancreas,* and *left colic flexure*; the *aorta* runs near the hilum of the left kidney.

A9 Ureter

Capsules of the Kidney

The capsules enclosing the kidney are important for fixing the organ in position. They consist of a pouch known as the renal fascia (**B10**) and a perirenal fat capsule (**BC11**). The **fascial pouch** is composed of a *thin anterior layer* and a *tough posterior layer*. The two layers are connected with each other at their superior and lateral borders, and surround the kidney, adrenal gland, and perirenal fat capsule. The *medial* side of the fascial pouch is open, and its *inferior* side is only closed by adipose tissue. The volume of the **perirenal fat capsule** varies, depending on the individual nutritional status; with extreme emaciation it may even be absent. Loss of the perirenal fat capsule can result in mobility of the kidney, which may descend toward the pelvis— an abnormal condition known as **floating kidney**.

Clinical note. Anatomic **variations** and **renal anomalies** are common. Common abnormalities include the presence of extra kidneys, kidney displacement, kidney fusion, and horseshoe kidneys. Renal aplasia is complete absence of a kidney, and renal hypoplasia signifies underdevelopment. Enlarged kidneys with duplication of the pelvis, ureter, or collecting system are called duplex kidneys. **Inflammation** of the kidney can involve the retrorenal subcostal, iliohypogastric, and ilio-inguinal nerves, with pain radiating to the groin and external genitalia.

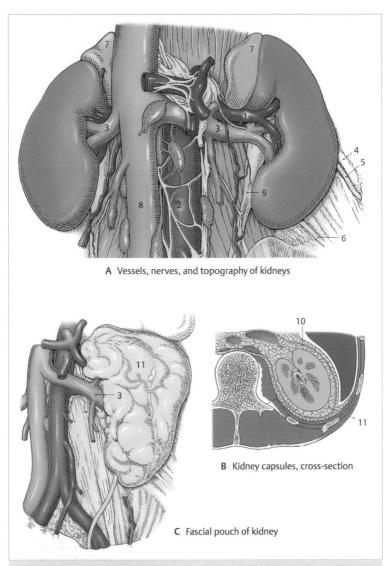

A Vessels, nerves, and topography of kidneys

B Kidney capsules, cross-section

C Fascial pouch of kidney

Fig. 5.5 Topography of the kidneys.

5.3 Excretory Organs

Renal Pelvis and Ureter

Gross Anatomy

Renal pelvis and calices (A). The **renal pelvis (AB1)** is a reservoir for the collection of urine formed by the union of the 8–10 **renal calices (A2)** that empty into it. *Minor calices (A2 a)* are small, trumpet-shaped renal calices that surround one (or occasionally two or three) renal papilla. They give rise to the 2–3 *major calices (A2 b)*, which open into the renal pelvis.

The **shape of the renal pelvis** varies (**A**) according to the branching pattern of the renal calices. If the minor calices consistently open into major calices, the renal pelvis is of the **branching** or **dendritic type**; if the minor calices also open directly into the renal pelvis, forming a widened saclike renal pelvis, it is considered an **ampullary type**. The volume of the renal pelvis is 3–8 mL.

Ureter (B3). The ureter is a slightly flattened, thick-walled tube that connects the renal pelvis with the urinary bladder. It is 25–30-cm long and is divided into two parts based on its course: an **abdominal part (B3 a)** and a **pelvic part (B3 b)**. Its terminal part follows an oblique course in the wall of the urinary bladder and is known as the **intramural part**.

B4 Kidney, **B5** Hilum of kidney, **B6** Renal artery, **B7** Renal vein, **B8** Aorta, **B9** Inferior vena cava, **B10** Ovarian artery, **B11** Internal iliac artery, **B12** Uterine artery

Microanatomy. The wall of the renal pelvis is thin, while that of the ureter is very thick. In cross section, the ureter has a star-shaped lumen (**C**). The walls of both organs are composed of three layers: the **mucosa (C13)** consists of the transitional epithelium, or *urothelium*, that is characteristic of the urinary excretory ducts and a layer of *loose connective tissue*; the **urothelium** consists of *5–7 layers of cells* and can adapt to the amount of distention of the ureter by altering the height and number of cell layers; the *thickened apical membrane* in the top layer of the cells that are visible in light microscopy protects the epithelial surface from hypertonic urine. In the renal pelvis, the **muscular layer** consists of an *inner longitudinal layer* and an *outer circular layer*. The muscle fibers

are interwoven to form *structures resembling sphincters* in the calices and at the junction of the renal pelvis with the ureter. The ureter possesses an especially strong muscular layer (**C14**). As it proceeds toward the urinary bladder, it is augmented by a *third outer longitudinal layer of muscle*. The *loose connective tissue* of the **adventitia (C15)** embeds the renal pelvis and ureter in their surroundings. The connective tissue of the renal pelvis, which contains abundant vessels and nerves, also contains smooth muscle cells that control its distention.

Vessels, Nerves, and Lymphatic Drainage

The vessels of the **renal pelvis (B)** arise from the **renal artery** and **vein (B6, B7)**. Lymphatic drainage corresponds to that of the kidneys. The renal pelvis receives sensory innervation and hence its distention is painful.

The **ureter** is supplied by branches from the large **surrounding arteries**: the *renal artery (B6)*, *testicular artery* or *ovarian artery (B10)*, *internal pudendal artery*, and *superior vesical artery*. The arteries are accompanied by veins of the same name. Lymph drains to the **lumbar nodes**. Innervation is by the **splanchnic nerves**, with parasympathetic fibers supplying the muscle wall and sympathetic fibers supplying the vessel wall. Sensory afferents travel in the splanchnic nerves.

Topography of the Renal Pelvis and the Abdominal Part of the Ureter

The greater part of the **renal pelvis (A)** lies hidden in the renal sinus. The **abdominal part of the ureter** begins at its exit from the renal pelvis, with the **first point of constriction of the ureter**. The ureter then proceeds caudally to the medial side of the psoas major (**B16**), where it lies between the muscle fascia (posterior to it) and the peritoneum (covering its anterior aspect). During its course, the path of the ureter is crossed over by the testicular or ovarian vein (**B10**), and the ureter itself crosses over the genitofemoral nerve. It enters the lesser pelvis at the level of the common iliac vessels or external iliac vessels. This is the site of the **second point of constriction of the ureter** (see also p. 244, for topography of the **pelvic part of the ureter**).

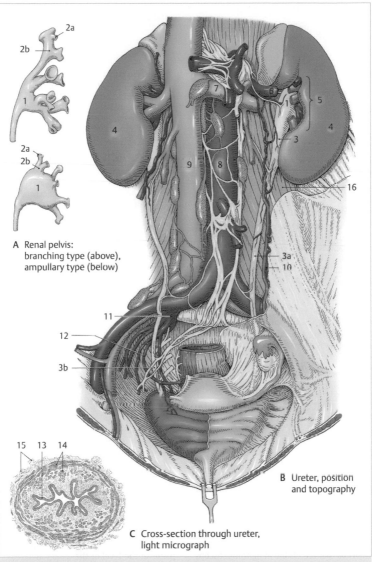

A Renal pelvis:
branching type (above),
ampullary type (below)

B Ureter, position
and topography

C Cross-section through ureter,
light micrograph

Urinary System

Fig. 5.6 Renal pelvis and ureter.

Urinary Bladder

The **urinary bladder** (**A1**) is a hollow, muscular organ whose size varies with the amount of contained urine. It is located behind the pubis (**A2**), in the subperitoneal connective tissue of the lesser pelvis.

Parts of the urinary bladder. The **body of the bladder** (**AB3**) constitutes the largest part of the organ. It is continuous anterosuperiorly with the *apex of the bladder* (**AB4**). The apex gives attachment to the obliterated urachus, which passes in the median umbilical ligament (**AB5**) (see p. 188) to the navel. Opening into the lateral and posterior aspects of the **fundus of the bladder** (**A6**), which empties posteriorly and inferiorly, are the ureters (**B7**). The **neck of the bladder** (**B8**) is continuous anteriorly with the **urethra** (**AB9**).

As the urinary bladder empties, the apex of the bladder and upper portion of the wall descend and the organ becomes bowl-shaped. As it fills, the apex and wall are drawn forward and upward between the peritoneum and abdominal wall, to form an ovoid shape. Depending on the amount of its contents, the urinary bladder can extend as far as the superior border of the pubic symphysis. The **capacity of the urinary bladder** is normally about 500 mL; the urge to void occurs at about 300 mL. It is possible, however, voluntarily to retain larger amounts of urine.

> **Clinical note.** The filled bladder can be punctured through the abdominal wall above the symphysis, without injuring, the peritoneal space (suprapubic urine drainage).

Internal surface (**C**). The inner surface of the urinary bladder is pale red in color. Two parts can be identified: throughout most of the urinary bladder, the mucosa contains folds due to its mobility against the underlying muscular layer. When the bladder is very full, the folds disappear. The triangular region formed on the fundus of the bladder, which is bounded by the two openings of the ureters known as the **ureteric orifices** (**CD10**) and the exit of the urethra called the **internal urethral orifice** (**C11**), is known as the **trigone of the bladder** (**CD12**). The mucosa of the trigone of the bladder is flat; it is firmly attached to the underlying muscular layer and thus does not contain folds. In the male, the *uvula of the bladder* (**D13**), a conical elevation produced by the underlying prostate, projects into the internal urethral orifice.

Microanatomy. The walls of the urinary bladder are made up of three layers. The **mucosa** consists of *transitional epithelium* (urothelium) overlying loose connective tissue (*lamina propria*), which is absent at the trigone of the bladder. Most of the **muscular layer** is made up of three distinct layers that are collectively known as the *detrusor muscle*. At the trigone of the bladder, the muscular layer constitutes a continuation of the muscular layer of the ureter and thus consists of only two layers. At the openings of the ureters into the bladder, the smooth muscle is organized in a complex *circular arrangement*. The **serosa**, which is accompanied by connective tissue of the subserosa, covers the superior surface of the urinary bladder and the portion of the posterior surface above the trigone of the bladder.

Vessels, Nerves, and Lymphatic Drainage

Arteries. The urinary bladder is nourished by branches from the bilateral **internal iliac arteries**, that is, the *superior vesical artery* (from the umbilical artery) and *inferior vesical artery*.

Veins. The **vesical venous plexus**, which surrounds the fundus of the bladder, collects blood from the urinary bladder, and usually empties directly into the *internal iliac veins*.

Nerves. Similar to the intestine, innervation of the urinary bladder is divided into **extrinsic** and **intrinsic nervous systems** (i.e., inside and outside of the wall of the urinary bladder). **Parasympathetic** fibers of the extrinsic system arise from S2–S4 and act to constrict the detrusor (micturition). **Sympathetic** fibers supply the smooth muscle of the vessel walls and presumably cause contraction of the muscle around the neck of the bladder and the upper portion of the urethra.

Regional lymph nodes. Lymph flows in various directions from the urinary bladder: the **external iliac nodes** collect lymph from the upper and lateral portions of the wall; **internal iliac nodes** collect lymph from the fundus and the trigone of the bladder. Lymph from the anterior wall of the urinary bladder also ultimately drains to the internal iliac nodes.

Urinary System

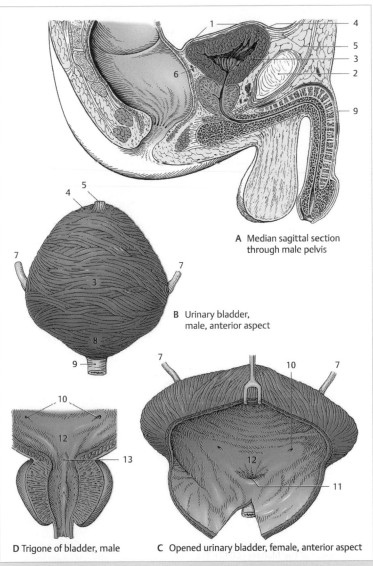

A Median sagittal section through male pelvis

B Urinary bladder, male, anterior aspect

D Trigone of bladder, male

C Opened urinary bladder, female, anterior aspect

Fig. 5.7 Urinary bladder.

Female Urethra

The female **urethra** (**A1**) is very short, only 3–5 cm, and lies behind the pubic symphysis (**A2**). It begins at the **internal urethral orifice** (**A3**) and passes upward in an anteriorly concave curvature, in close proximity to the anterior wall of the vagina (**A4**). It ends at a longitudinal slit, that is, the **external urethral orifice** (**A5**) in the *vestibule of the vagina* 2–3 cm behind the glans of the clitoris (**A6**).

Microscopic Anatomy

The walls of the urethra consist of a **mucosa** that lies in longitudinal folds and is lined by typical *transitional epithelium* resting on a highly vascularized *lamina propria* or *spongy layer* that contains abundant veins and glands (urethral glands); and a **muscular layer** that is derived from the muscular layer of the walls of the urinary bladder and is arranged in an *inner longitudinal layer* and an *outer circular layer*.

The urethra is surrounded by the **external urethral sphincter**, a circular arrangement of striated muscle that forms a type of loop of fibers that is open posteriorly and extends as far as the neck of the bladder.

The male urethra is discussed on p. 262.

Function of the excretory organs. Urine expelled from the renal papillae is first collected in the **renal calices** and then conveyed to the **renal pelvis**. After reaching a certain volume, the urine is ejected into the **ureter** by rapid movements. Once in the ureter, peristaltic waves transport the urine distally and empty it in portions into the **urinary bladder**. When the urinary bladder is filled to (individual) capacity, stimuli mediated by the nervous system initiate its emptying, or **micturition** (**urination**).

Topography of the Excretory Organs

Female pelvis. After exiting the renal pelvis (**first point of constriction of the ureter**) and completing its intra-abdominal course (see p. 241 B), the **ureter** enters the lesser pelvis in front of the sacroiliac joint,

at the level of the bifurcation of the common iliac artery (**B7**) or at the level of the external iliac artery. This is the site of the **second point of constriction of the ureter**. In the female lesser pelvis, the ureter runs superficially along the lateral wall of the pelvis immediately underneath the peritoneum. At about the level of the ischial spine, it leaves the lateral wall of the pelvis and runs in the base of the broad ligament of the uterus (**B8**), coursing medially and anteriorly. It crosses under the uterine artery (**B9**) and, at a variable distance from the vagina, reaches the posterolateral wall of the urinary bladder, which it penetrates diagonally from posterolateral to anteromedial. This intramural part of the ureter is approximately 2-cm long and forms the **third point of constriction of the ureter**.

The **urinary bladder** (**AB10**) lies in the subperitoneal connective tissue behind the pubic symphysis. The **retropubic space** (**A11**), a region of loose connective tissue, lies in front of it. The retropubic space extends between the anterior abdominal wall and the peritoneum as far as the navel and permits movement of the urinary bladder as it swells upward during filling. The superior part of the urinary bladder is covered by peritoneum; its inferoposterior surface is firmly attached to the surrounding structures.

The **female urethra** lies between the pubic symphysis and the anterior wall of the vagina (**A4**).

Male pelvis. In the lesser pelvis of the male (see p. 254 B), the **ureter** also passes immediately beneath the peritoneum along the lateral wall of the pelvis. It reaches the posterolateral wall of the urinary bladder at a point above the seminal vesicle, crossing below the ductus deferens.

Clinical note. Kidney stones can get stuck near the constricted parts of the ureter. The ureter attempts to pass the stone toward the bladder, by contracting the muscle in its walls, which is associated with violent pain (colic). Stenosis of the prevesical terminal ureter segment above the ostium causes ureter dilatation (megaureter).

A duplication of ureters occurs in about 2% of the population: ureter duplex = double ureter; ureter fissus = bifid ureter.

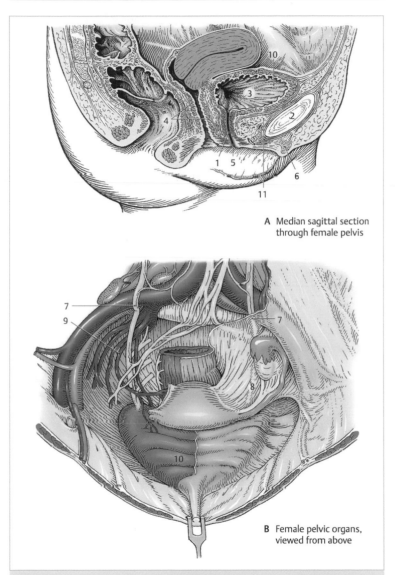

A Median sagittal section through female pelvis

B Female pelvic organs, viewed from above

Fig. 5.8 Urethra and topography of the urinary tract organs.

Urinary System

6 Male Genital System

6.1 Overview

Male Reproductive Organs

The organs of the **male genital system** can be divided topographically and developmentally into internal and external genitalia.

The **internal** genitalia consist of the *testis* (**A1**), *epididymis* (**A2**), *ductus deferens* (**A3**), and accessory sex glands, that is, the *prostate* (**A4**), *seminal vesicle/seminal gland* (**A5**), and *bulbourethral gland (Cowper glands)* (**A6**).

The **external** male genitalia include the *penis* (**A7**), *scrotum* (**A8**), and *tunics of the testes*.

The internal genitalia arise above the pelvic floor from the urogenital ridge, while the external genitalia are derived from the urogenital sinus below the pelvic floor.

Function. The male germ cells, or **spermatozoa**, are produced in the **testis** and transported through a system of small canals to the **epididymis**, where they mature. Mature spermatozoa are conveyed by the **spermatic cord** to the **male urethra**, through which they can leave the body cavity. As they travel through the seminal duct, the germ cells are mixed with secretions from the **accessory sex glands**. The ejaculate is the final product. Testosterone, the male hormone, is also produced in the testis and released into the circulation.

Peritoneal Relations of the Male Pelvis

The peritoneal cavity extends over the linea terminalis into the pelvic cavity. From the anterior abdominal wall, the **parietal peritoneum** continues along the wall of the lesser pelvis, covering the pelvic viscera projecting from it: it reflects from the *anterior abdominal wall* onto the *apex of the bladder* (**AB9**) and covers the entire *superior surface* (**AB10**) of the urinary bladder. Extending posteroinferiorly and laterally, the peritoneum passes to the level of the union of the ureters with the urinary bladder. The *upper portions of the seminal vesicles* extend along the posterior surface of the urinary bladder up to the level of the openings of the ureters, or sometimes higher, and are usually covered by parietal peritoneum. The *ductus deferens* is likewise covered by peritoneum up to its terminal portion, the ampulla of the ductus deferens. Occasionally, the peritoneum passes even deeper to cover a part of the *prostate*. It does not cover the fundus of the urinary bladder but rather forms the **rectovesical pouch** (**B11**), a peritoneal reflection from the *posterior wall of the urinary bladder* onto the *anterior wall of the rectum* (**B12**). It covers the anterior wall of the sacral flexure of the rectum and is continuous with the serosa of the sigmoid colon at the S3 level. In the male, the rectovesical pouch is the *lowest point in the abdominal cavity*. On either side, it is bounded by a nearly sagittal fold known as the *rectovesical fold*. The subserosal connective tissue of the rectovesical fold contains the autonomic nerves of the inferior hypogastric nerve plexus. When the urinary bladder is full, a peritoneal fold is also produced between the anterior abdominal wall and the apex of the bladder (the prevesical or retropubic space).

B13 Peritoneal fold produced by ureter

Clinical note. In patients with **urinary retention**, the distended urinary bladder can be punctured just above the border of the pelvic symphysis without injuring the peritoneum or opening the abdominal cavity.

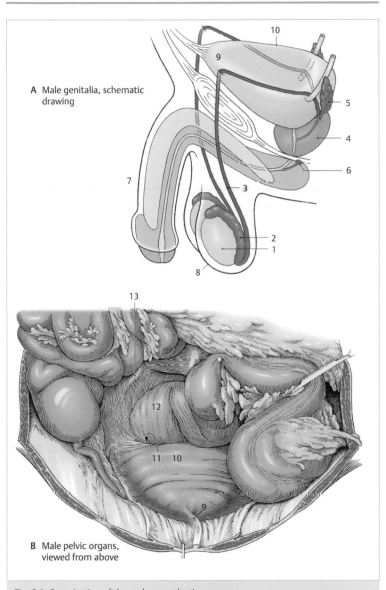

A Male genitalia, schematic drawing

B Male pelvic organs, viewed from above

Fig. 6.1 Organization of the male reproductive organs.

6.2 Testis and Epididymis

Gross Anatomy

Testes. The paired male gonads are the *site of production of spermatozoa* and are located outside of the body cavity in the *scrotum*. Each testis is an egg-shaped organ with a firm, elastic consistency, measuring 4–5 cm in length and 3 cm across. The left testis is usually somewhat larger than the right. Each testis has a **superior pole (A1)** and an **inferior pole (A2)**. The testis is flattened on its sides and has a **lateral surface (A3)** and a **medial surface (B4)**, which are continuous at the narrow, **anterior border (AB5)** and the wide, **posterior border (B6)**. The testes lie obliquely in the scrotum, with their superior poles directed anterolaterally and their inferior poles posteromedially. Investing each testis is a thick, white connective tissue capsule called the **tunica albuginea**. At the superior pole is a remnant of the embryonic *Müllerian duct*, known as the **appendix of the testis (B7)**.

Epididymis (AB8). Resting like a tail on the posteromedial surface of each of the testes is the epididymis. It consists of three parts: the **head of the epididymis (A8 a)** is the part that projects above the superior pole of the testis, while the **body of the epididymis (A8 b)** and the **tail of the epididymis (A8 c)** are completely in contact with the testis. Each epididymis has its own connective tissue capsule, which is distinct from that of the tunica albuginea of the testis and surrounds the roughly 5-m-long, tightly coiled **duct of the epididymis (AB9)**. Near the head of the epididymis is the **appendix of the epididymis (C10)**, a remnant of the *mesonephros*.

Coverings of the testis and epididymis. The testes first develop in the abdominal cavity and later descend during fetal development into the scrotum (*descensus testis*). As it travels from the abdominal cavity through the inguinal canal, the testis penetrates the layers of the abdominal wall (see Vol. 1), forming the **processus vaginalis testis**, a *peritoneal diverticulum*, which guides it into the scrotum. After birth, most

of the processus vaginalis testis is obliterated. Only its caudal end remains, forming the **tunica vaginalis of the testis (C11)**, a *closed serous sheath* that envelops the testis and epididymis. The **visceral layer (epiorchium)** lies on top of the tunica albuginea and covers those parts of the testis that are not covered by the epididymis. It also covers most of the epididymis and reflects onto the **parietal layer (periorchium)** at the exit site of the spermatic cord. Between the testis and epididymis is a narrow space called the *sinus of the epididymis (C12)*, which is bounded cranially and caudally by peritoneal folds known as the *superior* and *inferior ligaments of the epididymis (A13)*. The epiorchium and periorchium are separated by a fluid-filled serous pocket. Lying on the external surface of the parietal layer of the tunica vaginalis is the **internal spermatic fascia (C14)**, a continuation of the *transversalis fascia*. The internal spermatic fascia is covered by fibers from the cremaster **(C15)**, which make up the **cremasteric fascia**, an expansion of the *internal oblique muscle of the abdomen*. The **external spermatic fascia (C16)** is derived from an outer layer of fascia of the abdominal wall, that is, the fascia of the external oblique muscle of the abdomen, and forms the outer fascial sheath enclosing the testis, epididymis, and spermatic cord.

The testis, epididymis, and their coverings are contained in the **scrotum (C17)**. The thin skin of the scrotum is *continuous with the skin of the abdomen* and is heavily pigmented and covered with hair, and contains sebaceous glands. The subcutaneous tissue is devoid of fat. Consisting of connective tissue and smooth muscle cells, it is thus known as the **dartos fascia**. The scrotum is divided into two parts by the connective tissue **septum of the scrotum**. Its outer surface is marked by the **raphe of the scrotum**, a line in the skin that extends to the perineum.

Clinical note. The testes should be fully descended into the scrotum at the time of birth (**sign of maturity** in the male neonate). Congenital inguinal hernia is due to persistent patency of the peritoneal processus vaginalis (see p. 334).

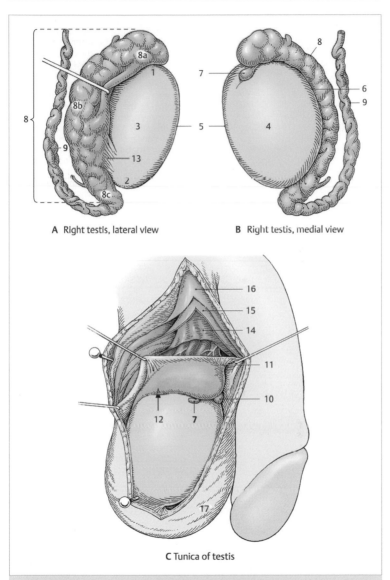

A Right testis, lateral view

B Right testis, medial view

C Tunica of testis

Fig. 6.2 Macroscopic structure of the testis and epididymis.

Microscopic Anatomy

Tissue framework of the testis and epididymis. The tunica albuginea sends numerous **septa testis** (**AB1**) into the interior of the organ, dividing the parenchyma into 250–370 conical **lobules of the testis** (**A2**) and converging to form the **mediastinum testis** (**A3**). Each lobule contains several **seminiferous tubules**, or *convoluted seminiferous tubules* (**B4**). These continue into the *straight tubules* (**B5**), which in turn are continuous with a network of tubules in the mediastinum testis known as the **rete testis** (**B6**). The rete testis is connected by **efferent ductules** (**AB7**) with the duct of the epididymis (**B8**). Each efferent ductule is about 20-cm long and is coiled to form a conical, 2-cm long **lobule of the epididymis**, whose apex is directed toward the rete testis and whose base faces the duct of the epididymis.

Seminiferous tubules (**C**). The seminiferous tubules, each with a diameter of 180– 280 μm, are surrounded by loose connective tissue called **interstitial tissue** (**C9**), which contains testosterone-producing, interstitial cells known as *Leydig cells* (see p. 376). A 7–10-μm layer of **myofibroblasts** and **fibroblasts** (**C10**) immediately surrounds the seminiferous tubules. The tubules are lined by **germinal epithelium**, which is composed of *spermatogenic cells* and supporting *Sertoli cells*. The entire length of the seminiferous tubules is estimated to be 300–350 m.

Spermatogenesis. Spermatozoa develop in the germinal epithelium (**D**), in a multistage process, arising from stem cells called spermatogonia.

Spermatogonia, which lie along the basement membrane, can be classified into two types. *Type A spermatogonia* are stem cells that are either resting or undergoing mitotic division to form more stem cells. *Type B spermatogonia* (**D11**) can be considered precursor cells of the spermatozoa, that is, they are involved in *meiosis* and subsequent differentiation processes, throughout which they remain connected by bridges of cytoplasm.

Mitotic division of type B spermatogonia gives rise to **primary spermatocytes** (**D12**). After duplicating their DNA content (to become 4n DNA), they enter the various stages of prophase of the first meiotic division. The meiotic prophase lasts up to 24 days and results in the recombination of genetic material. In histological preparations, primary spermatocytes can be identified by their large size. The remaining stages of the first meiotic division occur rapidly, at the conclusion of which two **secondary spermatocytes** (**D13**) (2n DNA) are formed. In the second meiotic division, the secondary spermatocytes divide to form **spermatids** (**D14**). Spermatids are the smallest cells in the germinal epithelium. They contain only a single set of chromosomes (22 autosomes and 1 sex chromosome, 1n DNA). They lie in bunches on the tips of the Sertoli cells (**D15**), from where they are secreted into the adluminal compartment of the seminiferous tubule (see below). After a long process of maturation, consisting of nuclear condensation and acrosome and flagella formation, the spermatids give rise to **spermatozoa capable of fertilization** (**D16**), which are released from the germinal epithelium in the final phase of spermiogenesis (**E**).

Spermatozoa. The mature spermatozoon (**F**) is about 60-μm long and consists of a **head** (**F17**) and a **tail** (**F18**). The tail can be further divided into a *neck* (**F18 a**), a *middle piece* (**F18b**), a *principal piece* (**F18 c**), and an *end piece*. The head is characterized by the presence of a dense *nucleus* (**F19**) surrounded by a cap called an *acrosome* (**F20**). The acrosome contains acrosin, an enzyme that plays an important part in fertilization.

Sertoli cells (**D15**). The Sertoli cells rest on the basement membrane, with their processes projecting into the lumen of the seminiferous tubules. Their basal portions are interconnected by numerous cell junctions, forming the **blood–testis barrier**, which divides the germinal epithelium into a **basal compartment** and an **adluminal compartment**. The germ cells travel through the intercellular spaces between the cell junctions of the Sertoli cells, as they slowly move toward the lumen of the seminiferous tubule. They are nourished by the Sertoli cells, for which they act as a support structure, and also secrete a fluid that transports the spermatozoa into the epididymis.

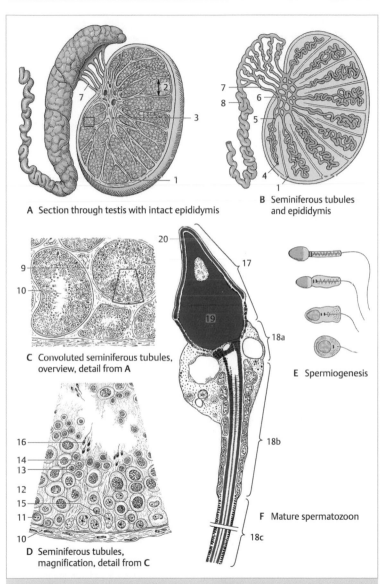

A Section through testis with intact epididymis

B Seminiferous tubules and epididymis

C Convoluted seminiferous tubules, overview, detail from **A**

D Seminiferous tubules, magnification, detail from **C**

E Spermiogenesis

F Mature spermatozoon

Fig. 6.3 Microscopic structure of the testis and epididymis.

Microscopic Anatomy, cont.

Rete testis, efferent ductules, and duct of epididymis. In histological sections of the testis and epididymis (**A**), the rete testis (**A1**) can be identified by its location in the mediastinum testis. The **rete testis** (**B**) is a system of channels lined by *simple squamous or cuboidal epithelium*, from which 12–20 **efferent ductules** (**A2**) lead to the duct of the epididymis (**A3**). The **efferent ductules** (**C**) are lined by *pseudostratified epithelium* with cells *of variable height*. They have alternating segments of columnar cells and flattened cells. The flat epithelial cells are absorptive, while the columnar cells possess *kinocilia* for transporting as yet nonmotile spermatozoa to more distal segments of the duct. Throughout the **duct of the epididymis** (**D**), the epithelium is characterized by *pseudostratified tall columnar epithelial cells that have stereocilia*. The epithelium of the duct of the epididymis produces steroid-5α-reductase, which converts testosterone to dihydrotestosterone, its more active form; neuroendocrine peptides; and secretory proteins that are important in maturation and storage of the spermatozoa. The walls of the duct of the epididymis are formed by a few layers of smooth muscle cells.

Function of the testis and epididymis. The production of **spermatozoa** in the seminiferous tubules of the testis lasts about 74 days. Movement through the epididymis takes an additional 8–17 days. There the spermatozoa undergo a **maturation process**, at the end of which they are capable of fertilization. The epididymis also serves as a **storage site** for mature spermatozoa. The endocrine and paracrine processes necessary for spermatogenesis are discussed in the chapter on the endocrine system (see p. 376).

Hormonal regulation and suitable **temperature**, at least 2°C below body temperature, are essential to the development of mature spermatozoa.

The **size of the testes** steadily increases during childhood, reaching its maximum between the ages of 20 and 30. In older age, the testes shrink. In the male child, the seminiferous tubules of the testis consist of cords of epithelial cells without lumen, containing only Sertoli cells and spermatogonia. Spermatogenesis, which commences during puberty, normally continues into advanced age.

> **Clinical note.** The higher temperatures in **inguinal** (**undescended**) **testes**, compared to testes that have descended into the scrotum, prevent production of spermatozoa.

Vessels, Nerves, and Lymphatic Drainage

Arteries. The *testes* are supplied by the **testicular artery**, which arises from the aorta directly below the renal artery and also sends a branch to the *epididymis*. It is relatively long, passing downward in the retroperitoneal space, and crossing the psoas and ureter. It anastomoses with the **artery to the ductus deferens**, a branch of the umbilical artery (see p. 256), and the **cremasteric artery** (← inferior epigastric artery), which supplies the *tunics of the testes*. The *scrotum* is nourished by branches from the **internal pudendal artery**.

Veins. Blood from the testes and epididymis drains into the *pampiniform venous plexus*, which in turn empties via the **right testicular vein** into the inferior vena cava and via the **left testicular vein** into the left renal vein. Drainage from the tunics of the testes and the scrotum is to the *great saphenous vein*, *inferior epigastric vein*, and *internal pudendal vein*.

Nerves. Sympathetic fibers from the **celiac plexus** accompany the supplying arteries to the testes and epididymides, as the testicular plexus. The scrotum is innervated by the **scrotal nerves** arising from the *ilioinguinal nerve* and *pudendal nerve*. Nerve supply to the cremaster muscle is provided by the genital branch of the genitofemoral nerve.

Regional lymph nodes. Lymph from the testes and epididymides drains to the **lumbar nodes**; that from the tunics of the testes and scrotum drains to the **inguinal nodes**.

> **Clinical note. Varicocele** is a condition of unknown etiology that involves abnormal dilatation of the large-caliber, valveless veins of the pampiniform venous plexus. The left testis is more often affected than the right.

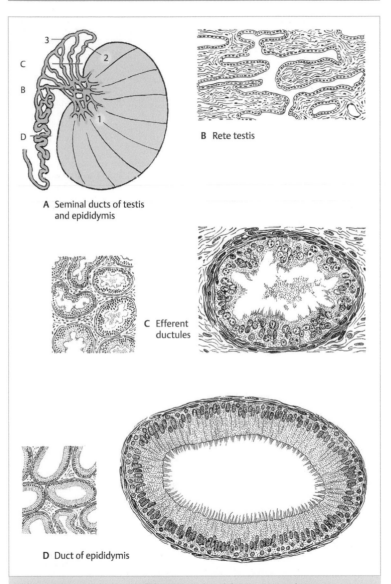

A Seminal ducts of testis and epididymis

B Rete testis

C Efferent ductules

D Duct of epididymis

Fig. 6.4 Microscopic structure of the testis and epididymis, continued.

6.3 Seminal Ducts and Accessory Sex Glands

Ductus Deferens (Vas Deferens)

Gross anatomy (**A**). The **ductus deferens/vas deferens** (**A1**) is a 35–40-cm long continuation of the duct of the epididymis that connects it to the urethra and **transports** spermatozoa. It is 3–3.5-mm thick and has a strong, muscular wall. After emerging from the head of the epididymis, its initial part is tortuous, followed by a straight segment, at the end of which is a spindle-shaped dilatation called the **ampulla of the ductus deferens** (**A2**). The ductus deferens opens into the **ejaculatory duct** (**A3**), which is located in the prostatic urethra.

Microanatomy (**B**). The disproportionately small star-shaped **lumen** of the ductus deferens has 3–4 longitudinal *folds allowing for its expansion*. It is lined by *pseudostratified, stereociliated, columnar* **epithelium** (**B4**) and a thin, underlying layer of connective tissue with abundant elastic fibers. The mucosal lining of the ampulla of the ductus deferens contains numerous folds. The thick **muscular layer** (**B5**) consists of bundles of smooth muscle cells traveling at various gradient angles. In cross section, this arrangement gives rise to an *outer longitudinal layer*, a *middle circular layer*, and an *inner longitudinal layer*. The ductus deferens is embedded in its surroundings by a connective tissue **adventitia** (**B6**).

Function. The ductus deferens **transports** spermatozoa and seminal fluid from the epididymis to the male urethra, by means of peristaltic waves.

Vessels, Nerves, and Lymphatic Drainage

Arteries. The ductus deferens (**C**) is supplied by the **artery to the ductus deferens** (**C7**), which springs from the patent part of the *umbilical artery*.

Veins. Venous drainage is via the **pampiniform venous plexus** (**C8**), as well as the **vesical** and **prostatic venous plexuses**.

Nerves. Innervation of the ductus deferens is provided by autonomic fibers from the **inferior hypogastric nerve plexus**.

Regional lymph nodes. Lymph drains through the inguinal canal to the retroperitoneal, para-aortic **lumbar nodes**.

Topography (A)

The first part of the ductus deferens, the **scrotal part**, travels along the *inner aspect of the epididymis*. The second part, the **funicular part**, lies surrounded by veins in the *spermatic cord* (see below). The third portion, the **inguinal part**, passes through the *inguinal canal* and traverses the *deep inguinal ring* (**A9**) medial to the vessels and nerves accompanying the ductus deferens. It proceeds *deep to the peritoneum* and crosses over the inferior epigastric and external iliac vessels. The **pelvic part** of the ductus deferens ultimately crosses the linea terminalis into the lesser pelvis.

Spermatic Cord (C)

The **spermatic cord** consists of the **ductus deferens** and its **accompanying vessels** (*testicular artery and vein, artery to the ductus deferens, pampiniform venous plexus, autonomic nerves*, and the *genital branch of the genitofemoral nerve*). It extends from the head of the epididymis to the deep inguinal ring, linking the testis with the abdominal cavity, and is covered by the following layers (from without): skin, dartos muscle, external spermatic fascia (**C10**), *cremaster* muscle (**C11**), and internal spermatic fascia (**C12**).

Clinical note. The muscular wall of the ductus deferens makes it readily palpable in the spermatic cord.
This makes it easily accessible for the surgical procedure of vasectomy, in which the ductus deferens is divided to induce male infertility.

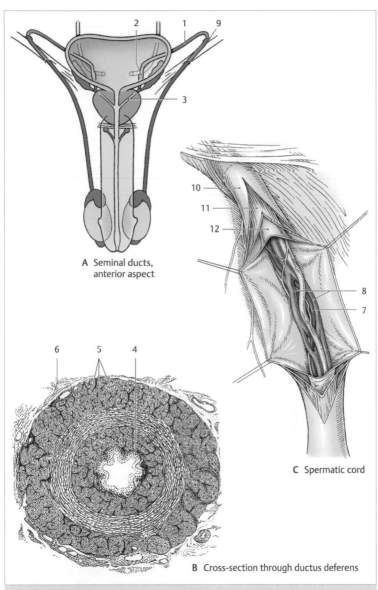

A Seminal ducts, anterior aspect

B Cross-section through ductus deferens

C Spermatic cord

Male Genital System

Fig. 6.5 Vas deferens.

Seminal Vesicles

The paired **seminal vesicles** (**A1**) lie against the posterior surface of the urinary bladder (**AC2**) lateral to the ampulla of the ductus deferens (**A3**). Only their lateral, uppermost portions are covered by peritoneum. Each seminal vesicle is about 5-cm long, has a bumpy surface, and contains a coiled duct that is about 15-cm long. The **excretory duct** unites with the ductus deferens and opens at the level of the prostatic urethra into the ejaculatory duct (**AC4**).

Microanatomy and function. The **surface architecture of the mucosa** is characterized by numerous mucosal folds, so that it appears to have a labyrinth of cavities in histological preparations. The variably tall **epithelial cells** are arranged in one to two layers and produce an *alkaline secretion rich in fructose* that makes up most of the volume of the seminal fluid. The seminal vesicles have strong, muscular walls.

A5 Ureter

Prostate

The chestnut-sized **prostate** (**A–C6**) lies below the urinary bladder on the pelvic floor. It measures roughly 3 cm × 4 cm × 2 cm. Its **anterior surface** (**B7**) faces the pubic symphysis, and its **posterior surface** faces the rectum. Its **inferolateral surface** faces the lateral pelvic wall and is adjacent to the (autonomic) inferior hypogastric nerve plexus. The **base of the prostate** (**B8**) is fused to the fundus of the urinary bladder, and the **apex of the prostate** (**B9**) faces the urogenital diaphragm. The prostate is penetrated by the initial portion of the *male urethra* (**BC10**) and by the *ejaculatory duct* (**AC4**). **The macroscopic** division into the *right* and *left lobes*, the *isthmus of the prostate*, and the *middle lobe* is less relevant than the embryological and pathological aspects of glandular tissue.

Microanatomy and function. The prostate is an **exocrine organ** made up of about **40 individual tubuloalveolar glands** that open by **prostatic ductules** around the seminal colliculus in the male urethra. It is surrounded by a tough connective tissue **capsule of the prostate** and contains typical **fibromuscular stroma**. The individual glands within the prostate are embedded in *connective tissue* containing large numbers of *smooth muscle cells*. The prostatic tubuloalveolar *epithelium* contains variably tall cells and is pseudostratified (two or more rows); the active cells of the gland are columnar. The thin **secretion** of the prostate is acidic (pH 6.4) and contains numerous enzymes, including acid phosphatase and proteases. It makes up 15–30% of the seminal fluid.

> **Clinical note.** The tissue of the prostate gland may be divided clinically into three overlapping zones (**D–F**) surrounding the urethra. The **transitional zone** (yellow) encloses the urethra to the level of the opening of the ejaculatory duct. It is surrounded by glandular tissue called the **central zone** (green), which also encloses the ejaculatory duct. The largest part of the gland is the outer, **peripheral zone** (red). In advancing age, the tissue of the central zone tends to become enlarged in a condition referred to as **benign prostatic hyperplasia**, which constricts the part of the urethra surrounded by the prostate, and impairs urination. **Prostate cancer**, one of the most common cancers in older men, usually starts in the peripheral zone.

Vessels, Nerves, and Lymphatic Drainage

Arteries. Arterial supply to the *seminal vesicles* is from the inferior vesical artery, the artery to the ductus deferens, and the middle rectal artery. The *prostate* is supplied by branches from the internal pudendal artery, inferior vesical artery, and middle rectal artery.

Veins. The veins around the prostate form a plexus, known as the **prostatic venous plexus,** which is connected with the vesical venous plexus. It receives blood from the seminal vesicles and empties into the internal iliac vein.

Nerves. Lying in close proximity to the tips of the seminal vesicles, as well as on the posterolateral side of the prostate, are parts of the **inferior hypogastric nerve plexus**, which sends numerous nerves to the gland.

Regional lymph nodes. Lymph from the *seminal vesicles* drains to the **internal iliac nodes**, while most of the lymph from the *prostate* drains to the **internal iliac nodes** and **sacral nodes**.

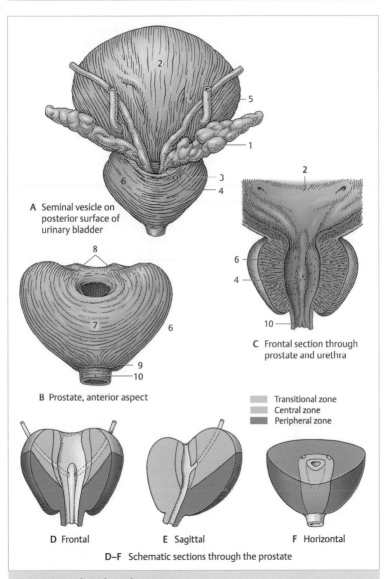

A Seminal vesicle on posterior surface of urinary bladder

B Prostate, anterior aspect

C Frontal section through prostate and urethra

Transitional zone
Central zone
Peripheral zone

D Frontal

E Sagittal

F Horizontal

D–F Schematic sections through the prostate

Fig. 6.6 Seminal vesicles and prostate.

Male Genital System

6.4 Male External Genitalia

Penis

The male sex organ is composed of a two-chambered cavernous body, called the **corpus cavernosum penis** (**A–C1**), and a cavernous body surrounding the urethra, known as the **corpus spongiosum penis** (**A–C2**). The penis consists of the **root of the penis** (**A3**), the part attached to the pubis and the perineum, and the freely movable **body of the penis** (**A4**). The flattened superior side of the body of the penis is known as the *dorsum of the penis*, and the inferior side is the *urethral surface*.

Root of the penis. The root of the penis arises from the inferior pubic rami by the right and left **crura of the penis** (**A5**), proximal extensions of the corpora cavernosa surrounded by the striated *ischiocavernosus muscle* (**A6**). The thickened end of the corpus spongiosum lying between the two crura of the penis is termed the **bulb of the penis** (**A7**). The bulb is firmly connected with the urogenital diaphragm (**A8**) and covered by the *bulbospongiosus* (**A9**) muscle. The root of the penis is attached to the abdominal wall and pubic symphysis by the *fundiform ligament of the penis* and the *suspensory ligament of the penis* (see Vol. 1).

Body of the penis. The two crura of the penis unite below the pubic symphysis to form the dual-chambered **corpus cavernosum penis**, which makes up most of the body of the penis. Each corpus cavernosum is enclosed in a thick connective tissue sheath called the **tunica albuginea of the corpora cavernosa** (**BC10**). A median partition known as the *septum penis* (**B11**) arises from the tunica albuginea and partially separates the two corpora cavernosa. Lying in the wide groove extending along the inferior surface of the corpus cavernosum to its conical end is the corpus spongiosum. The connective tissue sheath surrounding the corpus spongiosum, the **tunica albuginea of the corpus spongiosum** (**B12**), is relatively thin. The tough **fascia of the penis** (**B13**) surrounds the corpora cavernosa and corpus spongiosum collectively.

Glans penis. The corpus spongiosum of the penis receives the male urethra about 1cm from the bulb and terminates as the glans penis (**AC14**), an expansion of the corpus spongiosum projecting beyond the ends of the corpora cavernosa. On the tip of the glans penis is the slitlike opening of the male urethra known as the **external urethral orifice** (**C15**). The rounded margin encircling the base, the **corona of the glans** (**AC16**), is separated from the body of the penis by a furrow.

Penis coverings. The penis is covered by thin skin that does not contain any fat. Underneath is a thin subcutaneous fascia known as the **subcutaneous tissue of the penis** (**B17**). The skin overlying the body of the penis is freely movable and is attached at the corona of the glans (**C**), where it forms the **prepuce of the penis** (**foreskin**) (**C18**), a fold of skin that does not contain fat. The **frenulum of the prepuce**, formed by an inner layer of the prepuce, passes from its inferior aspect to the glans of the penis, attaching and tethering the foreskin to the glans.

Microscopic Anatomy of the Corpora Cavernosa and the Corpus Spongiosum

Corpus cavernosum of the penis (**C**). The **vascular spaces** (**cavernous spaces**) of the corpus cavernosum of the penis are lined by *endothelium* and are embedded in a framework of *collagenous* and *elastic fibers* as well as *networks of smooth muscle cells* called **trabeculae of the corpora cavernosa**. The spaces can hold variable amounts of blood, forming mere slitlike cavities when empty, and expanding during erection to a diameter of several millimeters. The smooth muscle between the spaces contracts and *stiffens the penis*. The vascular spaces are fed by the **helicine arteries** (from the deep artery of the penis, see p. 262), which act as *resistance vessels*. Blood is drained from the vascular spaces to subfascial and epifascial veins.

Corpus spongiosum of the penis. The corpus spongiosum of the penis also contains wide **vascular spaces** lined by *endothelium* which, however, are viewed as **continuations of the venous system**. In the body of the penis they parallel the course of the male urethra, and in the glans they are tortuous. The *connective tissue framework* and *trabeculae of the smooth muscle* are less prominent than in the corpora cavernosa. A filling of the cavernous spaces in the corpus spongiosum merely leads to *"soft"* swelling, permitting spermatozoa to be transported through the male urethra.

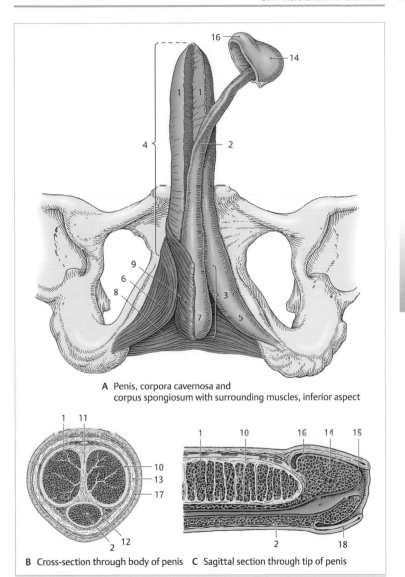

A Penis, corpora cavernosa and corpus spongiosum with surrounding muscles, inferior aspect

B Cross-section through body of penis   **C** Sagittal section through tip of penis

Fig. 6.7 Penis.

Penis, cont.

Vessels, Nerves, and Lymphatic Drainage

Arteries. The corpora cavernosa and the corpus spongiosum are supplied by three paired arteries arising from the internal pudendal artery: the **posterior artery of the penis** (**A1**), which passes deep to the fascia on the dorsum of the penis and supplies the glans, foreskin, and skin; the **deep artery of the penis** (**A2**), which passes in the middle of the corpora cavernosa, supplying them and giving off the *helicine arteries*; and the **artery of the bulb of the penis**, which supplies the corpus spongiosum and male urethra.

Veins. Venous drainage is mostly to the unpaired **superficial** (**A3**) and **deep posterior veins of the penis** (**A4**), which have numerous valves and open into the *prostatic venous plexus* and *vesical venous plexus*.

Nerves. Sensory innervation is provided by a branch from the dorsal nerve of the penis, a branch of the **pudendal nerve**. Autonomic fibers pass to the penis via the **inferior hypogastric nerve plexus** and arise from the *lumbar part of the sympathetic part* (L1–L3) and *sacral part of the parasympathetic part of the autonomic nervous system* (pelvic splanchnic nerves) (S2–S4).

Regional lymph nodes. Lymph drains from the penis to the **inguinal nodes**.

Function. The sequence of events that occur in **erection** is triggered by sexual stimuli that are processed by the autonomic nervous system, which is linked to centers in the central nervous system. The vascular spaces become engorged with blood, while the helicine arteries dilate and the outflow of blood is reduced. If sexual stimulation reaches a certain level, the center for the ejaculation reflex located at the L2/L3 spinal cord segments is stimulated, initiating the **orgasm phase**, which includes *emission* and *ejaculation*.

Male Urethra

Most of the approximately 20-cm long **male urethra** functions as a passage for both urine and semen. The short initial portion of the male urethra is contained in the wall of the urinary bladder, where it begins at the **internal urethral orifice** (**B5**). It continues as the 3.5-cm long **prostatic urethra** (**BC6**) through the prostate. The posterior

surface of the inner wall of the prostatic urethra presents a ridgelike projection called the *urethral crest*. In the middle, there is an expansion termed the *seminal colliculus* (**B7**). Opening on the lateral sides of the seminal colliculus are the ejaculatory ducts (**B8**), and on its summit there is a blind-ending sac called the prostatic utricle. Running along either side of the seminal collicula is a groove called the *prostatic sinus* (**B9**). At the inferior border of the prostate, the **intermediate part** (**BC10**) of the urethra begins. This short and narrowest part of the male urethra runs through the urogenital diaphragm and is continuous with its longest part, the **spongy urethra** (**BC11**). The proximal part of the spongy urethra is attached to the urogenital diaphragm and pubic symphysis. Its lumen is dilated to form an ampulla and contains the openings of the excretory ducts from the bulbourethral glands (**B12**) (see below). The second dilated part of the spongy urethra, known as the *navicular fossa* (**BC13**), is located within the glans of the penis. The navicular fossa is about 2-cm long and narrows to form the **external urethral orifice** (**B14**). Its roof often contains a fold known as the *valve of the navicular fossa*. The *internal urethral orifice*, *intermediate part of the urethra*, and the *external urethral orifice* are the **three narrow parts** of the otherwise wide male urethra.

> **Clinical note.** During **catheter insertion**, careful attention must be paid to the narrowed parts and bends present in the male urethra.

Microanatomy. The thin wall of the urethra has three layers. The **mucosa** contains longitudinal folds. As far as the middle of the prostatic urethra, the epithelium consists of *transitional epithelium*, which then transitions into *stratified, columnar epithelium*. The latter lines the spongy urethra as far as the navicular fossa, which is lined by *stratified, squamous epithelium*. Scattered throughout the spongy urethra are mucous *urethral glands* (*Littré glands*).

Bulbourethral glands. The bulbourethral glands are two pea-sized tubular glands (Cowper glands) lying in the urogenital diaphragm, that produce a stringy, mucous, slightly alkaline secretion, which is discharged through an excretory duct into the proximal portion of the spongy urethra.

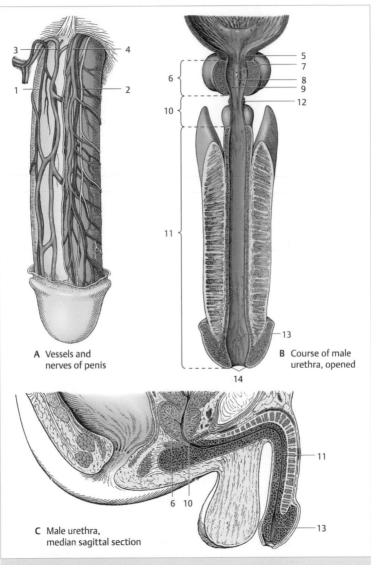

A Vessels and nerves of penis

B Course of male urethra, opened

C Male urethra, median sagittal section

Fig. 6.8 Penis and male urethra.

Male Genital System

6.5 Topographical Anatomy

Cross-Sectional Anatomy

Transverse Section at the Level of the Hip Joints (A)

The section cuts rather obliquely from anterosuperior to posteroinferior, with the anterior portion beginning above the level of the pubic symphysis. On the lateral pelvic wall, it cuts through the *obturator internus* (**AB1**) and *obturator vessels* (**A2**), as well as the *obturator nerve* (**A3**) just above the entrance to the *obturator canal*. In the lateroposterior part of the section, the attachment site of the *sacrospinal ligament* (**A4**) can be identified on the *ischial spine* (**A5**). In front of the *coccyx* (**A6**) is the *rectal ampulla* (**AB7**), whose lateral and posterior aspects are surrounded by a sparse covering of perirectal connective tissue and adipose tissue containing branches of the superior rectal vessels as well as rectal nerves and lymph nodes. In front of the rectum, the section is through the *seminal vesicles* (**A8**) and *ampulla of the ductus deferens* (**A9**). Lateral to the seminal vesicles are numerous vessels of the autonomic *inferior hypogastric nerve plexus* (**A10**) and *prostatic venous plexus* (**A11**). The section is through the *urinary bladder* (**A12**) at the level of the opening of the *ureters* (**A13**); on the left side, the intramural part of the ureter can be seen. The anterior and lateral aspects of the urinary bladder are surrounded by adipose tissue, permitting movement as it expands during filling.

AB14 Gluteus maximus, **AB15** Sciatic nerve, **AB16** Head of femur, **AB17** Neck of femur, **A18** Pectineus, **A19** Iliopsoas, **AB20** Femoral vessels, **AB21** Femoral nerve, **A22** Rectus abdominis

Transverse Section at the Level of the Ischial Tuberosities (B)

The section cuts anteriorly through the *pubic symphysis* (**B23**) and posteriorly through the *tip of the coccyx*. The lateral parts of the pelvic viscera rest on parts of the *levator ani* (**B24**). The posterior part of the rectum is surrounded by the *muscular sling formed by the puborectalis* (**B25**). Lateral to the puborectalis is the *fat body of the ischioanal fossa* (**B26**), which is bounded laterally by the *obturator internus* (**B1**) in

whose facial canal the *pudendal vessels* (**B27**) travel as well as the *pudendal nerve*. The posterior part of the ischioanal fossa is covered by the *gluteus maximus* (**B14**).

The *prostate* (**B28**), and *prostatic venous plexus* (**B11**) lying anterior and lateral to the gland can be seen in front of the rectum. The autonomic *inferior hypogastric nerve plexus* (**B10**) lies along the posterolateral border of the prostate and is accompanied by the *ductus deferens* (**B29**) coursing lateral to it. Between the prostate and the pubic symphysis is the *retropubic space*.

B30 Obturator externus

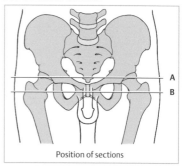

Position of sections

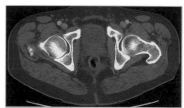

Fig. 6.9C Corresponding plane to Fig. 6.9A on CT.

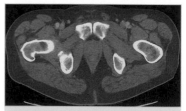

Fig.6.9D Corresponding plane to Fig. 6.9B on CT.

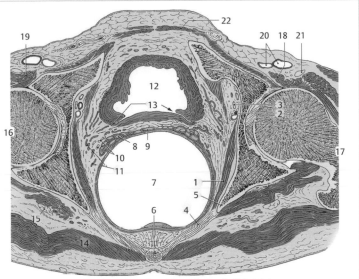

A Transverse section through male pelvis at the level of hip joints

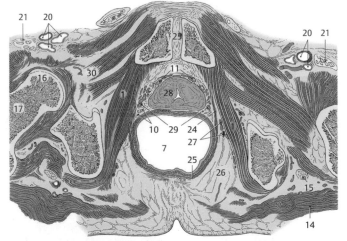

B Transverse section through male pelvis at the level of ischial tuberosities

Fig. 6.9 Cross-sectional anatomy.

Male Genital System

7 Female Genital System

7.1 Overview

Female Reproductive Organs

The **female genital system**, like that of the male, can be divided topographically and embryologically into internal and external genitalia.

The **internal** female genital organs are the *ovary* (**AC1**), *uterine tube* (**AC2**), *uterus* (**AC3**), and *vagina* (**A4**). The **external** female genitalia consist of the *labium majus* (**B5**), *labium minus* (**B6**), the *vestibule of vagina* (**B7**), the *vestibular glands* (**A8**), and the *clitoris* (**AB9**). In customary clinical usage, the term **vulva** refers to the *external genitalia* including the *urethral orifices* (**AB10**), *vagina*, and the *mons pubis* (**B11**), the fat pad overlying the pubic symphysis. The accessory genital organs consisting of the *uterine tubes* and *ovaries* are known as **adnexa**.

Function. The female reproductive cells, or egg cells (oocytes), mature in the **ovary**. Mature ova are released cyclically into the **uterine tube** and transported toward the **uterus**. If fertilization occurs, the young embryo (blastocyst) is implanted (nidation) in the prepared endometrium.

A12 Bulb of vestibule, **A13** Crus of clitoris

Peritoneal Relations of the Female Pelvis (C)

The peritoneal cavity continues, without any observable transition, from the abdominal cavity over the linea terminalis into the pelvic cavity. In the female pelvis, the uterus (**AC3**) is situated between the pelvic viscera, that is, the urinary bladder (**C14**) and the rectum (**C15**), resulting in different peritoneal relations from those observed in the male pelvis (see p. 248). As in the

male, the **parietal peritoneum** of the *anterior abdominal wall* passes to the urinary bladder, covering the *apex of the bladder* and the *superior surface of the bladder*. It reflects from the superior surface of the urinary bladder onto the *anterior surface of the uterus* at the junction between the cervix and body, covering the *fundus of the uterus* and the *adnexa* lateral to the uterus. From there it extends over the *posterior surface of the uterus*, passing from there as far as the posterior wall of the vagina, or *posterior part of the vaginal fornix*. The peritoneal covering of the uterus is called the **perimetrium**.

The uterus, uterine tubes, and ovaries are covered by peritoneum. Extending in the frontal plane from either side of the uterus to the lateral pelvic wall is a peritoneum-covered fibrous plate called the **broad ligament of the uterus** (**C16**). The broad ligament divides the peritoneal cavity of the female pelvis into anterior and posterior peritoneal pockets, known as the **vesicouterine pouch** (**C17**) and **rectouterine pouch** (**C18**). Depending on the fullness of the urinary bladder, the vesicouterine pouch may form only a very shallow recess. The rectouterine pouch (**pouch of Douglas**) is a true peritoneal pocket, marking the *deepest point in the female abdominal cavity*. It is bounded laterally by the *rectouterine fold* (**C19**), which contains subserous fibrous connective tissue known as the sacrouterine ligament, as well the (autonomic) inferior hypogastric nerve plexus.

Clinical note. Pathological accumulations of fluid in the peritoneal cavity collect in the **rectouterine pouch**. Fluid can be aspirated and drained by puncture of the vagina. The pouch of Douglas can also be palpated through the rectum.

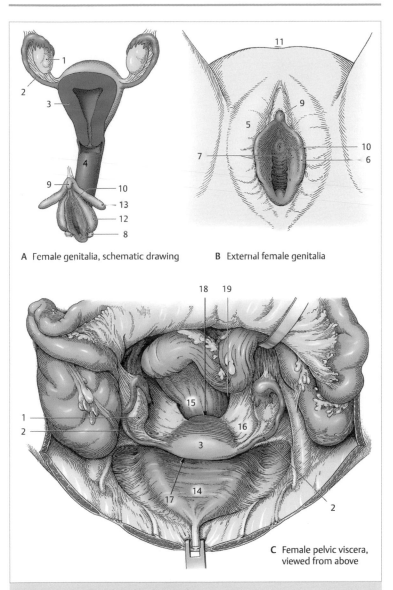

A Female genitalia, schematic drawing

B External female genitalia

C Female pelvic viscera, viewed from above

Fig. 7.1 Organization of the female reproductive organs.

7.2 Ovary and Uterine Tubes

The paired **ovaries** (**AB1**) are the **female reproductive glands** and the **site of maturation of the follicles and egg cells** (**oocytes**). They are normally located on either side of the body on the lateral wall of the pelvis in the *ovarian fossa* which is bounded by the division of the common iliac artery. The almond-shaped ovary is about 4-cm long, 1.5–2-cm wide, and 1-cm thick. Its **surface texture** changes with age: smooth in the child and bumpy in the sexually mature female. In the postmenopausal woman the ovary has an atrophic, wrinkled appearance.

Gross Anatomy of the Ovary

The **medial surface** (**B2**) of the ovary, which faces medially toward the pelvic viscera, is distinguished from its **lateral surface** (**B3**), which rests against the lateral wall of the pelvis. The superior pole of the obliquely oriented organ is referred to as the **tubal extremity** (**B4**) and the inferior pole as the **uterine extremity** (**B5**). The converging axes of the two ovaries intersect in front of the uterus. The ovary is located *intraperitoneally* and is anchored by a peritoneal fold called the *mesovarium* (**B6**), to the posterior side of the broad ligament of the uterus (**B7**). The *suspensory ligament of the ovary*, which contains vessels supplying the ovary, passes to the superior pole of the organ. The *ligament of the ovary* (**B8**) passes from its inferior pole to the tubal angle of the uterus. The **mesovarian border** (**B9**), to which the mesovarium is attached, contains the **hilum of the ovary** which allows vessels and nerves to enter and exit the organ. Opposite the mesovarian border is the convex **free border** (**B10**) facing a peritoneal fold produced by the ureter.

The position of the ovary is variable. In an adult (*nulliparous*) woman, it is in the **ovarian fossa**, a depression of the peritoneum between the internal and external iliac arteries. Beneath the peritoneum on the floor of the ovarian fossa are the obturator vessels and obturator nerve, and the fossa is bounded posteriorly by the external iliac vessels. The ureter is also closely related to the ovary and is separated from

it only by the parietal peritoneum. In *multiparous* women the ovary is usually somewhat lower. There may be loops of intestine below the ovary, with the sigmoid colon on the left and the cecum and appendix on the left.

Microscopic Anatomy of the Ovary

The ovary is surrounded by a tough connective tissue capsule called the **tunica albuginea** (**CD11**). The tunica albuginea has an **epithelial covering** that is often erroneously referred to as the *germinal epithelium*; it consists of mostly *cuboidal cells* that play an important role in restoring the surface of the ovary after ovulation. The interior of the organ is permeated by a tough, highly cellular, connective tissue called **ovarian stroma** and can be divided into an **ovarian cortex** (**CD12**) and an **ovarian medulla** (**CD13**). The ovarian medulla contains *abundant blood vessels and nerve fibers* as well as *endocrine cells* (see p. 378). The (endocrine) hilar cells resemble the Leydig cells of the testis.

The cortex of the **mature ovary** (**D**) contains *ovarian follicles* (**CD14**) in various stages of development during the menstrual cycle, as well as the *corpus luteum* and its remnants. The stroma of the cortex has a characteristic structure with parallel collagen fibers and spindle-shaped cells interlacing in different directions: spinocellular connective tissue.

The **ovarian cortex of a newborn female** contains *primordial follicles*, that is, *primary oocytes/egg cells* 30–50 μm in diameter surrounded by a single layer of flat, follicular epithelial cells. Although the ovary contains between 500,000 and 1,000,000 primordial follicles at birth, a significant number of these perish by the time of puberty. The oocytes remain in the prophase of meiosis until maturity. (Further information can be obtained from textbooks of embryology and biology.)

Clinical note. Ovarian cancer (80–90% of ovarian tumors) arises from the epithelial surface of the ovary (peritoneal epithelium), which can extend from the surface into the underlying ovarian stroma during ovulation.

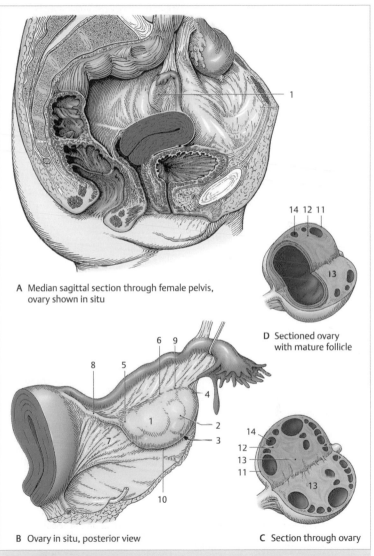

A Median sagittal section through female pelvis, ovary shown in situ

D Sectioned ovary with mature follicle

B Ovary in situ, posterior view

C Section through ovary

Fig. 7.2 Macroscopic and microscopic structure of the ovary.

Follicles

At puberty, a small number of follicles and their oocytes enter a hormonally regulated process of maturation. In histological preparations, follicles can be divided by developmental stage into primary, secondary, and tertiary follicles (**B**). During follicular maturation, the oocyte (**B1**) grows to a diameter of 15 μm.

Primary, secondary, and tertiary follicles develop from early childhood until menopause. Primary and secondary follicles are small, medium, and large **preantral** follicles, while tertiary follicles are described as small, medium, and large **antral** follicles. During the period of sexual maturity, 99.9% of maturing oocytes perish (**follicle atresia**). At puberty, there are about 400,000 oocytes, and 300–400 oocytes are capable of fertilization during a woman's childbearing years.

The **primordial follicle** (**B2**) develops into a **primary follicle** (**B3**), in which the primary oocyte is surrounded by a closed ring consisting of a single layer of cuboidal follicular epithelium. Between the ring of epithelium and the oocyte, a homogenous zona pellucida (**B4**) forms, which subsequently becomes a sperm receptor via anchoring proteins. In the **secondary follicle** (**B5**) (diameter above 400 μm), the oocyte is surrounded by a ring of cuboidal stratified follicular epithelial cells (**B6**), also known as granulosa cells. The spaces between adjacent follicular epithelial cells, known as lacunae, contain follicular fluid. The connective tissue surrounding the follicle forms the theca interna (**B7 a**), containing steroid-producing cells, and the theca externa (**B7 b**), consisting of contractile cells. In the **tertiary follicle**

(antral follicle) (**B8**) (diameter 0.4–1 cm), the intercellular spaces merge to form a large, fluid-filled cavity called the follicular antrum (**B9**); the oocyte is now positioned off to one side of the follicle in the cumulus oophorus (**B10**). The granulosa cells touching the oocyte form the corona radiata (**B11**). The stratified epithelium lining the antrum is called the granular layer (**B12**). The theca interna (**B7 a**) and theca externa (**B7 b**) are well developed.

In each **cycle**, a tertiary follicle grows over a period of a few days to five times its original size, developing into a mature **Graafian follicle** (see p. 270 **D**) that resembles a blister on the tunica albuginea of the ovary and is ready for ovulation. **Ovulation** (day 12–15, see p. 378) occurs when the Graafian follicle releases the oocyte with its corona radiata into the uterine tube.

After release of the oocyte, the walls of the follicle collapse to form the corpus rubrum, which later becomes the yellow body or **corpus luteum** (**A13**) (diameter about 3 cm). The cells of the granular layer undergo differentiation to become granulosa lutein cells, and the cells of the theca interna become theca lutein cells. The cells of the corpus luteum produce progesterone and estrogen. The secretory stage lasts about 8 days. If fertilization does not occur, acute vasoconstriction heralds **luteolysis**, the regression stage. Luteal cells degenerate, leaving a connective tissue scar known as the **corpus albicans**. If impregnation occurs, the corpus luteum continues to develop and becomes the **corpus luteum of pregnancy**, which is necessary for maintaining pregnancy until the 3rd month. For information on hormonal regulation of simultaneous maturation of the follicle and ovum, (see p. 378).

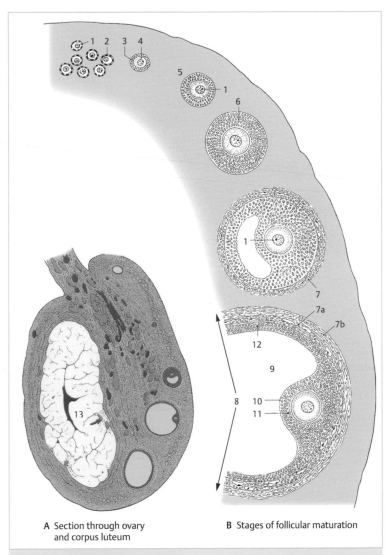

A Section through ovary and corpus luteum

B Stages of follicular maturation

Female Genital System

Fig. 7.3 Follicular maturation.

Gross Anatomy of the Uterine Tube

The **uterine tubes** (**AB1**) extend from either side of the uterus in the *superior border of the broad ligament of the uterus* (**B2**). Each uterine tube (salpinx) is 10–18-cm long and opens at its free end through the **abdominal ostium** (**B3**) into the abdominal cavity. The funnel-shaped opening, the **infundibulum of the uterine tube** (**AB4**), possesses fringelike processes approximately 15 mm in length, known as *fimbriae of the uterine tube* (**AB5**), one of which, the *ovarian fimbria* (**B6**), is especially long and is attached to the ovary. The infundibulum is continuous with the **ampulla of the uterine tube** (**AB7**), which makes up the lateral two-thirds of the uterine tube. The narrow part closer to the uterus is known as the **isthmus of the uterine tube** (**A8**). The **intramural part of the uterine tube** (**A9**) passes through the upper corner of the uterine wall and opens into the uterine cavity through the narrow ostium of the uterine tube. The uterine tubes lie *intraperitoneally* and are connected by the *mesosalpinx* (**B10**) to the *broad ligament of the uterus*. The inner surface of the uterine tubes contains longitudinal mucosal folds.

Microscopic Anatomy of the Uterine Tube

The **walls** of the uterine tube are composed of three layers. The **mucosa** (**CD11**) bears a *single layer of columnar epithelium with ciliated and glandular cells*. The *tubal lining produces fluid* that consists of glandular cell secretion and absorbed peritoneal fluid. The **muscular layer** (**CD12**) can be divided into several components consisting of a *subperitoneal layer*, a *perivascular layer*, and the *autochthonous muscles of the tube itself*. The complex configuration of the muscle layers permits independent movement of the uterine tube, assists the flow of tubal fluid, and helps to move the oocyte forward while transporting spermatozoa in the opposite direction. The outer surface of the uterine tube is covered by the **serosa** (**CD13**), which permits its movement against its surroundings.

Function of the ovary and uterine tube. The **ovary** contains the **female gametes**, which are released as mature ova at a certain point in the menstrual cycle. It also produces **hormones** (estrogens, gestagens, and other steroid hormones) and regulates the **ovarian and menstrual cycles** (see p. 378).

The **uterine tube** catches the oocyte as it is released from the ovary and transports it to the uterus; it also serves as a **site of fertilization** since the egg and spermatozoa can meet and unite in it.

Vessels, Nerves, and Lymphatic Drainage

Arteries. The *ovary* receives most of its blood supply from the **ovarian artery** (**B14**) (from the abdominal aorta) and the **ovarian branch** (**B15**) of the **uterine artery** (**B16**). The *uterine tube* is supplied by anastomosing branches of the ovarian and uterine arteries. The uterine artery crosses the ureter. Within the mesosalpinx, the tubal branches of the ovarian artery and the tubal branch of the uterine artery form the **ovarian arcade**.

Veins. The veins draining the *ovaries* connect to form the **ovarian plexus**, which gives rise to the *ovarian vein*. The veins from the *uterine tube* drain via the **uterine venous plexus**.

Nerves. Parasympathetic and sympathetic nerves from the **superior mesenteric nerve plexus** and **renal nerve plexus** accompany the ovarian vessels to the ovaries and uterine tubes. The uterine tubes are also supplied by the **uterovaginal nerve plexus** (← inferior hypogastric nerve plexus) whose parasympathetic nerve fibers originate from the sacral spinal cord.

Regional lymph nodes. Lymph from the *ovary* drains to the **lumbar nodes**. Lymphatic drainage from the *uterine tube* also flows to the **internal iliac nodes**.

B17 Ureter

Clinical note. Extrauterine or ectopic pregnancy occurs if the blastocyst implants outside the uterus; 98% of all extrauterine pregnancies are tubal pregnancies, when the blastocyst implants in the mucosa of the tube. The tube cannot adapt to the growing fetus as the uterus does, so, without surgery, local blood vessels rupture, resulting in fatal internal bleeding.

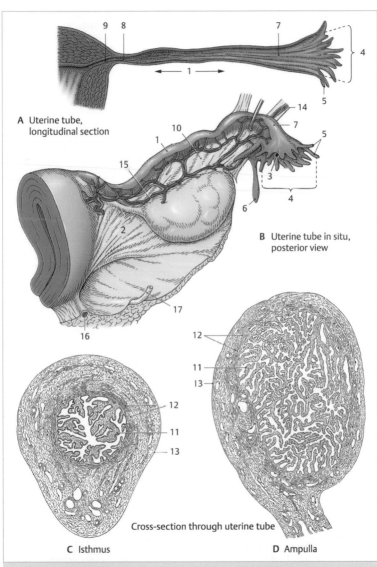

A Uterine tube, longitudinal section

B Uterine tube in situ, posterior view

Cross-section through uterine tube

C Isthmus

D Ampulla

Fig. 7.4 Macroscopic and microscopic structure of the uterine tube.

Female Genital System

7.3 Uterus

Gross Anatomy

The **uterus** (**AD1**) is a thick-walled muscular organ situated near the center of the lesser pelvis between the urinary bladder and rectum. Tilted slightly forward, it is 7–8-cm long, weighs 50–70 g in the sexually mature female and resembles an anteroposteriorly flattened pear. In terms of external structure, it can be divided into a **body of the uterus** (**B2**) and **cervix of the uterus** (**AB3**).

Body of the uterus. The upper two-thirds of the organ have a flattened **anterior surface** (**A4**) and a convex **posterior surface** (**A5**), both of which are lined by peritoneum (see p. 280). In the sexually mature female, the **fundus of the uterus** (**BC6**) projects beyond the *right uterine horn* (**B7**) and *left uterine horn* (**B8**), where the uterine tubes join the uterus. The narrow portion at the junction of the uterus and the cervix is known as the **isthmus of the uterus** (**B9**). It can be identified on the outer surface of the organ as a shallow constriction.

Cervix of the uterus (**AB3**). The thin, round, lower one-third of the uterus is directed posteriorly and inferiorly. The **vaginal part of the cervix** (**A10**) protrudes into the vagina (**AB11**), and the **supravaginal part of the cervix** (**A12**) lies above the vagina. The cervical end of the vaginal part contains an aperture in the uterine cavity, known as the **external os of the uterus** (**AC13**), which is bounded anteriorly by the *anterior lip* (**B14**) and posteriorly by the *posterior lip* (**B15**).

Uterine cavity (**C**). The slitlike, mucosa-lined **uterine cavity** (**C16**) resembles an inverted triangle lying in the frontal plane, with the paired uterine tubes extending from each of its upper corners. The lower apex of the triangle continues as the canal of the isthmus through the **histological**

internal os (**C17**) to the cervical canal, opening by the **external os of the uterus** (**AC13**) into the vagina. The **cervical canal** (**C18**) is spindle-shaped, and its surface structure is marked by *palmate folds* (**C19**). Its mucosa contains *cervical glands*, which produce a mucus that closes the cervical canal like a plug. In the uterine cavity, the distance from the external os of the uterus to the fundus is about 6 cm.

Position of the uterus. The position of the uterus depends on the contents of the nearby hollow organs (urinary bladder and rectum). When the urinary bladder is empty, the uterus as a whole is generally tilted forward (**anteversion**), while its body is flexed anteriorly toward the cervix (**anteflexion**). The term **uterine position** refers to the position of the uterus or its deviation from the median sagittal plane.

> **Clinical note.** In clinical practice, the vaginal part of the cervix is sometimes referred to as the "**portio**" of the cervix; the "**external os**" is distinguished from the "**internal os**," which refers to the canal of the isthmus. During pregnancy, the isthmus of the uterus widens and is known as the "**lower uterine segment**." The internal vertical diameter from the portio to the fundus is 6–7 cm. This distance can be measured with a graduated probe.

Age-related uterine changes. In the **neonate**, the uterus is a tubular organ that extends beyond the lesser pelvis. The cervix of the uterus is relatively long compared with its body. The organ does not assume the typical shape described above until **sexual maturity**. During **menstruation**, the uterus is slightly enlarged and more highly vascularized, and during **pregnancy** it becomes so enlarged that it extends into the epigastric region. In **advanced age**, the uterus atrophies; its body remains large, while the cervix shrinks markedly. In a woman who has never had a vaginal birth, the **external os** is round; after the first vaginal birth, it becomes a horizontal, slitlike opening.

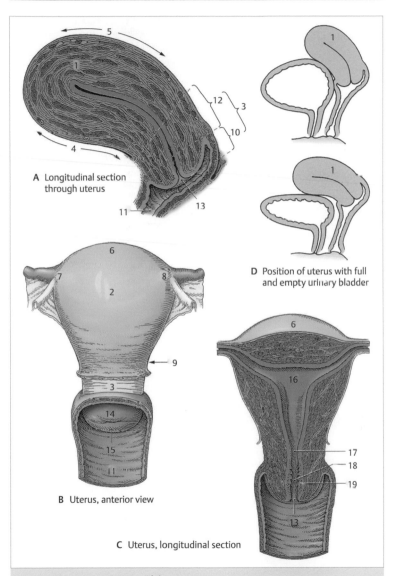

A Longitudinal section through uterus

B Uterus, anterior view

C Uterus, longitudinal section

D Position of uterus with full and empty urinary bladder

Fig. 7.5 Macroscopic structure of the uterus.

Microscopic Anatomy
Layers of the Uterine Wall (A)

The mucosal layer that lines the luminal surface of the uterine cavity is known as the **endometrium** (**AC1**). The thickest layer in the walls of the uterus is the strong muscular layer, or **myometrium** (**AC2**). Parts of the body and fundus of the uterus are lined by parietal peritoneum, known as the **serosa** or **perimetrium** (**AC3**). Lying alongside the lateral *borders of the uterus* (**A4**) is connective tissue known as the **parametrium** (**AC5**). The connective tissue to the right and left of the cervix is known as the **paracervix**.

Microscopic Anatomy of the Body of the Uterus

Endometrium. The endometrial lining of the body of the uterus rests directly on top of the muscular layer. It contains *cell-rich connective tissue with few fibers.* Its *simple columnar epithelium* contains *ciliated cells* and invaginates to form the tubular *uterine glands.* The endometrium can be divided into two layers: a **functional layer** (**II + III**), or "functionalis," which undergoes cyclic changes, and a **basal layer** (**I**), or "basalis," which is not shed during menstruation and gives rise to cyclical regeneration of the endometrium.

Menstrual cycle (**B**). During childbearing years, the functional layer of the endometrium is subject to cyclic changes brought about by ovarian hormones. In the **proliferative phase** (days 5–14) (**B7**, **B8**), the rejected functional layer is restored under the influence of *estradiol* and the glands increase in size. This is followed by the **secretory phase** (days 15–28) (**B9**, **B10**), in which the glands continue to grow under the influence of *progesterone and estrogen* and produce a viscous secretion; blood vessels multiply and extend. The zone containing the tubular parts of the glands becomes the *spongy layer* (**II**). Superficial to this zone is a dense zone called the *compact layer* (**III**), in which large, epithelioid stromal cells, or *pseudodecidual cells,* appear. If the ovum is not fertilized, "hormone withdrawal" occurs and the endometrium degenerates. This is known as the **ischemic phase**, which lasts several hours and leads to tissue damage followed by bleeding and sloughing off of the functional layer in the **desquamation phase**, or menstruation (days 1–4) (**B6**).

> **Clinical note. Curettage** removes the functional layer, leaving intact the basal layer, which is closely interlinked with the *subvascular layer* of the myometrium. Endometrial tissue can migrate from the uterine cavity to the ovary or pelvic peritoneum, producing the clinical condition of **endometriosis**.

Myometrium. The myometrium is by far the thickest part of the uterine wall. It is composed of *smooth muscle cells, connective tissue,* and *vessels.* **Three layers of muscle** can be distinguished in the body and the fundus of the uterus, of which the **middle layer** is the thickest. The middle layer has a very rich blood supply, lending it a spongelike appearance. Its muscle cells form a three-dimensional meshwork that mostly parallels the surface of the uterus. The middle layer is the *main layer helping to expel the fetus* during birth. The **inner** (subvascular) and **outer** (supravascular) muscle layers are thin.

> **Clinical note.** During **pregnancy**, enlargement of smooth muscle cells enables rapid growth of the uterus to about 7–10 times its original size. Benign tumors of the myometrium are called leiomyomas, myomas for short, or fibroids.

Microscopic Anatomy of the Cervix

The **mucosa of the cervix of the uterus** is not subject to the cyclic degeneration and restoration of the uterine mucosa; it does not have functional and basal layers. Its *columnar epithelium* overlies a layer of *fibrocellular connective tissue.* The **cervical glands** are branching, tubular epithelial invaginations (**D11**) that produce an alkaline mucus. Unlike other regions of the cervix, the **vaginal part** is covered by *stratified, nonkeratinized squamous epithelium.*

> **Clinical note.** The abrupt transition between the columnar epithelium of the cervical canal and the portio forms a **transformation zone** that in women of childbearing age can be readily visualized and examined by colposcopy. With increasing age, this area extends *into* the cervical canal. The transformation zone is the most common site of **cervical carcinoma**.

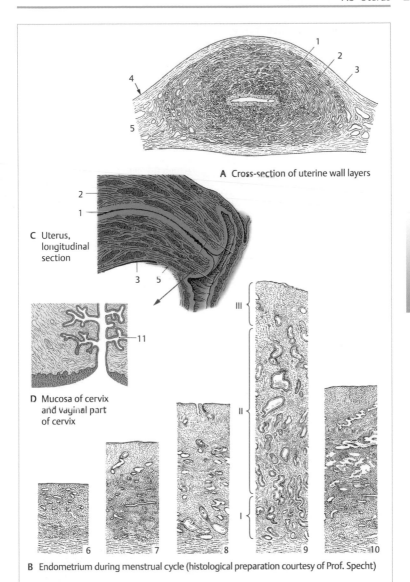

A Cross-section of uterine wall layers

C Uterus, longitudinal section

D Mucosa of cervix and vaginal part of cervix

B Endometrium during menstrual cycle (histological preparation courtesy of Prof. Specht)

Fig. 7.6 Microscopic structure of the uterus.

Vessels, Nerves, and Lymphatic Drainage

Arteries. The uterus (**AB1**) mainly receives its blood supply from the **uterine artery** (← internal iliac artery) (**A2**). It courses in subperitoneal connective tissue over the ureter (**A3**), to the base of the broad ligament of the uterus (arrow), and reaches the wall of the uterus near the cervix. After dividing, it runs along the lateral uterine wall as the tortuous *ascending main branch* and the *descending vaginal artery* (**A4**). At the fundus of the uterus, the ascending main branch joins its counterpart from the opposite side and gives rise to an *ovarian branch* (**A5**), which in turn joins the *ovarian artery* (**A6**) and a *tubal branch* (**A7**) to the uterine tube.

Veins. A network of valveless veins forms the **uterine plexus** (**A8**) around the body and cervix of the uterus. It drains via the *uterine veins* (**A9**) into the *internal iliac veins* and is located in the parametrium.

Lymphatic drainage. Lymph from the body and fundus mostly flows in *three* directions: along the *suspensory ligament of the ovary* to the **lymph nodes along the aorta**; along the *round ligament of the uterus* to the **superficial inguinal nodes**; and via the *broad ligament of the uterus* to the **lymph nodes along the division of the common iliac artery**, which also collect a part of the lymph from the cervix of the uterus. Additional lymphatic vessels pass from the cervix to the parietal lymph nodes along the internal iliac artery and posteriorly to the sacral nodes.

Nerves. Autonomic innervation is via the *inferior hypogastric plexus* (*pelvic plexus*) and *pelvic splanchnic nerves* (S2–S4), which form a plexus lateral to the cervix with large ganglion cells known as the **uterovaginal plexus** (**A10**) (Frankenhäuser ganglion).

Functions. In the nonpregnant state, the uterus prevents bacteria from entering the uterine and abdominal cavities through the vagina. It also undergoes cyclical preparations to receive the ovum, and during pregnancy is the **site of development of the embryo and fetus**. At birth it **expels the fetus**.

Support of the Uterus

The **peritoneal relations** of the uterus are described in the section on peritoneal relations in the female pelvis (see p. 268).

The anatomical and clinical literature describes various connective tissues as **"ligaments"** attaching the uterus to adjacent structures. They are attributed with a *supporting function*. In the official nomenclature, these are known as the round ligament of the uterus (**B11**), the broad ligament of the uterus (**AB12**), the rectouterine ligament, and the rectouterinus muscle.

The **round ligament of the uterus** arises near the uterine horns. It has smooth muscle cells and runs through the inguinal canal, ending in the subcutaneous fat tissue of the labia majora. It is *derived from the gonadal fold* and is a continuation of the *suspensory ligament of the ovary*.

The **broad ligament of the uterus** is a *peritoneal fold* between the lateral margin of the uterus and the lateral pelvic wall. It contains connective tissue, vessels, and nerves.

The **rectouterine fold** is a *peritoneal fold bounding the rectouterine pouch*. It is formed by dense subperitoneal connective tissue and nerves of the (autonomic) inferior hypogastric nerve plexus. Its connective tissue originates alongside the cervix and ascends to the posterolateral pelvic wall. It is also known as the **rectouterine ligament** or **sacrouterine ligament**. There is disagreement in the literature about whether it contains the smooth **rectouterinus** muscle.

A band called the **cardinal ligament** (Mackenrodt ligament) is frequently described in clinical practice. It consists of a condensation of connective tissue that presumably fixes the cervix to the lateral pelvic wall. Of the structures named above, the literature agrees only on the existence of the round ligament of the uterus and the broad ligament of the uterus. The uterus is mainly *supported* by the *pelvic floor muscles*, not by the above-mentioned ligaments.

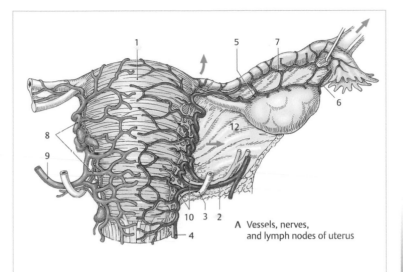

A Vessels, nerves, and lymph nodes of uterus

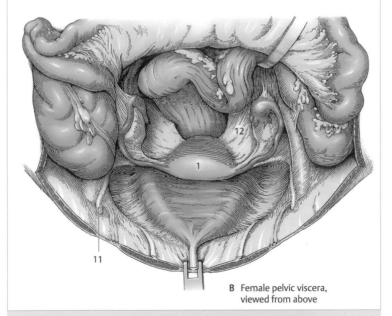

B Female pelvic viscera, viewed from above

Fig. 7.7 Vessels, nerves, and lymphatic drainage of the uterus, uterine suspensory ligaments.

Female Genital System

7.4 Vagina and External Genitalia

Gross Anatomy

The **vagina** (**AB1**) is a thin-walled, hollow fibromuscular organ. It extends from the cervix of the uterus (**A2**) to the **vaginal orifice** (**A3**) in the **vestibule of the vagina**. Located just *anterior* to the vagina are the urinary bladder (**A4**) and urethra (**AB5**); *posterior* to it are the rectum (**A6**) and anal canal (**A7**). The vagina extends approximately along the pelvic axis. Its frontal aspect is flattened, and its anterior and posterior walls touch, bounding an H-shaped crevice (**B**). The posterior wall of the vagina is 1.5–2-cm longer than its anterior wall. The superior end of the vagina surrounds the cervix of the uterus (**A**), forming the **vaginal fornix**, which has a flat *anterior part* (**A8**), a deep *posterior part* (**A9**), and a *lateral part*. The widest part of the vagina is at the vaginal fornix. The posterior part of the fornix extends to the deepest point of the rectouterine pouch (**A10**). The rather narrow lower one-third of the vagina is below the levator hiatus. The **vaginal orifice** is bounded by the **hymen** or **hymenal caruncles** (see below).

Mucosal landmarks (**C**). The vaginal mucosa contains transverse folds called **vaginal rugae** (**C11**), as well as longitudinal folds called **vaginal columns** produced by well-developed *venous plexuses* in the walls of the vagina. The anterior vaginal column is continuous with the prominent **urethral carina of the vagina** (**C12**) which is produced by the nearby urethra.

Microscopic Anatomy

Vaginal wall. The wall of the vagina is composed of a thin **muscular layer** chiefly consisting of a *meshwork of smooth muscle* and *elastic fibers*. The vagina is embedded in the surrounding tissues by its connective tissue adventitia known as the **paracolpium**.

Mucosa. The vaginal mucosa is composed of **glycogen-rich, stratified, nonkeratinized squamous epithelium** lying on top of a lamina propria. The vaginal epithelium, consisting of basal, parabasal, intermediate, and superficial layers, undergoes *cyclic changes*, which are expressed, for instance, by the varying levels of glycogen stored in the epithelial cells evident in histological preparations. There are no glands in the walls of the vagina. **Vaginal fluid** is made up of a *transudate from the venous plexuses* in the vaginal walls, *cervical secretion*, and *exfoliated epithelial cells*. Its slightly acidic pH of 4.0–4.5 results from *lactic acid* produced by the breakdown of glycogen in exfoliated epithelial cells, by lactic acid (*Döderlein*) bacteria.

Vessels, Nerves, and Lymphatic Drainage (D)

Arteries. The vagina is supplied by the **vaginal branches** (**D13**) from the *uterine artery* and by branches from the *inferior vesical artery* (**D14**) and *internal pudendal artery* (**D15**).

Veins. Venous drainage is to the **vaginal venous plexus** lying adjacent to the vagina. The vaginal venous plexus is connected to the venous plexuses of the adjacent urogenital organs and drains to the *internal iliac veins*.

Nerves. Autonomic innervation of the vagina, like that of the uterus, is provided by the **uterovaginal nerve plexus**. The inferior parts of the vagina are innervated by the **pudendal nerve**.

Lymphatic drainage. Lymph from the vagina drains to the **external and internal iliac nodes** as well as to the **superficial inguinal nodes**.

Functions. The vagina acts as an *organ of sexual intercourse* and also serves as a channel for drainage of *cervical secretion* and *menstrual blood*. During childbirth, it is the last, most distal portion of the *birth canal*.

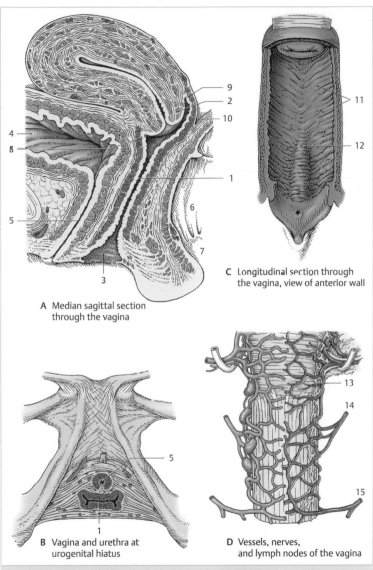

A Median sagittal section through the vagina

C Longitudinal section through the vagina, view of anterior wall

B Vagina and urethra at urogenital hiatus

D Vessels, nerves, and lymph nodes of the vagina

Fig. 7.8 Macroscopic and microscopic structure of the vagina.

Female Genital System

External Genitalia

Mons pubis and labia majora. The female external genitalia are located below, or outside of, the pelvic floor. The anterior portion consists of the **mons pubis** (**A1**), a *skin-covered fat pad* overlying the pubic symphysis, which is covered with terminal hair after puberty. The **pubic hair** continues caudally onto the **labia majora pudendi** (**A2**), prominent longitudinal folds that extend from the mons pubis to the perineum (**A3**) and cover the **pudendal cleft**. They correspond to the scrotum in the male. The labia majora meet anteriorly at the **anterior commissure of the labia majora** (**A4**) and posteriorly at the **posterior commissure of the labia majora** (**A5**). Their outer surfaces are lined with pigmented skin containing smooth muscle cells, hair, and sebaceous and sweat glands. The epithelium lining their inner surfaces is poorly keratinized; the skin contains sebaceous glands, but is devoid of hair. The labia majora are basically composed of *fat pads* and *venous plexuses*. The **bulb of the vestibule** (**B6**) is a large venous plexus invested in fascia and covered by the *bulbospongiosus muscle* (**B7**). It forms a mass of erectile tissue and corresponds to the corpus spongiosum of the penis in the male. The two bulbs of the vestibule are connected anteriorly by the thin *commissure of bulbs*.

Labia minora. The **labia minora of the pudenda** (**AB8**), thin folds of skin that are devoid of fat, bound the *vestibule of the vagina* (**AB9**). They are connected posteriorly by the **frenulum of the labia minora** (**A10**), which is obliterated by the first vaginal birth. Anteriorly, the labia minora taper into two folds each: the two inner folds form the **frenulum of the clitoris** (**A11**), passing to the clitoris, and the two outer folds unite in front of the clitoris to form the **prepuce of the clitoris** (**A12**). The labia minora consist of a thin epidermal covering overlying *connective tissue* and *sebaceous glands*.

Vestibule of the vagina. The urethra opens into the anterior portion of the **vestibule of the vagina** via the **external urethral orifice** (**AB13**), and the vagina opens in the posterior portion through the **vaginal orifice** (**AB14**), which may be partially closed off by the **hymen**. There is great individual variation in the size of the hymen. It ruptures upon initial intercourse, but its remnants remain and after vaginal birth are known as the **hymenal caruncles** (**A15**). On either side of the vaginal orifice, at the termination of each of the vestibular bulbs here, are the bean-sized **greater vestibular glands** (Bartholin glands), which open via a 1.5–2-cm long excretory duct into the vestibule of the vagina. The **lesser vestibular glands** secrete a mucoid discharge.

Clitoris. The clitoris is an erectile, sensory organ (corpuscular nerve endings, tactile corpuscles) made up of the **crus of the clitoris** (**B16**), **body of the clitoris** (**B17**), and **glans of the clitoris** (**B18**). The bulk of the clitoris is formed by the *right and left corpora cavernosa of the clitoris* which arise from paired crura that are attached to the inferior pubic rami, unite to form the unpaired *body of the clitoris*, and end in the *glans of the clitoris*. In the body of the clitoris, the two corpora cavernosa are partially divided by the *septum of the corpora cavernosa*. In a similar fashion to the penis, the clitoris is attached to the inferior border of the pubic symphysis by the **suspensory ligament of the clitoris** (see Vol. 1) (**B19**). The crura of the corpora cavernosa are covered by the *ischiocavernosus muscle* (**B20**).

Vessels, Nerves, and Lymphatic Drainage

Arteries. The terminal branches of the *internal pudendal artery* supply the female external genitalia.

Veins. Venous drainage is via the internal pudendal vein, external pudendal veins, and deep posterior vein of the clitoris (to the vesical venous plexus).

Nerves. Innervation is by branches from the *pudendal nerve*, *ilio-inguinal nerve*, and *genitofemoral nerve*.

Lymphatic drainage. Lymph from the external genitalia drains to the *inguinal nodes*.

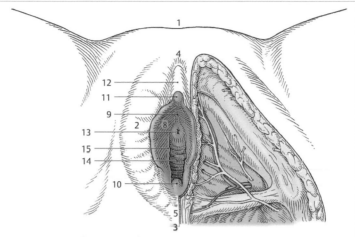

A Female external genitalia and superficial perineal compartment

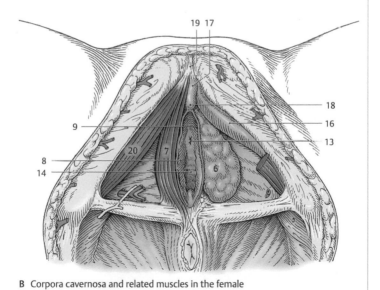

B Corpora cavernosa and related muscles in the female

Fig. 7.9 External genitalia.

7.5 Topographical Anatomy

Cross-Sectional Anatomy

Transverse Section at the Level of the Hip Joints (A)

The section cuts anteriorly through the *superior pubic rami* (**A1**) and posteriorly through the *top of the coccygeal vertebrae* (**A2**). On the lateral pelvic wall, the section cuts through the *obturator internus* (**A3**) covering the entrance to the *obturator canal* (**A4**). Laterally and posteriorly, the *sacrospinal ligament* (**A5**) can be seen, including its attachment on the *ischial spine* (**A6**). The *rectum* (**A7**) lies in front of the coccyx and is surrounded by an adventitial layer of adipose and connective tissue containing numerous *superior rectal vessels* (**A8**), which are also visible. Anterior to the rectum is the *rectouterine pouch* (pouch of Douglas) (**A9**), the deepest point in the female peritoneal cavity. Its peritoneal lining covers the posterior side of the *cervix of the uterus* (**A10**). Numerous *uterine vessels* (**A11**) can be identified in the connective tissue alongside the cervix of the uterus. Passing posterolaterally from the cervix is a band of dense connective tissue known as the *rectouterine ligament* (**A12**). The *urinary bladder* (**A13**) can be seen in front of the uterus just above the site where the *ureter* (**A14**) joins the urinary bladder. The anterior and lateral surfaces of the urinary bladder are covered by abundant adipose tissue. Irrespective of their structure and origin, the connective tissues alongside the rectum are known in clinical practice as the *paraproctium*, those alongside the cervix as the *paracervix*, and those alongside the urinary bladder as the *paracystium*.

A15 Gluteus maximus, **A16** Sciatic nerve, **A17** Ligament of head of femur, **A18** Head of femur, **A19** Neck of femur, **A20** Pectineus, **A21** Iliopsoas, **A22** Femoral vessels, **A23** Femoral nerve

Transverse Section at the Level of the Ischial Tuberosities (B)

The section cuts anteriorly through the *pubic symphysis* (**B24**) and posteriorly through the *tip of the coccyx*. Laterally, the pelvic viscera rest against parts of the

levator ani (**B25**) (*pubococcygeus* **B25 a**, *iliococcygeus* **B25 b**). The section cuts through the *rectum* (**B7**) above the *anorectal flexure* and thus diagonally through its posterior wall. Anterior to the rectum is the *vagina* (**B26**); lateral to the vagina, the numerous vessels of the *vaginal venous plexus* (**B27**) can be seen. The section is through the *urethra* (**B28**), which is surrounded by striated muscle of the *external urethral sphincter* (**B29**). The *retropubic space* (**B30**) contains adipose tissue with abundant vessels also visible in the section. Outside of the pelvic cavity, the *ischioanal fossa* (**B31**) can be observed. Lying in its lateral wall is the *pudendal canal* (**B32**) containing the *pudendal vessels* and *pudendal nerve*.

B33 Obturator externus

> **Clinical note.** Modern imaging techniques are used, for instance, to assess tumor size and spread. In female patients, this can include an evaluation of *rectal and bladder tumors*, as well as other malignancies involving the *body and cervix of the uterus* and the *ovaries*. Imaging procedures are a necessary part of surgical preparation for correctly determining malignant spread to subperitoneal connective tissue and adjacent organ systems.

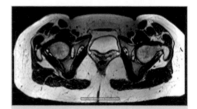

Fig. 7.10C Corresponding plane to Fig. 7.10A on MRI.

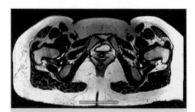

Fig. 7.10D Corresponding plane to Fig. 7.10B on MRI.

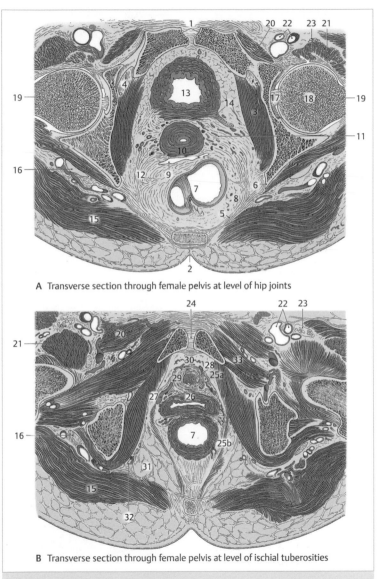

A Transverse section through female pelvis at level of hip joints

B Transverse section through female pelvis at level of ischial tuberosities

Fig. 7.10 Cross-sectional anatomy.

7.6 Comparative Anatomy of the Female and Male Pelves

Soft Tissue Closure of the Pelvis

The pelvic outlet is covered by the muscles of the **pelvic floor** in such a manner that the rectum and urogenital organs can still open properly.

The pelvic floor consists of the levator ani (**AB1**) and ischiococcygeus (**AB2**) muscles. The levator ani can be further subdivided into three major components: the *pubococcygeus* (**C1 a**) and *iliococcygeus* (**C1 b**), which form a muscular sheet that closes the pelvis and supports the pelvic and abdominal viscera in their normal anatomical position; and the *puborectalis* (**A–C1 c**), which arises from the pubis and forms a sling around the rectum at the level of the anorectal flexure. It supports rectal continence and, along with the medial fibers from the other levator muscles, compresses portions of the urogenital organs passing through the *levator hiatus* (**C3**). The muscle fascia covering the levator ani on the side facing the pelvis is known as the **superior fascia of the pelvic diaphragm**, and that covering the muscle on its outer surface is known as the **inferior fascia of the pelvic diaphragm**.

Similar to the bony pelvis, whose features differ between men and women, the levator ani also exhibits **sex-specific differences**. In the woman (**A**), the levator ani contains more connective tissue than in the man (**B**), in whom the pelvic floor muscles are on the whole better developed, which, in particular, results in a higher puborectalis.

AB4 Coccyx, **AB5** Femur, **AB6** Sacrum with coccyx, **AB7** Piriformis, **AB8** Obturator internus with superior and inferior gemelli, **AB9** Quadratus femoris, **AB10** Ischial tuberosity, **AB11** Ischial spine, **AB12** Anococcygeal body, **AB13** Anus, **A14** Pudendal canal, **A15** Sciatic nerve, **A16** Hamstrings

> **Clinical note.** Especially in women who have had multiple vaginal births, the pelvic floor muscles have a tendency to become lax with age under the pressure of the viscera resting on them. The result is a pelvic floor dysfunction or insufficiency, which may lead to organ **prolapse or incontinence**, that is, the inability to maintain closure of the excretory passages.

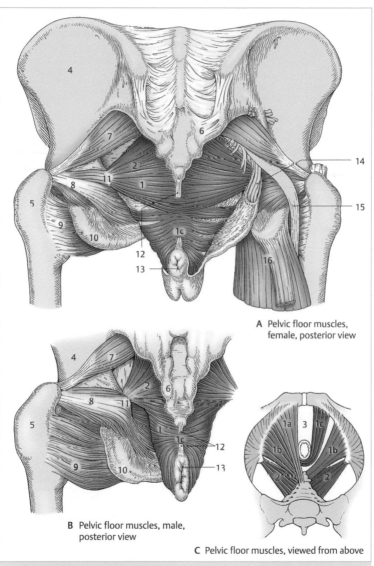

A Pelvic floor muscles, female, posterior view

B Pelvic floor muscles, male, posterior view

C Pelvic floor muscles, viewed from above

Fig. 7.11 Pelvic soft tissue floor.

Female Genital System

290 **Female Genital System**

Transverse Section through the Perineal Region in the Male (A)

The posterior part of the section is through the *anal opening* (**A1**) and surrounding *external anal sphincter* (**AB2**). Lateral and anterior to the anal opening is the fat body of the *ischioanal fossa* (**AB3**). In front of the anal canal, the section cuts through the transverse striated muscle fibers and connective tissue of the *superficial transverse perineal muscle* (**A4**). Arising on either side from the *inferior pubic ramus* (**AB5**) is the *ischiocavernosus muscle* (**AB6**), which encloses the *crus of the penis* (**A7**). Between the crura of the penis is the *bulb of the penis* (**A8**), in which the *male urethra* is visible anteriorly (**A9**).

The surrounding striated *external urethral sphincter* is visible in the section. Alongside the tangential section through *part of the penis*, the *spermatic cord* (**A10**) can be seen on either side.

AB11 Adductor muscles

Transverse Section through the Perineal Region in the Female (B)

The section lies above the anal opening, cutting through the *anal canal* (**B12**), which is surrounded by the sphincter complex consisting of the *internal anal sphincter* (**B13**), *longitudinal muscle*, and *external anal sphincter* (**B2**). Anterior to the anal canal is the *vagina* (**B14**), the anterior wall of which is firmly joined to the *urethra* (**B15**). As in sections through the male pelvis, the origin of the *ischiocavernosus muscle* (**B6**), which encloses the *crura of the clitoris* (**B16**), can be identified on either side. The *bulb of the vestibule* (**B17**) surrounds the *vaginal and urethral openings*.

Ischioanal Fossa

Lying outside of the pelvic floor on either side of the anal canal is the *ischioanal fossa* (green in the figure shown in the text, **AB3**), a pyramidal space filled by the *fat body of the ischioanal fossa*. The **base** of the ischioanal fossa is covered by *perineal skin* (**18**), and its **apex** is near the union of the *levator ani* and *obturator internus*. The space is bounded **medially** by the *external anal sphincter* (**2**) and *levator ani* (**19**), that is, its fascia, the *inferior fascia of the pelvic diaphragm* and **laterally** the *ischial tuberosity* (**20**) and *obturator fascia*. **Posteriorly**, the space is covered by the *gluteus*

maximus (**21**) and *sacrotuberous ligament;* **anteriorly**, it extends to the posterior border of the *urogenital diaphragm.*

Clinical note. The *internal pudendal vessels* and the pudendal nerve course in the lateral wall of the ischioanal fossa. They lie protected in a fascial sheath of the obturator internus known as the *pudendal canal (Alcock canal).*

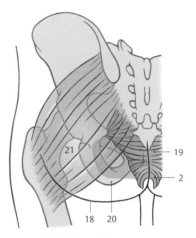

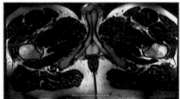

Fig. 7.12C Corresponding plane to Fig. 7.12A on MRI.

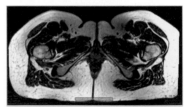

Fig. 7.12D Corresponding plane to Fig. 7.12B on MRI.

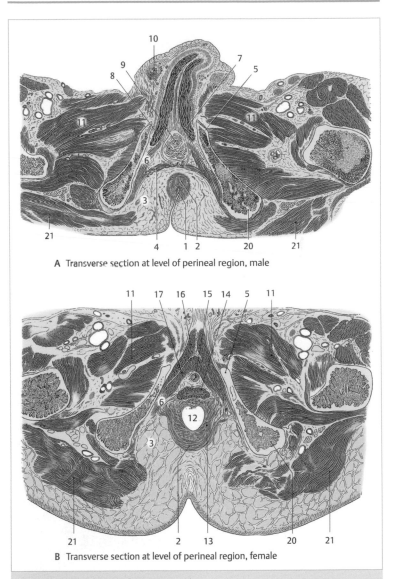

A Transverse section at level of perineal region, male

B Transverse section at level of perineal region, female

Fig. 7.12 Pelvic soft tissue floor, continued.

Female Genital System

8 Pregnancy and Human Development

8.1 Gametes

All cells contain genetic information in threadlike DNA (deoxyribonucleic acid) molecules consisting of a double helix. Genetic information is carried in the cells of the human body in a diploid set of chromosomes consisting of 46 chromosomes, that is, 44 autosomes, and two sex chromosomes (heterosomes). Before cell division (**mitosis**), the DNA is replicated so that the division produces two identical daughter cells, each with a diploid set of chromosomes.

Fertilization (conception), the *union* of an egg cell and a sperm cell, involves fusion of the two cell nuclei, which carry genetic material from the father and mother. Since all members of a given species have the same number of chromosomes, the number of chromosomes carried by the uniting gametes must be halved (to yield a haploid set of chromosomes) before fertilization. This process of reduction is known as **meiosis**, producing **gametes** (**oocytes** and **spermatozoa**) for the purpose of sexual reproduction, each of which possesses a haploid set of chromosomes (23 X or 23 Y). The union of the male and female haploid gametes produces a diploid zygote that can undergo cell division, or mitosis. The nucleus of the zygote contains one set each of the mother's and father's chromosomes (46 XX or 46 XY).

In the *first stage of meiosis* the homologous chromosomes are divided, and in the *second stage of meiosis* the chromatids are divided.

Spermatocyte meiosis occurs in the convoluted seminiferous tubules in the testes and results in four gametes (*spermatids*) of equal size.

The **oocyte** undergoes the first meiotic division before ovulation. The resulting cells are *unequal* in size; the smaller daughter cell is known as the **polar body** (**A1**). At the time of *impregnation* (penetration of the egg cell by a **spermatozoon [AB2]**), the egg cell is still in the second meiotic division, during which a further rudimentary cell, the **second polar body** (**B–D3**), arises as well as the large, haploid **oocyte** that contains the **pronucleus** (**BC4**). (A third polar body may occasionally be present, presumably arising from a second meiotic division of the first polar body.)

The mature ovum (**A5**) has a thick, acellular glycoprotein coat known as the **zona pellucida** (clear membrane) (**A–E6**), which is mostly a product of the **follicular epithelial cells** (**AE7**). This pushes the follicular epithelial cells (granulosa cells), in this stage also known as **corona radiata cells** (**AE7**), away from the surface of the egg cell; yet, via their long, thin processes (**E8**) passing through the zona pellucida, they form a nexus (connexin 37) and remain in contact with the cell membrane (**E9**). In some areas, the processes project into the surface of the oocyte producing nodular elevations (**E10**).

Biological sex is genetically determined at the time of fertilization, by the combination of chromosomes: two X chromosomes (XX) produce a female offspring and the combination XY produces a male offspring. After meiosis, during which a single set of chromosomes is halved, the "mature" (haploid) oocyte has an X chromosome and the "mature" spermatozoon has either an X or a Y chromosome. At the time of fertilization, the spermatozoon determines the sex of the gamete.

C13 Male pronucleus, **E11** Oocyte cytoplasm, **E12** Nucleus of oocyte

Ejaculate (semen, seminal fluid) is composed of a cellular part and a fluid part. The *cellular component* consists mainly of **spermatozoa**, as well as sloughed-off epithelial cells from the genital tract. The *fluid component* of semen, known as **seminal plasma**, consists of fluid secreted in the epididymis and accessory sex glands (prostate, seminal vesicle). The *ejaculate volume* is 2.0 mL or more, and the *total sperm count* is 40×10^6 per ejaculation or more. The chances of fertilization are significantly diminished at levels below 20×10^6 sperm per milliliter.

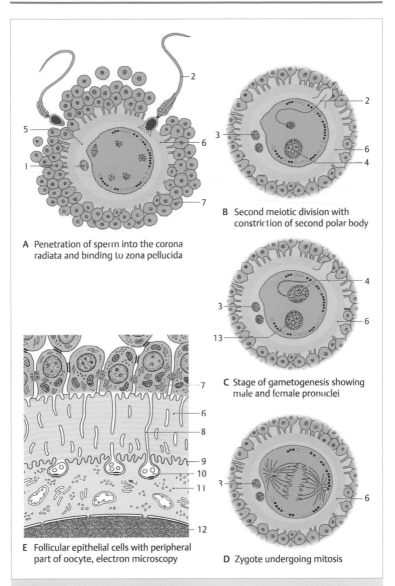

A Penetration of sperm into the corona radiata and binding to zona pellucida

B Second meiotic division with constriction of second polar body

C Stage of gametogenesis showing male and female pronuclei

D Zygote undergoing mitosis

E Follicular epithelial cells with peripheral part of oocyte, electron microscopy

Fig. 8.1 Gametes.

8.2 Fertilization

Before **fertilization** can occur, the *spermatozoa must travel* through the female reproductive tract. Their migration is chiefly influenced by the hormonal milieu of the female genital tract. A woman's fertility depends on the ability of the spermatozoa to successfully traverse the cervical canal and reach the *ampulla of the uterine tube*, where fertilization can take place under physiologic conditions.

For most of the menstrual cycle, the cervical canal is closed by thick *cervical mucus*, preventing ascension of the spermatozoa. Increasing estrogen levels cause the cervical mucus to become watery, stringy, and alkaline, which assists migration of sperm cells. Most importantly, the mucosal plug stopping the external os becomes passable.

Capacitation and Acrosome Reaction

After migration, sperm cells undergo **capacitation**, a process that is also assisted by estrogen. Capacitation is a biochemical and physiological "maturation process" that allows the sperm cell to penetrate an egg cell. The resulting changes to the plasma membrane of the spermatozoa are necessary for the subsequent **acrosome reaction**. Perforation and vesiculation of its plasma membrane and outer acrosomal membrane causes leakage of *lysosomal enzymes*, including a protease called acrosin. This enables the sperm cell to penetrate the *corona radiata* and *zona pellucida:* the spermatozoon (**B1**) first binds to **receptors** (**B2**) in the zona pellucida (**B3**) and, after penetrating the zona pellucida, enters the narrow **perivitelline space** (**C4**) between the zona pellucida and the surface of the egg cell. The acrosome reaction consists of fusion of the inner acrosomal membrane with the plasma membrane of the egg cell. After this, the penetrating sperm cell lies without a cell membrane, within the cytoplasm of the egg cell. The acrosome thus resembles a large lysosome that envelops the apex of the cell nucleus.

Formation of the Zygote

After the sperm cell penetrates the egg cell, the second polar body is expelled, a sign of completion of the second meiotic division. The egg cell itself reacts to contact with the sperm cell and penetration in various ways. Membrane receptors trigger a cortical reaction: **cortical vesicles** (**B5**) in the egg cell release their contents (cortical granules, enzymes) into the perivitelline space (**CD4**), causing structural changes to the egg cell that block fertilization by more than one sperm cell (**D1**).

B–D3 Zona pellucida, **B–D4** Perivitelline space, **B–D6** Plasma membrane of egg cell, **D7** Emptied cortical vesicles

At the same time, *decondensation of sperm chromatin* occurs, visible as swelling of the sperm head. Under the influence of *growth factors*, a male pronucleus develops and the haploid nucleus of the oocyte swells to form a female pronucleus. The union of the two pronuclei produces a zygote with a diploid set of chromosomes (see Fig. **CD**, p. 295).

Contact between the sperm and egg cells immediately *depolarizes* the oocyte membrane and induces *activation of egg metabolism*. Translation of preformed RNA begins and new RNA is formed; *protein synthesis* increases. The process of mitosis begins and biological sex is genetically determined. Upon fertilization, genetically programmed development begins.

Figure **A** summarizes important reactions before and during the process of fertilization.

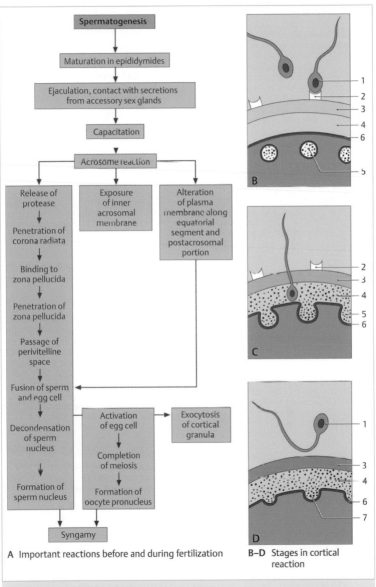

A Important reactions before and during fertilization

B–D Stages in cortical reaction

Pregnancy and Human Development

Fig. 8.2 Spermatozoal reactions, zygote formation.

8.3 Early Development

Ovulation is the release of the egg cell with its surrounding **zona pellucida** and **corona radiata** (= follicular/granulosa cells), and reception by the **infundibulum of the uterine tube** via the **abdominal ostium of the uterine tube**. Fertilization must occur within 6–12 hours, after which the egg cell is no longer viable. Fertilization normally occurs in the **ampulla of the uterine tube**. The zygote is transported to the uterus within 4 or 5 days, propelled by ciliary action of the tubal epithelial cells, the production (flow) of tubal fluid, and contractions of the muscular wall of the uterine tube. All these actions are regulated by hormones.

Zygote development is also regulated by hormones. The zygote is nourished by substances found in tubal fluid, including pyruvate, lactate, and amino acids.

Cleavage. As it moves through the uterine tube, the zygote undergoes a series of mitotic divisions termed **cleavage**. With each cleavage, the dividing cells, **blastomeres**, become smaller, since they remain encased in the inelastic zona pellucida (**A–C1**), cf. pre-embryonic period (see p. 312).

Morula. By around the 3rd day after conception, the zygote reaches the 16-cell stage, at which point it resembles a mulberry and hence is termed a **morula** (**A**). The morula can be divided into a central, inner cell mass called the **embryoblast** (**BC4**) (embryonic disc) and a covering layer called the **trophoblast** (**BC2**), which later gives rise to the fetal portion of the placenta. In the blastomere stage, the cells resemble each other. In terms of cytology, they are *omnipotent* cells and are indeterminate; thus, as late as the 8-cell stage, complete separation can produce multiple offspring.

Blastocysts. In subsequent stages of development, a fluid-filled cavity arises from the confluence of widened intercellular spaces containing fluid secreted by the blastomeres. The zygote is now referred to as a **blastocyst** (**B**), and the fluid-filled cavity is the **blastocyst cavity** (**BC3**). The cells of the inner cell mass (embryoblast) now lie on one side, and the cells of the outer layer (trophoblast) flatten to form the epithelial wall of the blastocyst (**BC2**).

At the same time, the **endometrium** (**C7**, **C8**) is prepared for blastocyst implantation by progesterone secreted by the **corpus luteum**. The lining of the uterus thickens and becomes more vascularized and receptive to implantation, allowing the blastocyst to burrow into it and receive nourishment. Implantation (**C**) (nidation) of the blastocyst in the endometrium occurs at a favorable site (from which it will not be easily moved), usually in the posterior (**D9**) or anterior wall (**D10**) of the uterine cavity.

C7 Functional layer of endometrium, **C8** Uterine epithelium, **D15** Rectum

Implantation. Implantation (nidation, day 6–7 after conception) involves a series of phases. In the first phase, **apposition**, the blastocyst comes into contact at its **embryonic pole** (**BC4**) (implantation pole) with the epithelium of the *endometrium*. The second phase is **adhesion**, requiring *adhesion molecules*, which are only available for 24 hours (the so-called *window of implantation*). Only then can **invasion** occur: the trophoblast of the embryonic pole proliferates and forms villi, erodes the uterine epithelium, and invades the endometrium (**C6**). Trophoblast cells that come into contact with endometrial cells form the **syncytiotrophoblast**, which contains multiple nuclei without identifiable cell boundaries. Nonfused trophoblast cells produce the inner layer known as the **cytotrophoblast**. The cytotrophoblast consists of a single layer of cuboidal epithelial cells. The previously single-layered trophoblast now consists of two layers (see p. 312).

Clinical note. Implantation outside of the uterine cavity resulting in extrauterine pregnancy (ectopic pregnancy) can occur in the abdominal cavity (**D11**) or ovary (**D12**), demonstrating that the sperm cells can travel into the abdominal cavity and fertilize an egg cell there (abdominal pregnancy). Most ectopic pregnancies are **tubal pregnancies** (**D13**) (in the uterine tube). Implantation of the blastocyst in the uterine tube can erode the mother's vessels and cause life-threatening hemorrhage. Implantation in the isthmus (**D14**) of the uterus results in placenta previa, in which the placenta obstructs the birth canal.

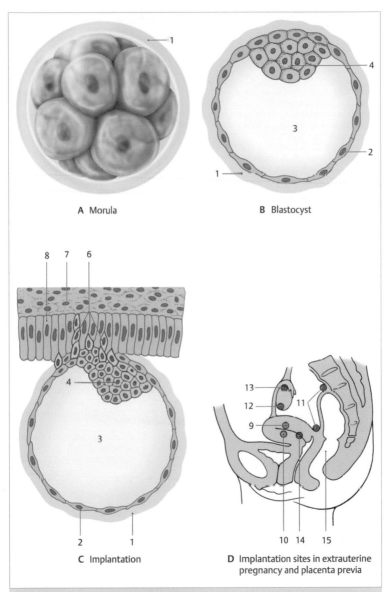

A Morula

B Blastocyst

C Implantation

D Implantation sites in extrauterine pregnancy and placenta previa

Fig. 8.3 Cleavage, morula, blastocyst, implantation.

Pregnancy and Human Development

Implantation and deciduation. After the zona pellucida disintegrates, the nourishing **trophoblast** (in later stages known as the "chorion") (**AB1**) divides to form trophoblast cells which, assisted by the action of enzymes, send projections (implantation, see also **C**, p. 299) into the **endometrium** (**AB2**). The trophoblast cells form the fetal part of the **placenta** (**C3**). At the same time, the *corpus luteum* secretes progesterone which transforms the endometrial cells into edematous, enlarged cells storing glycogen and lipids. This process is known as the **decidual reaction**. It begins in the stromal cells surrounding the implanted blastocyst and later spreads throughout almost the entire endometrium. The portion of the endometrium underlying the implantation site—that is, the portion between the blastocyst and the myometrium—becomes the **decidua basalis**, the maternal part of the placenta (**C4**). The thin endometrial layer overlying the implanted blastocyst becomes the **decidua capsularis**. The endometrial lining of the rest of the uterine cavity forms the **decidua parietalis**. As pregnancy progresses, the decidua capsularis disappears completely.

Amniotic cavity. A cavity, yolk sac, and amniotic cavity develop in the embryoblast above and below the blastocyst. The **yolk sac** (**C5**) degenerates to form a vesicle, and the **amniotic cavity** (**BC6**) grows with the **embryo** (**A–C7**). From the 3rd month of development onward, the embryo is known as a *fetus*. The amniotic cavity contains *amniotic fluid*, approximately one liter by the final stages of pregnancy. The fetus swims in the amniotic fluid, connected to the mother by the umbilical cord. Amniotic fluid prevents adhesion of the fetus to the amnion, cushions it against mechanical trauma, and allows it to move about.

A–C8 Uterine cavity, **A–C9** Myometrium

Clinical note. From week 14 of pregnancy, amniotic fluid can be obtained for testing by **amniocentesis**. Under ultrasound control, a needle is passed through the mother's abdominal wall to aspirate the amniotic cavity via the wall of the uterus.

Pregnancy

Hormones. After ovulation, gonadotropin secretion by the pituitary gland decreases and is taken over by trophoblast cells which synthesize **human chorionic gonadotropin** (**HCG**). Among other functions, HCG maintains the corpus luteum and the prepared endometrial lining. Menstruation does not occur. The *corpus luteum of pregnancy* inhibits contraction of the uterus until the 5th month, after which placental hormones assume this function and the corpus luteum regresses. Immunological protection of the embryo is provided in part by *"early pregnancy factor,"* which is released within a few hours after fertilization.

Pregnancy tests. Human chorionic gonadotropin can be detected in blood and urine samples within 5–6 days after fertilization and is commonly used as the basis for (chemical, biological, or immunological) pregnancy tests. Pregnancy can be detected before a missed menstruation.

Contraception. A vast array of contraceptive measures is currently available. Among the best known are *hormonal contraceptives*, which use substances such as estrogens and gestagen. Oral contraceptives work by inhibiting the release of gonadotropin by interrupting the signal for hormone secretion to the hypothalamus and in turn the pituitary gland, thereby eliminating the mid-cycle luteinizing hormone/follicle-stimulating hormone (LH/FSH) peak and ovulation (**ovulation inhibitors**).

Other options include **intrauterine contraceptive devices** (IUDs), chemical or mechanical **barrier methods** (e.g., spermicides, diaphragm, cervical cap, or condom), and inhibition of sperm motility by gestagens (**mini pill**).

Figure **D** shows the position of the uterus in various stages of pregnancy.

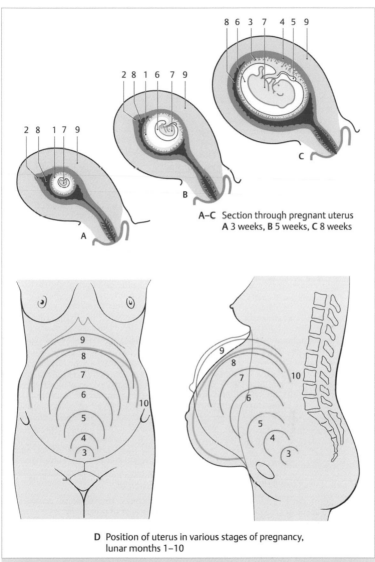

A–C Section through pregnant uterus
A 3 weeks, B 5 weeks, C 8 weeks

D Position of uterus in various stages of pregnancy,
lunar months 1–10

Fig. 8.4 Decidualization, amniotic cavity, pregnancy.

8.4 Placenta

The placenta (**A1**) is composed of an embryonic/fetal part known as the **chorion frondosum** (**BC2**) and a maternal part known as the **decidua basalis** (**BC3**). The **chorion** (**BC2**) is initially entirely covered by villi, but ultimately only its basal plate remains villous. The villous portion is known as the chorion frondosum, with a villous surface area of 9–14 m²; the remainder of the surface, the nonvillous **chorion laeve**, later fuses with the decidua to form the amnion, which is about 250-μm thick.

At birth the placenta is discoid, approximately 20 cm in diameter and 3–4-cm thick at its center (**A1**), and weighs 350–700 g. The floor of the disk is made up of the *decidua basalis* (consisting of uterine mucosa, maternal decidual cells) and *"extravillous" trophoblast cells*, whose upper part is referred to as the **basal plate** (**BC3**). It bounds the **intervillous space** (**BC7**) on the uterine side. The upper surface of the disk is formed by the **chorionic plate** (**BC2**) and forms the boundary between the placenta and the **amniotic cavity** (**A14**). The chorionic plate is composed of a single layer of amniotic epithelium (**BC15**), amniotic and chorionic connective tissue, and extravillous trophoblast cells with branching umbilical vessels (**C16**). The placental septa (**decidual septa**) (**BC4**) projecting from the basal plate toward the chorionic plate divide the discoidal placenta into smaller, convex units known as **placentomes**, which form **fetomaternal circulatory units**.

Projecting from the chorionic plate (**BC2**) into these convex areas are 30–50 intricately branching villous trees (**C5**). They are attached by **anchoring villi** (**C17**) to the basal plate and anchor the chorionic villous trees to the wall of the uterus (decidua). The space between the chorionic plate, basal plate, and villi is referred to as the **intervillous space** (**BC7**). The intervillous space is a *circulatory compartment* containing approximately 150 mL of the mother's blood, which circulates, bathing the villi from the fetal part of the placenta. The human placenta is thus a *hemochorial placenta*.

Until the end of the 4th month, the villi are covered by a bilayered epithelium, a syncytiotrophoblast, and a cytotrophoblast. The **syncytiotrophoblast** (**BD6**), whose free surface is covered by microvilli surrounded by maternal blood circulating in the intervillous space, is formed by the fusion of cells and does not have any lateral intercellular gaps. It forms the critical barrier between the maternal and fetal circulations, absorbing oxygen, nutrients, hormones, and other substances from the mother's blood and releasing waste products, hormones, and carbon dioxide into it. Oxygen (**BC**, red vessels) is transported by the mother's vessels to the fetal blood, and carbon dioxide is released into the maternal blood (**BC**, blue vessels). The **cytotrophoblast** (*Langhans cells*) (**D8**) initially consists of a continuous layer of cells. It begins to break up during the second half of pregnancy and is reduced to 20% of its original size by the end of pregnancy (see p. 381).

The *uteroplacental arteries* lying in the uterine wall and decidua basalis release maternal blood into the intervillous spaces (**BC7**), through some 200 openings (**BC9**). The blood flows up toward the chorionic plate and into the *subchorial lake* and then back down between the villi to the wide venous outlets (**C10**) of the basal plate.

Placental barrier. The fetal circulation is separated from the maternal circulation by the **placental barrier** (**D11**). (Mother and fetus can have different blood groups.) All nutrients exchanged between maternal and fetal blood cross the placental barrier. In the early stages of placentation, the barrier consists of six layers: the syncytiotrophoblast (**BD6**), cytotrophoblast (**D8**), basal plate, connective tissue of the villi (**D12**), basal lamina of the fetal capillaries (**D13**) and endothelium. Later, it consists of only the syncytiotrophoblast, cytotrophoblast, basal plate, and endothelium.

Clinical note. Lesions or microlesions in the villi can result in leakage of fetal blood into the maternal blood. If the mother is Rh-negative and the fetus is Rh-positive, the mother's immune system can become sensitized, possibly threatening the fetus in later Rh-positive pregnancies by development of Rh antibodies.

C16 Umbilical vessels, umbilical vein shown in red

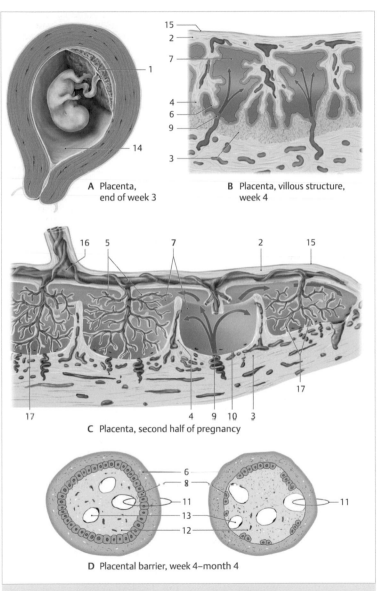

A Placenta,
end of week 3

B Placenta, villous structure,
week 4

C Placenta, second half of pregnancy

D Placental barrier, week 4–month 4

Fig. 8.5 Placenta, placental barrier.

Pregnancy and Human Development

8.5 Birth (Parturition)

Hormones involved in parturition. Delivery of the fetus is regulated by hormones. The fetal adrenal cortex produces *cortisol* and precursors for *estrogen* synthesis and thus plays an important role in the hormonal control of birth. Progesterone, which is produced during the first 4 months of pregnancy by the corpus luteum of pregnancy, and afterward by the placenta, as well as relaxin, inhibit uterine contractions during pregnancy. Birth is immediately preceded by a drop in *progesterone levels*. The resulting increased proportion of estrogen to progesterone depolarizes the myometrial cells, which, until then, have been hyperpolarized by progesterone. Falling progesterone levels also lead to the formation of *gap junctions* between smooth muscle cells, which rapidly transmit impulses between myometrial cells throughout the entire myometrium. There is also an increasing formation of receptors for *oxytocin* and *a-adrenergic* hormones produced in the paraventricular and supraoptic nuclei of the hypothalamus and stored in the posterior lobe of the pituitary gland; the uterus becomes increasingly sensitive to these hormones. The myometrium, sensitized to oxytocin, contracts at regular intervals (**labor**). Delivery requires a **"ripened" cervix**, which **remains closed** for the duration of pregnancy. The strong and firm consistency of the cervix containing *collagen fibers* and *ground substances* softens during the last 2–3 weeks before birth because of the steadily increasing volume of fluid. "Softening" of the cervical connective tissues results in greater elasticity and distensibility. The cervix dilates, allowing the fetal head and body to form the birth canal for delivery. The baby is "packaged" for birth, with its head bent down and its arms and legs crossed (**A**). The head has the largest diameter of all of the fetal body parts; its passage through the birth canal thus enables the rest of the body to pass the cervix easily.

A1 Uterus, **A2** Placenta (umbilical cord hidden from view), **A3** Internal os, **A4** External os, **A5** Urinary bladder, **A6** Rectum, **A7** Vagina

Mechanism of birth. The head is the most helpful part of the fetus' body during birth, leading the body and forming the birth canal around its path. **Cephalic presentation** is the most common delivery presentation (96%); 3% are breech births; oblique or transverse presentation occurs in 1% of births.

The fetal head enters the pelvic inlet (engages) toward the end of pregnancy or at the beginning of labor. The bony pelvis and the soft tissues of the cervix, vagina, and pelvic floor make up the birth canal. In the normal female pelvis, the **pelvic inlet** (indicated by the linea terminalis (**B8**), the boundary between the greater and lesser pelves, see Vol. 1), is an oval aperture that is widest in the transverse plane, while the oval-shaped pelvic outlet (between the pubic symphysis (**C9**), ischial tuberosities (**B10**), and posteriorly convex coccyx (**C11**), see Vol.) is widest in the sagittal plane. The fetal head enters at the largest diameter of each with its largest diameter, that is, the *sagittal* diameter; in other words, it must complete a rotation of about 90°as it passes through the pelvis. After rotation, the head follows the concave path of the pelvis and its soft tissues (**C12**). Before passing below the pubic symphysis (**C9**), the head extends from the flexed position. The shoulders pass through the transverse diameter of the pelvic inlet and then the sagittal diameter of the pelvic outlet; the head, which has already been delivered, makes another 90°turn in the same direction. The obstetrician assists this part of delivery by holding the head and raising and lowering it, allowing the anterior and posterior shoulders to emerge one at a time.

The **soft tissues**—cervix, vagina, and pelvic floor—change shape during birth to form a **soft-tissue tube**.

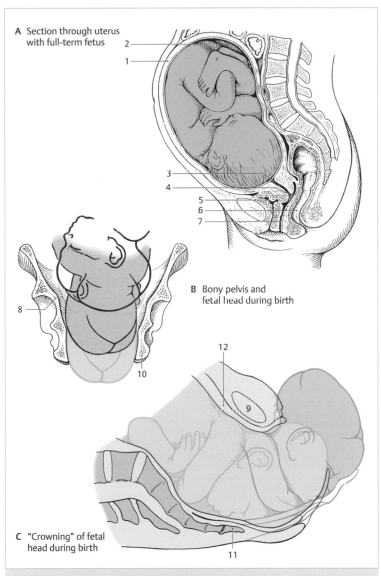

A Section through uterus
with full-term fetus

B Bony pelvis and
fetal head during birth

C "Crowning" of fetal
head during birth

Fig. 8.6 Hormonal control, mechanism of birth.

Dilation Stage

In the **dilation stage** of active labor, the uterus contracts at regular intervals three times every 10 minutes (**labor contractions**). The soft tissues that have kept the uterus closed—the cervix, vagina, and pelvic floor—are distended and stretched to form an anteriorly curving **soft-tissue passageway**. The *levator hiatus* and the *bulbospongiosus* (**F11**) muscle sling stretch and become lax. The pain associated with cervical dilation is due to myometrial contractions and hypoxia, as well as distension of cervical tissue and the tissues of the lesser pelvis. The dilation stage, which generally need not be assisted by active maternal pushing, lasts about 8–12 hours in nulliparous women, and is shorter in multiparous women.

Contractions push the **amniotic sac** ("bag of waters") (**C1**), consisting of the *amnion* and *chorion* ("extraembryonic membranes") and filled with **amniotic fluid** ("the waters"), through the cervix. A part of the sac precedes the head of the fetus (**B–D2**), supporting the elastic stretching of the soft tissues, which were softened by fluid retention during pregnancy. The amniotic sac is pushed further through the cervical canal, passes the dilated external os, and finally appears in the vagina. At the end of the dilation stage, the *bag of waters ruptures*, there is cervical "show," and the frequency of contractions increases. The next stage, the **expulsion stage**, begins.

Cervix of the uterus. Cervical dilation (**A–C4**) involves active and passive factors. *Passive* widening is caused by secretions (**C3**) from the greatly enlarged **cervical glands** (cf. **A4** cervical glands in the nonpregnant state) and venous plexuses. *Active* dilation is produced by tension from the descending bundles of muscle fibers from the uterus into the cervix and ascending bundles of muscle fibers from the vaginal wall, as well as reconfiguration of its more circular arrangement of muscle fibers. In women giving birth for the first time, cervical dilation proceeds gradually from the **internal os** (**C–E5**) toward the **external os** (**A–E6**); multiparous women may have a patulous external os, even in the nonpregnant state.

Vagina. Distention of the vagina, which is approximately 10-cm long (**A–E16**) with a much wider lumen than the cervix, is mostly *passive*. The vagina stretches as fluids in its tissues and vessels are squeezed out and circular muscle fibers and connective tissue structures are realigned.

AB7 Rectouterine pouch, **A–E8** Posterior vaginal fornix

Pelvic floor. The pelvic floor, softened during pregnancy by fluid retention, *passively* stretches (*"crowning"*). The greatest stretch occurs in the **levator ani** (**F9**), with reorientation of muscle fibers. The **levator plate**, which bounds the **levator hiatus** on either side with its **levator crura**, is forced downward during birth so that its upper surface is placed against the birth canal. The sagittally oriented bulbospongiosi **muscles** (**F11**) also widen to form a ring. This causes considerable muscle tension in the perineum (**central tendon of perineum** [**F12**]). The obstetrician can protect the muscles against perineal tearing (manual perineal support) by using two fingers to hold back the fetal head during contractions, and slowly guiding it out of the vagina; in extreme circumstances, an **episiotomy**, a perineal incision, can prevent tearing. After birth, the pelvic floor structures return to their original position.

F13 External anal sphincter, **F14** Fetal head, **F15** Gluteus maximus, **A–E16** Vagina

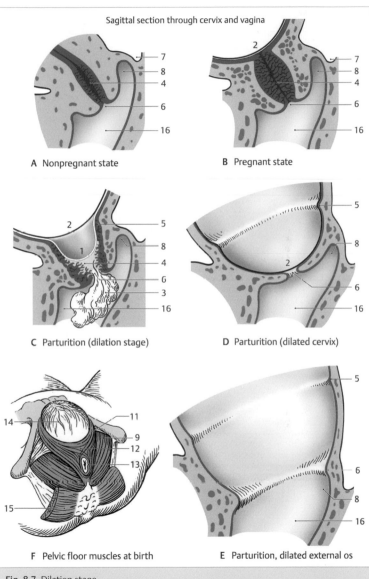

Sagittal section through cervix and vagina

A Nonpregnant state

B Pregnant state

C Parturition (dilation stage)

D Parturition (dilated cervix)

F Pelvic floor muscles at birth

E Parturition, dilated external os

Fig. 8.7 Dilation stage.

Expulsion Stage

The expulsion stage begins with full dilation of the external os. During this stage, the intensity and frequency of contractions increases, and the mother uses rhythmic abdominal compressions (**abdominal contractions, bearing down**) to help expel the fetus. Contractions now greatly shorten the uterine muscle, moving the uterus over the fetus (shaping it into a "fetal cylinder" for easier passage through the birth canal) toward the fundus (**retraction**). The **fixed point** of the uterine muscle, or that part providing resistance, is "anchored" to the cervix and the round ligament of uterus (**A1**) on either side.

A2 Uterine tube, **B3** Urethra, **B4** Vulva, **B5** Anus, **B6** External os, **B7** Internal os, **B8** Placenta, **BC9** Vagina

During expulsion, the fetus must pass the bend in the birth canal (**B**). Led by the smaller fontanelle, the fetus lies with its neck in contact with the pubic angle and extends its head from the flexed position so that its face is directed toward the mother's sacrum (**BC** on p. 304). The back of the head passes first beneath the pubic symphysis through the vaginal opening, followed by the face, which faces the perineum (**occiput anterior position**). Delivery of the head is quickly followed by the shoulders, one at a time, and then the rest of the body. Next, the **umbilical cord**, connecting the neonate to the in utero placenta, is clamped and cut (**cutting the umbilical cord**).

Delivery causes hypoxia and metabolic acidosis in the neonate. The accumulation of carbon dioxide in its blood activates the respiratory center in the brain, and the neonate begins to breathe with its first cry. At the same time, fetal circulation is converted into postnatal circulation (see p. 8).

Expulsion of the placenta. After delivery, the myometrium contracts, producing the first **afterpains**. The uterus retracts to a length of 15 cm and the fundus is located near the level of the umbilicus. The placenta separates from the uterus, disrupting the large uteroplacental vessels and

resulting in blood loss, or *retroplacental hematoma*. Complete separation of the placenta is indicated by the shape and firmness of the uterus, which "rises." The placenta is delivered within 1–2 hours after the fetus by pushing, and, if needed, manual assistance by the obstetrician or midwife. Postpartum uterine contractions also compress the uterine vessels, controlling the bleeding in the region of the placental bed and shrinking it to an area the size of the palm of a hand.

Postpartum changes. About 2 hours after delivery, the entire soft-tissue tube forming the birth canal remains soft and distensible, including the portion formed by the bulbospongiosus muscle sling and levator hiatus, which do not return to their original anatomic positions for several hours. The cervix returns to its normal state by about 1 week after birth.

The time between delivery of the placenta and complete return of the genital organs to their nonpregnant state—as well as resolution of other changes associated with pregnancy—takes about 5–6 weeks. This stage is referred to as the **postpartum period** (puerperium, childbed). During this time, the uterus undergoes *involution* (apoptosis, atrophy, and breakdown of the extracellular matrix; the uterus loses about 1 kg) and quickly shrinks. After 10 days, the fundus of the uterus is at the level of the pubic symphysis; the epithelium has been regenerated and the endometrium restored; and the internal os is closed. The healing uterus secretes a postpartum discharge called **lochia**, consisting of blood, decidual tissue, leukocytes, and bacteria. The body mobilizes regional and systemic immune system functions against ascending infections that could lead to puerperal fever.

Similar to the myometrium, uterine blood vessels also undergo **involution**, adapting to the decreased demand for nourishment. A part of the vessels perishes.

C Size of the uterus: red = immediately after delivery; violet = day 5, black = 12 days after delivery

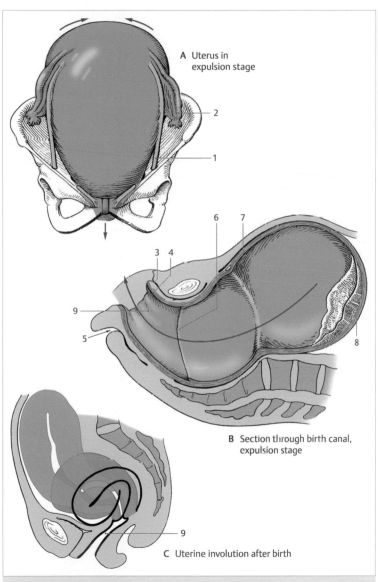

A Uterus in expulsion stage

B Section through birth canal, expulsion stage

C Uterine involution after birth

Fig. 8.8 Expulsion stage, delivery of the placenta.

8.6 Overview and Prenatal Period

Human development begins with **fertilization** and proceeds as a continuum of morphological and functional developments, which may be divided into stages, culminating in death. The stages of human development can be roughly divided into a **prenatal** and a **postnatal** period. Birth is the event dividing the two, but it is merely a temporal boundary and does not constitute the end of development. Before birth, the morphological and structural changes occurring in the growing *embryo* (the unborn offspring in weeks 3–8 of development) or *fetus/fetuses* (the unborn offspring from week 9 of development until birth) are not visible to the outside world. Postnatal morphological and structural changes are visible and thus generally recognized.

In diagnostic gynecology and obstetrics, the *age* and *size* of the developing embryo or fetus are calculated from the 1st day of the mother's last menstruation. The period of *gestation* is also calculated from the 1st day of the mother's last menstrual cycle. Since ovulation occurs around day 12 or day 14 of the cycle, however, the estimated gestation period is about 14 days too long (**A**). Clinical calculations are based on a typical gestation period of about 40 weeks (corresponding to 10 *lunar months* of 28 days each). Yet the actual process of human development begins with fertilization when the egg cell and sperm cell unite. The timeline of embryological and morphological development used in the rest of this chapter is therefore based on a gestation period of 38 weeks, or 9.5 lunar months (**B**). It should be noted that because the exact date of fertilization is usually only an estimate, any assessment of prenatal size and age always involves a level of uncertainty, not least because no timeline can take into account individual structural development with complete accuracy.

Prenatal Period

Prenatal development from gamete to neonate is a complex process of growth and differentiation that can be subdivided into different **periods** (**C**): the **pre-embryonic period** consists of the first 2 weeks, lasting from the union of the gametes (fertilization) to nidation, or *implantation* of the fertilized oocyte in the uterine lining.

The **embryonic period** covers weeks 3–8, which are characterized by formation of the *primordia*.

The **fetal period** lasts from week 9 until birth. It is mainly characterized by *growth* and *increasing weight* of the fetus.

The **neonatal period** extends from delivery until 28 days afterward. It is divided into an *early neonatal* period (until day 7) and a *late neonatal* period (until day 28). The *perinatal period* spans the latter part of the prenatal period and the early neonatal period, beginning before birth at the end of week 24 of fetal development, covering the early neonatal period, and ending with the beginning of the late neonatal period. Infants born during the *perinatal period* are considered preterm or full-term neonates; loss of the fetus due to natural causes before week 24 is termed spontaneous abortion or miscarriage.

Ultrasound evaluation of the developing embryo or fetus requires sound knowledge of the major stages of prenatal human development for early identification of any abnormalities involving the pregnancy or fetal/embryonic development.

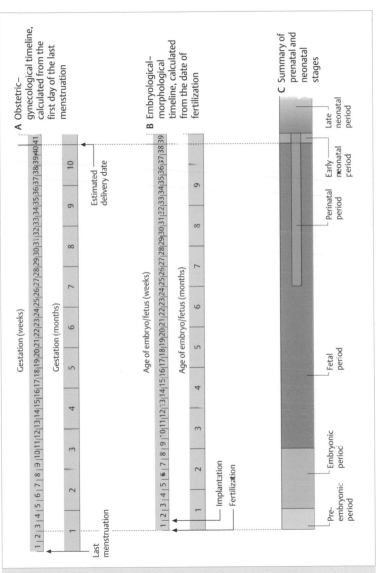

Fig. 8.9 Overview and prenatal period.

Pregnancy and Human Development

Stages in Prenatal Development

The early developmental stages of the gamete (embryo) can be described and classified according to *Carnegie stages 1–23*. The Carnegie stages are based on morphological descriptions of outer and inner structures of the developing gamete and placenta and are the accepted basis for subdividing early human development into phases. The following sections briefly highlight the main developmental events occurring in these stages, chiefly focusing on the *embryonic primordia*.

Pre-embryonic Period

Stages 1–3 (**week 1**). The first stage of human development, lasting 24 hours, consists of fertilization. In stage 2, mitotic cell division (A), or *cleavage*, begins. Mitotic divisions give rise to daughter cells known as **blastomeres**, which form a cluster of cells referred to as a **morula** (**B**) (mulberry) once it reaches a size of 12 cells or more. All of these developments occur while the gamete is migrating through the uterine tube. After reaching the uterine cavity, a fluid-filled cavity known as the **blastocyst** (**C**) appears in the morula on the 4th day (stage 3). Cell differentiation in the morula produces an outer cell mass called the **trophoblast** (**C1**) and an inner cell mass called the **embryoblast** (**C2**).

Stages 4–6 (**week 2**). In stage 4, the blastocyst attaches to the uterine lining. Stage 5 begins with the start of implantation, a process lasting from about day 7 through day 12 (**D**). The embryoblast forms the bilaminar embryonic disc, which is composed of an upper cell layer called the **epiblast** (**D2 a**) and a lower cell layer called the **hypoblast** (**D2 b**). The **amniotic cavity** (**D3**) arises in the embryoblast and is the first structure that can be visualized on a pregnancy ultrasound. The embryonic disc has a *posteroanterior polarity*. The primary yolk sac forms on the hypoblast side (**D4**).

Stage 5 is characterized by differentiation of the trophoblast into the cytotrophoblast and the syncytiotrophoblast on the placental side. Extraembryonic mesenchyme develops and, together with the trophoblast, forms the *chorion* in which the chorionic cavity arises.

During stage 6 (**E**), formation of the **primitive streak** (**E4**) begins. The primitive streak is a band of proliferating epiblastic cells at the caudal end of the embryonic disc that develops along the longitudinal axis of the embryo. The *bilateral symmetry* of the developing organism is thus established.

Stage 6 is characterized on the placental side by formation of chorionic villi.

Embryonic Period

Stages 7–9 (**week 3**). In stage 7, the development of the primitive streak continues, and it becomes thicker at its cranial end, to form the **primitive knot** (**E5**). The *trilaminar embryonic disc*, consisting of the ectoderm (**E2 a**), **mesoderm** (**E2 c**), and endoderm (**E2 b**), begins forming (*gastrulation*), as epiblastic cells from the primitive streak and primitive knot migrate anteriorly and laterally and differentiate to produce new embryonic cell layers. The hypoblast is replaced in the process. A portion of the cells migrate from the primitive knot cranially, becoming the *notochordal (head) process*, which extends as far as the *prechordal plate* (or *buccopharyngeal membrane*). At the caudal end of the embryonic disc is the *cloacal membrane*. The cloacal membrane and the buccopharyngeal membrane remain devoid of mesoderm. In stage 8, the embryo consists of a trilaminar disc. A furrow called the *primitive groove* forms in the median plane of the primitive streak and ends with the *primitive pit*. The *primitive pit* expands into the notochordal process and forms the *chordal canal*. In a sequence of complex events, the *notochord* arises around this canal, forming the primitive axial skeleton.

In stage 9 (**F, G**), *neurulation* begins. During this stage, the **neural plate** (**FG6**) forms, containing the lateral thickened parts known as the **neural folds** (**FG7**) and an unpaired groove in the midline of the plate called the **neural groove** (**FG8**). Midway along the neural groove, the first segmental units known as **somites** (**1–3**) (**G9**) appear. At the end of the 3rd week of development, the primordial heart, consisting of the heart tubes, is connected to the embryonic circulatory system.

C3 Blastocyst cavity, **D1** Trophoblast, **FG4** Primitive streak, **FG5** Primitive knot

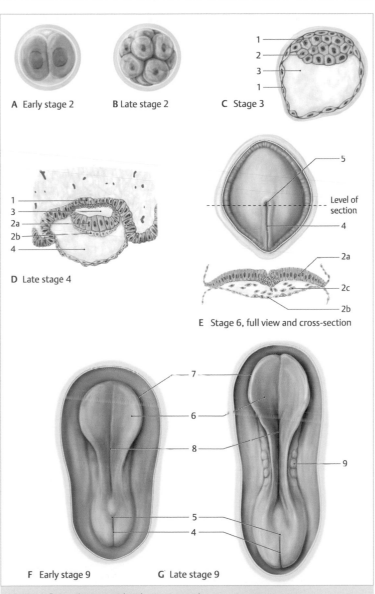

A Early stage 2

B Late stage 2

C Stage 3

D Late stage 4

Level of section

E Stage 6, full view and cross-section

F Early stage 9

G Late stage 9

Fig. 8.10 Pre-embryonic and embryonic periods.

Pregnancy and Human Development

Stages 10–12 (**week 4**). Somite formation continues in stages 10–12: there are 4–12 somites in stage 10, 13–20 somites (**AB1**) in stage 11 (**AB**), and 21–29 somites in stage 12. In stage 10, the neural folds (**AB2**) begin to close to form the **neural tube**. The brain develops at the anterior end, and the spinal cord forms at the posterior end. The cranial and caudal ends of the neural tube remain open, as the **superior neuropore** (**AB3**) and **inferior neuropore** (**AB4**). In stage 11, the embryo is curved and has a cephalic (**B5**) and a caudal folding (**B6**). The first two pairs of branchial arches (**B7**) appear, and the optic vesicles are visible. The superior neuropore closes. In stage 12, there are three pairs of branchial arches. The inferior neuropore closes and the otic pit is visible. The primordial heart is composed of a loop in which contractile activity begins. The limb buds of the upper limbs appear.

Stages 13–15 (**week 5**). The embryo becomes markedly curved and has 30 or more somites (the exact number is difficult to ascertain). In stage 13, four pairs of branchial arches can be seen; the lens placode has been established, and the limb buds of the lower limbs appear. In stage 14, the lenses and nasal pit are visible; the optic cup has formed; limb differentiation continues. In stage 15, the cerebral vesicles are present and the hand plates have developed.

Stages 16–18 (**week 6**). Stages 16–18 are characterized by continued differentiation of the limbs and development of the foot plate (**C8**) and finger rays (**C9**). In stage 18, the elbow is visible and the toe rays appear. Ossification of the mesenchymal condensations begins. Facial development includes formation of the auricular hillocks, the nasolacrimal groove, the apex of the nose, the eyelids, and retinal pigmentation.

Stages 19–20 (**week 7**). The flexure of the embryo decreases, since its trunk is

lengthening and straightening and its head is becoming larger relative to its trunk. The limbs are also becoming longer, growing anteriorly beyond the primordial heart. Restricted space in the abdominal cavity causes the intestinal loop of the midgut to herniate into the umbilical cord.

Stages 21–23 (**week 8**). The stages in the last week of the embryonic period are characterized by differentiation of the typical human features. The head flexure reduces, and the neck is established (**DE10**). The external ear (**D11**) develops and the eyelids (**D12**) appear. The limbs become longer and the fingers (**D13**) divide into separate digits. The toes establish and chondral ossification begins. Sex-specific differences begin to become apparent on the external genitalia.

Fetal Period (Overview)

The fetal period is characterized by differentiation and maturation of organ systems, as well as a rapid growth of the fetus. The size of the fetus is measured in centimeters or millimeters, as crown–rump length (CRL) (sitting height) or crown–heel length (CHL) (standing height). In ultrasound examinations, the biparietal diameter (BPD) of the cranium and the femur length can also be determined, to help more precisely assess size and age. The fetus weighs about 10 g at the beginning of week 9 and about 3,400 g by birth.

Major changes taking place during the fetal period are measured in months. A main feature is the apparent disproportionate growth of the head in relation to the trunk and limbs. At the beginning of the fetal period, the head makes up nearly one half of the length of the body; at the end of the fetal period, it makes up only one quarter.

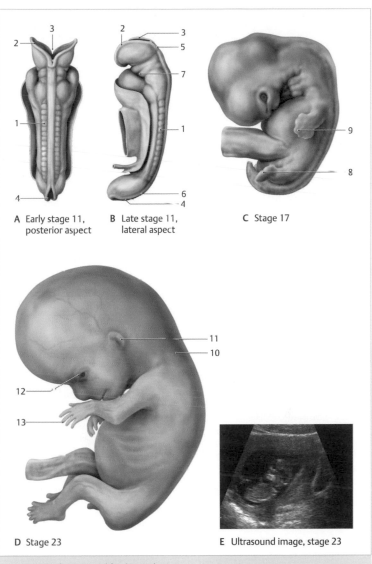

A Early stage 11, posterior aspect

B Late stage 11, lateral aspect

C Stage 17

D Stage 23

E Ultrasound image, stage 23

Fig. 8.11 Embryonic and fetal periods.

Pregnancy and Human Development

Fetal Period (Monthly Stages)

Weeks 9–12. This is a stage of rapid fetal growth. By the end of week 12 of development, the CRL has doubled. The neck and limbs, in particular the upper limbs, increase in size relative to the trunk (**A**). The face takes on a more human appearance, as the eyes move from their original position on the sides of the head to the front, and the ears reach their final position on the sides of the head. The eyelids stick together, closing the palpebral fissure. The intestinal loops lying in the umbilical cord return to the now enlarged abdominal cavity by week 11 or 12. In week 12, final differentiation occurs between external male and female genitalia.

Weeks 13–16. This period is marked by an extremely rapid growth of the trunk, neck, and limbs. The head becomes more erect. *Lanugo hair* appears on the body and the pattern of hair growth on the head becomes recognizable. Ossification progresses and the bones of a 16-week-old fetus (**B**) are visible on radiographs.

Weeks 17–20. Fetal growth slows and weight gain is minimal during this period. The lower limb segments have now also reached their final fetal position (**C**). The sebaceous glands secrete a fatty, cheese-like material called *vernix caseosa*, which protects the skin of the fetus from the macerating effect of being surrounded by amniotic fluid. Hair appears on the head of the fetus, and eyebrows on the face. The mother can now perceive fetal movements. Regular ultrasound examinations are recommended (**D**).

Weeks 21–25. The fetus continues to gain weight. However, because the layer of subcutaneous fat has not yet formed and the skin of the fetus is growing quickly, it still has a reddish, wrinkled appearance. The fingernails are established, and the face and body already resemble those of a full-term fetus. Normally the fetus is not capable of survival if delivered before week 25, when the respiratory system becomes sufficiently mature to support life.

Weeks 26–29. With formation of a layer of fat beneath the skin, the body of the fetus becomes more rounded and plumper. There is a marked weight gain during this period. The eyelids separate and the eyes re-open (**D**). The eyebrows and eyelashes are well developed. The hair on the head of the fetus grows. At this stage, the fetuses can survive outside the womb.

Weeks 30–34. The proportion of subcutaneous fat to total body weight continues to increase. The arms and legs become more rounded, and the body becomes fatter. The skin has a pinkish hue. Although the fingernails already extend to the tips of the fingers, the toenails are just beginning to develop. In the male fetus, the testes descend (*descensus testis*).

Weeks 35–38. In the final month of pregnancy, the girth of the trunk of the fetus becomes even larger. The attachment site of the umbilical cord has moved to the center of the abdominal wall. The toenails extend to the tips of the toes, and lanugo is shed, leaving only the *vernix caseosa* covering the skin. In the male fetus, the testes descend into the scrotum; in the female, the ovaries remain above the lesser pelvis.

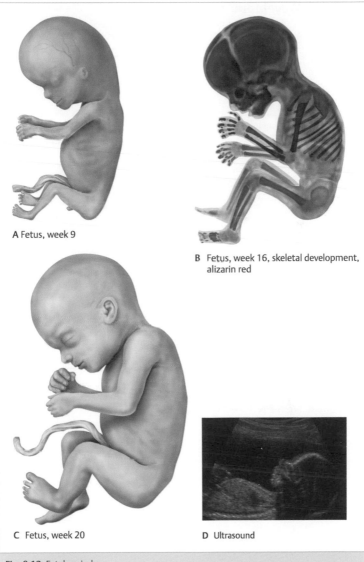

A Fetus, week 9

B Fetus, week 16, skeletal development, alizarin red

C Fetus, week 20

D Ultrasound

Fig. 8.12 Fetal period.

Pregnancy and Human Development

8.7 Organ Development

Body Cavities

At the end of the 3rd week, intercellular spaces appear in the lateral plate mesoderm (**A1**), which merge to produce the **intraembryonic coelom cavity** (**AF2**). This divides the lateral plate mesoderm into the dorsal **somatopleure** (somatopleural mesoderm) (**ADF3**) and ventral **splanchnopleure** (visceropleural mesoderm) (**ADF4**). The intraembryonic coelom is lined by a single layer of serosal epithelium. The parietal layer of the serous cavities develops from the somatopleural epithelium, and the visceral layer from that of the splanchnopleure.

The intraembryonic coelom develops initially in the region of the primordial heart (**B5**) and forms a single **pleuropericardial cavity** for the heart and lungs (**B6**). The intraembryonic coelom enlarges as a result of the folding of the embryo and now extends from the thorax to the pelvic region. The mesodermal **septum transversum** (**C7**), between the floor of the pleuropericardial cavity and the root of the yolk sac, divides the pleuropericardial cavity incompletely from the **peritoneal cavity** (**DE8**); these remain connected via the **pericardioperitoneal duct** (**C9**). The peritoneal cavity (**DE8**) is connected to the yolk sac and extraembryonic (chorionic) coelom via the umbilical coelom. This connection becomes obliterated only after the developing bowel loops (**E10**) have moved from the umbilical cord into the peritoneal cavity. The primordial liver grows into the septum transversum, which ultimately becomes the central tendon of the diaphragm. The two body cavities become separate during subsequent development.

Heart

Early development (**week 3**). Development of the heart and vessels begins in the 3rd week, when the embryonic disc can no longer be nourished only by diffusion. Blood islands (**FG11**), which will give rise to blood cells and primary vessels, develop in the visceral layer of the lateral plate mesoderm on either side of the neural plate. Cardiac muscle precursor cells migrate from the epiblast lateral to the primitive streak and ascend cranial to the buccopharyngeal membrane (**GH12**). Blood islands in the vicinity of the cardiac myoblasts (angiogenetic material) merge to form a horseshoe-shaped tube lined with endothelium; together with the muscle precursor cells, this constitutes the **cardiogenic zone** (**G13**). Because of the craniocaudal folding of the embryo at the end of the 3rd week, the primordial heart moves initially to the anterior cervical region and then to its final anterior thoracic position in the (pleuro-) pericardial cavity in the cranial part of the coelom. Lateral folding of the embryo causes the paired endothelial heart primordia to become an **endocardial tube** (**H14**) with **myocardium** (**H15**) on the outside. **Cardiac jelly**, a broad gelatinous basement membrane, develops between the two layers, and the primordial heart later becomes covered with serosal epithelium, the **epicardium**. The primordial heart bulges more and more into the pericardial cavity, where it is initially fixed by **dorsal mesocardium** (**H16**), which ultimately degenerates so that the originally paired pericardial cavities become a single cavity communicating through the **transverse sinus of the pericardium**.

A–F, H17 Neural tube, neural groove
A–E18 Amniotic cavity

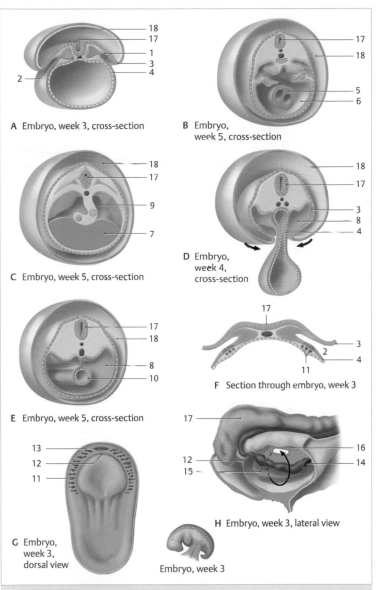

A Embryo, week 3, cross-section

B Embryo, week 5, cross-section

C Embryo, week 5, cross-section

D Embryo, week 4, cross-section

E Embryo, week 5, cross-section

F Section through embryo, week 3

G Embryo, week 3, dorsal view

H Embryo, week 3, lateral view

Embryo, week 3

Fig. 8.13 Body cavities and heart.

Heart, cont.

Looping of the heart tube (week 4). The **truncus arteriosus (A1)** is at the cranial end, and the **sinus venosus (A2)** at the caudal end of the tubular primordial heart, which starts to beat at the end of the 3rd week. The tube bends more as it grows and the cranial end moves ventrally, caudally and to the right (**BC**). The caudal end moves dorsally, cranially, and to the left. The resulting **cardiac loop** now consists of the **bulbus cordis (BC3)**, with the **truncus arteriosus (BC1)** and **conus arteriosus (infundibulum) (BC4)**, a joint **ventricle (BC5)**, a joint **atrium (BC6)**, and the **sinus venosus (BC2)**. Development of the heart loop is complete on day 28.

Development of intracardiac septa (weeks 5–7). The junction between the joint atrium and primordial ventricle is narrow and forms the **atrioventricular canal (CG7)**. Endocardial cushions **(C8)** develop on its dorsal and ventral walls. These fuse with smaller lateral endocardial cushions, to divide the atrioventricular canal into right and left segments. Parts of the atrioventricular valves develop from the endocardial cushions. An **interventricular sulcus (C9)** can be seen on the surface of the heart between the ascending and descending limbs of the ventricle. This marks the location on the inside of the myocardial trabecula **(D10)** and the muscular **interventricular septum (EFG11)**, which grows toward the endocardial cushions **(DE8)**. An opening between the ventricles persists initially–the **interventricular foramen (E12)**. It is closed by the membranous part of the septum **(F13)**, which arises from the endocardial cushions.

The half-moon shaped **septum primum (D14)** grows down from the roof of the single atrium toward the endocardial cushions at the end of the 5th week but does not fuse with them, thus forming a **foramen** (or ostium) **primum (arrow in D)**. The septum primum later fuses with the endocardial cushions to close the foramen primum. Before then, perforations in the upper part of the thin septum merge to produce the **foramen secundum (arrow in E)**. The **septum secundum (EF15)**, a further semilunar partition, develops to the right of the septum primum and grows toward the endocardial cushions but never divides the atrium completely. The septum secundum overlaps the foramen secundum, and the remaining opening, the **foramen ovale (F16)**, allows right-to-left blood flow in the fetal circulation.

In the 5th week, paired spiral ridges **(G17)** appear in the proximal **bulbus cordis** and distal **truncus arteriosus** in the initially undivided ventricular outflow tract. Growth of the truncal ridges results in the **aortopulmonary septum (G18)**, which divides the two coiled outflow channels, the **aorta (divided arrow)** and **pulmonary trunk (solid arrow)**. The growing ridges in the bulbus cordis divide the smooth-walled outflow tracts of the two ventricles.

Remodeling of the sinus venosus (weeks 5–10). In the 4th week, the sinus venosus receives blood from large embryonic veins, through roughly equal-sized right and left **horns (H19)**. The junction between the sinus venosus and primitive atrium is wide and central at first. As a result of remodeling of embryonic veins and the development of right-to-left short circuits, the right sinus horn and right veins grow very large. Finally, the right sinus horn is drawn into the atrium, and its opening moves to the right. The boundary between the smooth-walled sinus and trabecular right atrium is later marked by the **crista terminalis** and **terminal sulcus**. The left horn of the sinus becomes the small coronary sinus.

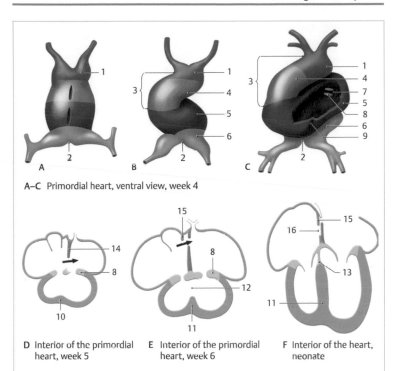

A–C Primordial heart, ventral view, week 4

D Interior of the primordial heart, week 5

E Interior of the primordial heart, week 6

F Interior of the heart, neonate

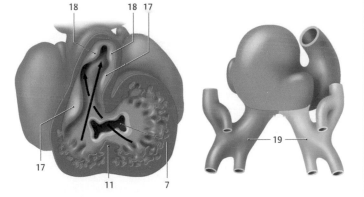

G Opened primordial heart, week 6

H Primordial heart, dorsal view, week 4

Fig. 8.14 Heart.

8.8 Vessel Development

Overview. A distinction is made between **vasculogenesis**, in which **vessels** develop from blood islands, and **angiogenesis**, in which new vessels sprout from existing ones. The first blood islands appear in the extraembryonic mesoderm of the yolk sac in the 3rd week, and in the intraembryonic lateral plate mesoderm a short time later. Simple endothelial tubes arise from the blood islands and fuse to form a mesh. The other structures of the vessel wall develop from the surrounding mesenchyme. As soon as the primary vascular network has appeared, further vessels are produced by vasculogenesis stimulated by VEGF (vascular endothelial growth factor).

Arterial system. The final human arterial system develops from a complex paired early embryonic aortic system. This consists of the paired dorsal aortae (**A1**), the paired ventral aortae (**A2**) (broadened part of the truncus arteriosus or aortic sac), and the aortic arch arteries (**AI–VI**) (pharyngeal arch arteries), which link the dorsal and ventral systems. The paired dorsal aortae accompany the foregut and fuse just below the sixth aortic arch artery, to form an unpaired vessel that descends in front of the vertebral column. Six aortic arches develop cranially in proximity to the pharyngeal arches, though not all are present at the same time. While the sixth aortic arch develops, the first two have already dwindled. This segmental system is converted to the definitive arterial system by the end of the embryonic period. The most important arteries derived from it include (**B**):

First aortic arch → maxillary artery

Second aortic arch → hyoid artery and stapedial artery

Third aortic arch → common carotid artery (**B3**) and first part of the internal carotid artery (**B4**)

Fourth aortic arch → arch of the aorta on the left (**B5**), right subclavian artery on the right (**B6**)

Fifth aortic arch → rudimentary and only temporary

Sixth aortic arch → ductus arteriosus (**B7**) and left pulmonary artery on the left (**B8**), pulmonary trunk on the right (**B9**)

Venous system. At the end of the 4th week, three large pairs of veins open into the embryo's cardiac tube through the horns of the sinus (**C**): the vitelline (yolk sac) veins (**C10**), which transport deoxygenated blood to the heart from the yolk sac; the umbilical veins (**C11**), which convey oxygenated blood from the placenta; and the cardinal veins (**C12**), which return deoxygenated blood to the heart from the embryo's body. At the level of the future duodenum, the vitelline veins form liver sinusoids, which form the basis for the portal vein. The left vitelline vein regresses as the left horn of the sinus becomes smaller.

The umbilical veins are paired at first but the right one shrinks while the left one transports oxygenated blood from the placenta to the right atrium (see fetal circulation, p. 8).

The cardinal vein system is symmetrical at first. Paired anterior (superior) cardinal veins (**D13**) and posterior (inferior) cardinal veins (**D14**) drain through common cardinal veins (**D15**) into the sinus horns in the 4th week. The superior cardinal veins are joined by an anastomosis. Further anastomosing cardinal veins appear in the 5th week: supracardinal veins (**D16**), subcardinal veins (**D17**), and sacrocardinal veins (**D18**). The majority of the posterior cardinal veins disappear. The cardinal veins contribute to the final major veins as follows:

Superior vena cava (**D19**) ← right common cardinal vein, right superior cardinal vein

Left brachiocephalic vein (**D20**) ← anastomosis between anterior cardinal veins

Inferior vena cava (**D21**) (hepatocardiac part) ← right vitelline vein

Inferior vena cava (**D22**) (renal part) ← subcardinal vein

Inferior vena cava (**D23**) (sacrocardinal part) ← right sacrocardinal vein

Left common iliac vein (**D24**) ← anastomosis between sacrocardinal veins

Azygos vein (**D25**) ← right supracardinal vein

Hemiazygos vein (**D26**) ← left supracardinal vein

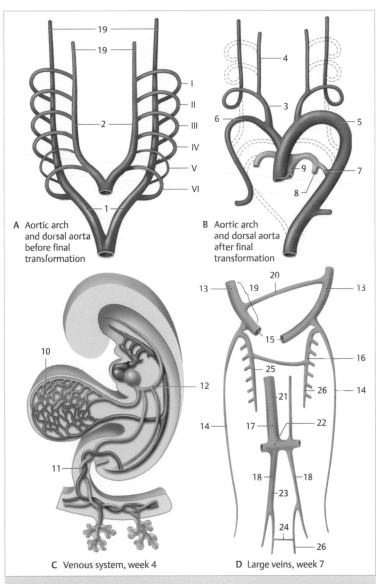

A Aortic arch and dorsal aorta before final transformation

B Aortic arch and dorsal aorta after final transformation

C Venous system, week 4

D Large veins, week 7

Fig. 8.15 Vessels.

8.9 Respiratory System

While the nose and paranasal sinuses develop with the face, the other segments of the respiratory tract arise from the foregut.

Nose and paranasal sinuses. The face of a 5-week embryo has elevations of superficial ectoderm and neural streak mesenchyme at the site of the future nose (**A**): frontonasal elevation (**A1**), medial (**A2**) and lateral (**A3**) nasal elevation (**A4**), and mandibular prominence (**A5**). The nasal elevations surround the olfactory pit, which becomes deeper to form nasal sacs in week 6 and becomes the primordial nasal cavity (**B6**). This is initially separated from the primordial oral cavity by a thin oronasal membrane (**B7**). Perforation of this membrane at the end of the 6th week leads to a connection between the nasal and oral cavities via primary choanae (**C8**) located directly above the primary palate. The final nasal cavities and choanae, which are now at the junction of the nasal cavity and pharynx, develop from the secondary palate, nasal conchae on the lateral wall of the nose, and a nasal septum from the medial nasal elevations (**D9**). The paranasal sinuses develop in the fetal period as diverticula from the lateral wall of the nose; they continue to develop postnatally from superficial ectoderm and neural streak mesenchyme.

Larynx, trachea, and bronchial tree. The **laryngotracheal groove**, a diverticulum from the ventral wall of the foregut, develops in the 4-week-old embryo and widens to form a **tracheobronchial diverticulum** (**E10**). This provides the epithelial lining of the larynx, trachea, and bronchial tree. The diverticulum has a direct connection to the foregut at first.

Longitudinal growth produces two longitudinal folds (**E11**), which fuse to form the **esophagotracheal septum** (**F12**). This divides the ventral respiratory part from the dorsal esophageal part. The respiratory portion remains open to the pharynx cranially through the T-shaped laryngeal inlet. The laryngeal cartilages and muscles develop from the mesenchyme of branchial arches IV–VI (**G**).

The lung buds grow out from the tracheobronchial diverticulum (**FH13**) and develop into main bronchi at the beginning of the 5th week. The proliferating lung buds grow into the pleuropericardial canals (**H14**), which form bilateral pleural cavities with a visceral (**I15**) and parietal layer (**I16**), separate from the pericardial and peritoneal cavities.

Continuing proliferation produces three lobar bronchi on the right and two on the left. The segmental bronchi (HI) and further generations of bronchi and bronchioles develop according to this pattern of division. Development of the air-conducting segments initially resembles growth of a gland and is called the **pseudoglandular phase**. In the **canalicular phase** (**J**), smaller and smaller canals are produced up to the 7th week and increasing numbers of blood vessels (**J17**) develop beside them from the splanchnopleure. Terminal sacs (**K18**), the precursors of alveoli, develop only in week 26, the **terminal sac phase**. The capillaries become closely related to the terminal sacs, where cells differentiate into two different types, with type II alveolar epithelial cells that produce surfactant detectable at the end of the 6th month. In the **alveolar phase** in the final months before birth, the alveoli grow and form the blood–air barrier with the neighboring capillaries (**K**).

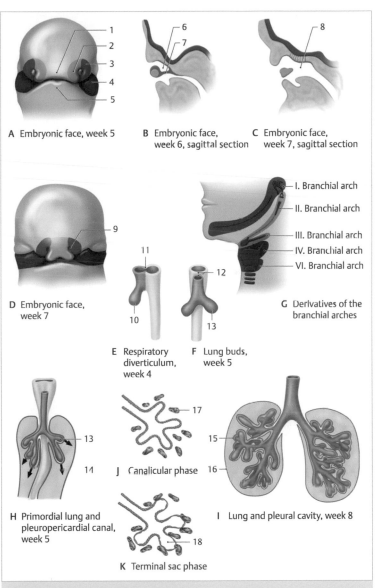

A Embryonic face, week 5

B Embryonic face, week 6, sagittal section

C Embryonic face, week 7, sagittal section

D Embryonic face, week 7

G Derivatives of the branchial arches

- I. Branchial arch
- II. Branchial arch
- III. Branchial arch
- IV. Branchial arch
- VI. Branchial arch

E Respiratory diverticulum, week 4

F Lung buds, week 5

H Primordial lung and pleuropericardial canal, week 5

J Canalicular phase

I Lung and pleural cavity, week 8

K Terminal sac phase

Fig. 8.16 Respiratory system.

Pregnancy and Human Development

8.10 Gastrointestinal System

Foregut

In the course of the folding that takes place in the 4th week, some of the entoderm-lined yolk sac is incorporated in the embryo, to form the primordial gut. This is divided into foregut (**A1**), midgut (**A2**), and hindgut (**A3**). The foregut and hindgut each end blindly in the buccopharyngeal (**A4**) or cloacal membrane (**A5**), where the tube of entoderm meets the body surface, and thus the superficial ectoderm.

Foregut. Parts of the mouth and pharynx, the respiratory system, esophagus, stomach, upper duodenum, and liver, including the biliary tract, develop from the foregut, which extends from the buccopharyngeal membrane to the outlet of the yolk sac.

Mouth and pharynx. The buccal cavity and pharynx develop in tandem with the branchial arches, and therefore with the face and neck. The stomatodeum (**BC6**) or primitive mouth arises at the level of the first branchial arch; in week 5, it is bounded initially by the paired maxillary elevations (**BC7**), the medial nasal elevations (**BC8**), the frontonasal elevation (**BC9**), and a mandibular prominence (**BC10**). The maxillary processes fuse with the medial nasal elevations, to form the premaxilla (**D11**), which produces parts of the upper lip, maxilla, upper incisor teeth, and primary palate. However, most of the final palate develops from two plates originating from the maxillary processes (**D–F12**). Initially, these are on either side of the tongue bud, but

by week 7 they are in horizontal position above the tongue, where they fuse with one another and with the primary palate and nasal septum (**EF13**). The lower lip, Meckel (mandibular) cartilage, and masticatory muscles develop from the mandibular process or bar (see p. 325). The mandible develops by desmal osteogenesis in close proximity to the Meckel cartilage. Various elevations present as early as week 4 contribute to the development of the tongue: these include two lateral tongue buds (**GH14**) and a median tongue bud, the tuberculum impar (**GH15**), which arise from the first branchial arch and fuse to form the presulcal part of the tongue (**H16**); the copula, another median elevation (**G17**), arises from the second and third branchial arch and becomes the postsulcal part (**H18**). The union between the different parts of the tongue is marked throughout life by the foramen cecum (**H19**) and terminal sulcus (**H20**). The thyroid gland originates in the foramen. The epiglottis (**H21**) and its connections with the tongue are produced from elements of the fourth branchial arch, where the pharyngeal muscles also develop.

Starting from the esophagus, the actual foregut develops from the tube of entoderm, and the adjacent mesenchyme from the splanchnopleure. The esophagus is divided from the primordial respiratory system by the esophagotracheal septum (see p. 324). It is short at first but elongates rapidly because of the caudal movement of the primordial heart and lungs. Striated muscle develops in the upper one-third of the esophagus, with smooth muscle below this.

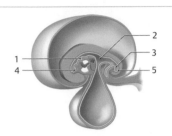

A Embryo, week 4, sagittal section

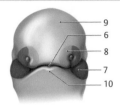

B Embryonic face, week 5

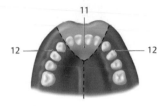

D Parts of the premaxilla

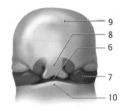

C Embryonic face, week 7

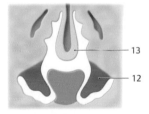

E Buccal cavity, week 7, frontal section

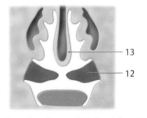

F Buccal cavity, week 8, frontal section

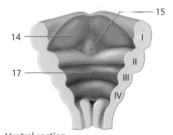

G Ventral section
through branchial arches, week 5

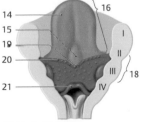

H Ventral section
through branchial arches, 5th month

Fig. 8.17 Digestive system.

Foregut, cont.

The **stomach** can be recognized in the 4th week as a fusiform dilatation of the foregut. Because the different parts of the stomach grow at different rates, the position of the stomach and duodenum changes as a result of rotation around the long axis (**A**) and anteroposterior axis (**B**). The left wall of the stomach faces ventrally, while the right wall faces dorsally. The vagus nerve, which innervates the stomach, follows this rotation. Greater growth of the originally posterior part of the stomach results in the greater curvature (**C1**) and lesser curvature (**C2**). This causes the pylorus to ascend toward the right (**C3**) and the cardia moves to the left (**C4**). The stomach is connected to the posterior body wall by the dorsal mesogastrium (**DE5**) and to the anterior wall by the ventral mesogastrium (**DE6**); gastric rotation causes the dorsal mesogastrium to move to the left, resulting in the omental bursa (**EG7**) behind the stomach, while the ventral mesogastrium moves to a position to the right of the midline. The dorsal mesogastrium projects below the greater curvature like an apron, owing to further growth and rotation (**F8**). This grows to cover the transverse colon (**FG9**) and small intestine (**FG10**). The four layers ultimately fuse to form the greater omentum (**G11**).

The **duodenum** (**DEH12**) develops from the foregut and upper part of the midgut. The boundary between the two is distal to the origin of the liver bud and is indicated by the dual vascular supply from the celiac trunk and superior mesenteric artery. Gastric rotation causes the C-shape of the duodenum, which is retroperitoneal because of growth of the surrounding organs and pancreas (**H13**); only the superior (first) part of the duodenum remains intraperitoneal. The lumen of the upper part of the duodenum becomes temporarily occluded by proliferating cells in the 2nd month.

The entodermal **liver diverticulum** appears at the caudal end of the foregut at the start of week 4. It grows into the septum transversum as liver trabeculae (**H14**), and projects caudally into the abdominal cavity (**HI15**). The ventral mesogastrium between the stomach, superior part of the duodenum, and liver bud becomes the lesser omentum (**DE6**), and the portion between the liver bud and the anterior abdominal wall becomes the falciform ligament of the liver (**E16**). The bile canaliculi develop from the distal liver trabeculae. The gallbladder (**IJ17**) and bile duct originate in the caudal part of the liver diverticulum (**IJ18**).

The **ventral primitive pancreas** is the most caudal outgrowth from the liver diverticulum (**IJ19**). The **dorsal primitive pancreas** (**IJ20**) develops directly opposite it from the duodenal tube. As a result of growth and rotation of the duodenal loop, the ventral pancreas and bile duct move dorsally, with the ventral part finally located below and behind the dorsal pancreas (**J**). The excretory ducts of both pancreatic primordia usually fuse to form a single pancreatic duct (**J21**). The endocrine islets of Langerhans develop throughout the gland from the epithelium, during the 3rd month.

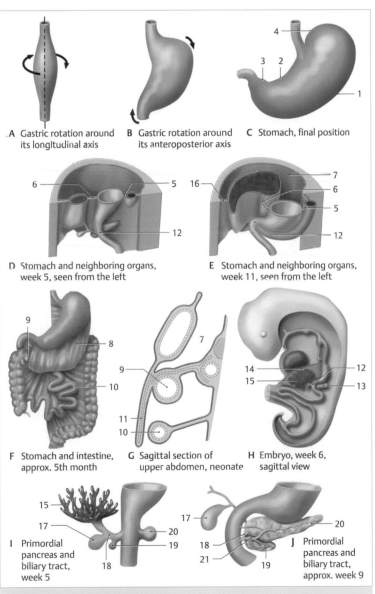

A Gastric rotation around its longitudinal axis

B Gastric rotation around its anteroposterior axis

C Stomach, final position

D Stomach and neighboring organs, week 5, seen from the left

E Stomach and neighboring organs, week 11, seen from the left

F Stomach and intestine, approx. 5th month

G Sagittal section of upper abdomen, neonate

H Embryo, week 6, sagittal view

I Primordial pancreas and biliary tract, week 5

J Primordial pancreas and biliary tract, approx. week 9

Fig. 8.18 Digestive system, continued.

Midgut and Hindgut

Like the caudal sections of the duodenum, the **jejunum** and **ileum** (**A–C1**) develop from the midgut. The small intestine is connected to the posterior abdominal wall by a dorsal mesentery; there is no ventral mesentery. The midgut communicates with the yolk sac via the **vitelline duct** (**A–C2**). The midgut grows rapidly, resulting in a ventral-facing primary loop (**B**) enclosing the superior mesenteric artery (**B3**). The cranial limb of the loop becomes the small intestine (**BC1**) and the caudal limb develops into the cecum (**BC4**), ascending colon, and proximal two-thirds of the transverse colon. With the rapid growth of the cranial limb, the intestinal tube elongates and no longer fits in the embryonic coelomic cavity. In week 6, the loops of the small intestine (**D1**) move into the extraembryonic coelom of the umbilical cord (**D5**), to produce a physiological hernia. While it is elongating, the intestinal loop rotates anticlockwise through approximately 270° (**BC**). The superior mesenteric artery marks the axis of rotation. The jejunum and ileum form several loops in the course of longitudinal growth, and the proximal jejunum loops (**E–G6**) are the first to return to the coelomic cavity in week 10, where they are located on the right, with the remaining loops accommodated on the right (**E–G7**); this is reflected in the final line of the root of the mesentery (**G8**). The vitelline duct becomes obliterated after the small intestine has returned to the abdomen and the anterior abdominal wall is formed.

> Clinical note: In 2%–4% of persons, the vitelline duct does not become obliterated, resulting in a **Meckel diverticulum** in the ileum.

The **cecum**, **ascending colon** and the proximal two-thirds of the **transverse colon** develop from the caudal limb of the primary umbilical loop (**BC4**) and are also supplied by branches of the superior mesenteric artery. The colon segments are involved in the "hernia," and elongate but do not form loops. The cecum usually develops in week 6 as a bud from the cranial primary loop (**CD9**); on its return to the coelomic cavity, it is first located below the liver (**E9**) but then migrates downward to the right iliac fossa (**FG9**). The ascending colon and right colic flexure (**G10**) lie on the right dorsal wall and are secondarily retroperitoneal, owing to fusion of the mesentery. The transverse colon (**G11**) retains its mesentery, which fuses with the posterior layer of the greater omentum. The vermiform appendix (**FG12**) begins as a diverticulum from the cecum and is usually in a retrocecal location.

The distal third of the **transverse colon** (**G13**), the **descending colon** (**G14**), **sigmoid colon** (**G15**), **rectum** (**G–I16**), and **anal canal** develop from the hindgut, which at the same time provides the epithelial lining of the bladder and urethra. The arterial supply by the inferior mesenteric artery (hindgut artery) starts in the distal third of the transverse colon and ends at the anal canal, where it is provided by the inferior rectal artery from the internal pudendal artery. The descending colon is retroperitoneal along the left dorsal abdominal wall (**G14**), whereas the sigmoid colon remains intraperitoneal (**G15**). The rectum develops from the **cloaca** (**H17**), a sac at the ventrocaudal end of the embryo lined with entoderm, which is initially closed by the **cloacal membrane** (**H18**). Growth of the mesodermal urorectal septum (**H19**) toward the cloacal membrane divides the cloaca into the ventral urogenital sinus (**H20**), which will become the bladder and urethra, and the dorsal anorectum. In week 7, the cloacal membrane perforates to produce the urethral (**I21**) and anal openings (**I22**). The opening of the anal canal is closed again briefly for a short time by an anal membrane, produced by epithelial proliferation.

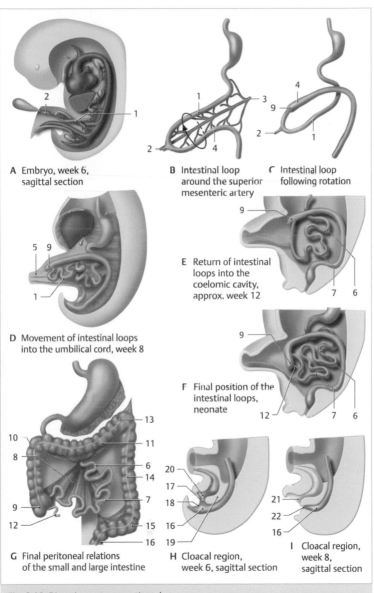

A Embryo, week 6,
sagittal section

B Intestinal loop
around the superior
mesenteric artery

C Intestinal loop
following rotation

D Movement of intestinal loops
into the umbilical cord, week 8

E Return of intestinal
loops into the
coelomic cavity,
approx. week 12

F Final position of the
intestinal loops,
neonate

G Final peritoneal relations
of the small and large intestine

H Cloacal region,
week 6, sagittal section

I Cloacal region,
week 8,
sagittal section

Fig. 8.19 Digestive system, continued.

Pregnancy and Human Development

8.11 Urinary System

Development of the Urinary System

The urinary system develops with the reproductive system from intermediate mesoderm (**A1**), in which three generations of primordial kidney are found from cranial to caudal: **pronephros**, **mesonephros**, and **metanephros**. The rudimentary and non-functioning segmental pronephros (**B2**) develops in the neck in week 3; only the pronephric duct (**B3**) plays a part in subsequent development. The mesonephros appears in week 4 and extends from the thoracic to lumbar region (**B4**). It consists of mesonephric canaliculi, vascular loops, and the mesonephric (Wolffian) duct (**BC5**), which grows in a caudal direction as a continuation of the pronephric duct. S-shaped mesonephric tubules form close to the mesonephric duct (**C6**), accompanied by medial capillary loops (**C7**), with a glomerular capsule derived from tubule epithelium. The resulting functional units (nephrons) of the mesonephros drain laterally through tubules into the mesonephric duct. While mesonephric nephrons are still appearing caudally, they are degenerating cranially (**B**). The mesonephric duct opens into the cloaca at the end of week 4 (**B8**). The large, oval genital ridge (**C9**) develops in week 6, medial to the mesonephric duct.

The permanent kidney starts to develop in week 6, with the appearance of the metanephros (**B10**). Metanephric and mesonephric nephrons develop similarly, but development of the draining system differs. The **ureter bud** (**B11**) sprouts from the mesonephric duct close to where it opens into the cloaca. The blind end of this bud projects at first into the as yet unsegmented metanephric blastema. The ureter bud is the origin of the ureter, renal pelvis,

and collecting tubules, and epithelial renal vesicles (**D12**) arise from the mesenchymal metanephric blastema in proximity to the collecting tubules (**D13**). Different segments of the tubules develop from these vesicles (**E14**). One end establishes a connection with the collecting tubule (**arrow in E**), and the other end becomes the glomerular capsule (Bowman capsule) (**F16**), containing capillary loops (**F15**).

The metanephros (**G10**) is located in the pelvis at first but ascends into the abdomen as it develops (**H10**). The blood supply of the primordial kidney changes from branches of the iliac arteries to separate branches from the aorta, the renal arteries.

The **urinary bladder** (**G–I17**) and **urethra** (**HI18**) develop from the urogenital sinus (**G–I19**), the ventral part of the cloaca, which is divided into three regions. The wide upper segment becomes the urinary bladder, which is at first connected with the umbilicus through the allantoic duct (**GH20**). This channel is obliterated and becomes the urachus in the median umbilical fold on the anterior abdominal wall. During bladder differentiation, the terminal part of the mesonephric duct (**JK21**), with the ureter rudiment arising from it (**J22**), becomes incorporated in the dorsal bladder wall (**JK23**); the ureter and mesonephric duct retain separate openings. The ureter openings move cranially, owing to ascent of the kidney (**IK24**); the now caudal openings of the mesonephric ducts move together and mark the bladder trigone and the start of the prostatic urethra in males (**K25**). In the female, the middle or pelvic segment of the urogenital sinus becomes the urethra, and in the male it is the origin of the prostatic and intermediate parts of the urethra. The vaginal vestibule in females, and spongiose part of the urethra in males, develop from the lower segment of the urogenital sinus.

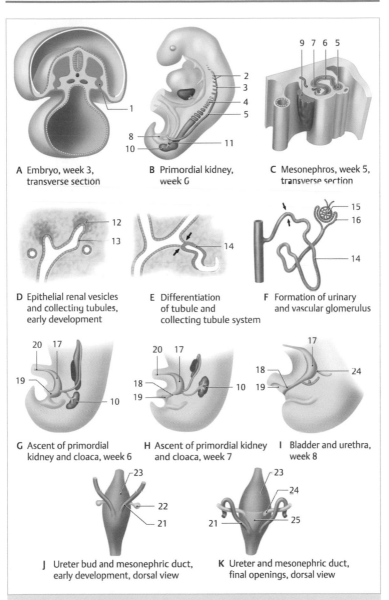

A Embryo, week 3, transverse section

B Primordial kidney, week 6

C Mesonephros, week 5, transverse section

D Epithelial renal vesicles and collecting tubules, early development

E Differentiation of tubule and collecting tubule system

F Formation of urinary and vascular glomerulus

G Ascent of primordial kidney and cloaca, week 6

H Ascent of primordial kidney and cloaca, week 7

I Bladder and urethra, week 8

J Ureter bud and mesonephric duct, early development, dorsal view

K Ureter and mesonephric duct, final openings, dorsal view

Pregnancy and Human Development

Fig. 8.20 Urinary system.

8.12 Genital System

Development of the Genital System

Although the embryo's sex is determined genetically, the early rudiments of the genital system, that is, the gonads, genital ducts, and external genitalia, are indifferent. It is therefore useful to compare and contrast the development of the male and female genital systems.

Indifferent gonads. In week 5, the coelomic epithelium at the medial border of the mesonephros thickens to form the **genital ridge** (**A1**). The epithelial cells form cords surrounded by mesenchyme and contain mesonephric cells (**A2**). **Primordial sex cells** (**AB3**) migrate into this **indifferent gonad** (**B**) in week 6. These probably originate from the epiblast and pass to the yolk sac and thence to the hindgut (**A4**). The cells migrate along the dorsal mesentery by ameboid movement to the coelomic epithelium, and enter the genital ridge (**B1**).

Testis. In an embryo with XY chromosomes, SRY (*sex-determining region on Y chromosome*), the master gene, produces TDF (*testis-determining factor*), thereby initiating testis development. By the end of the 7th week, the testis can be distinguished from the ovary. The testicular cords (**CD5**) develop in the center of the testis and are connected with the hilum (**CD6**) through the rete testis. The testicular cords consist of primordial germ cells and Sertoli cell precursors. They remain compact until puberty, when they obtain a lumen and become seminiferous tubules. The fibrous tunica albuginea (**CD7**) develops beneath the surface epithelium of the testis, and Leydig cells are produced from interstitial connective tissue; these produce testosterone from week 8 onwards, which influences differentiation of the genital ducts and external genitalia.

Ovary. In an embryo with XX chromosomes, and thus in the absence of TDF, the gonad develops into an ovary, in which the primary germ cords in the center first form meshlike collections of cells and are finally replaced by vascular ovarian stroma (**EF8**). The cortex becomes broader and thicker, owing to the development of secondary germ cords (**E9**) from the coelomic epithelium. The germ cords are interlinked with the cortical stroma but degenerate in the 4th month into clusters of cells containing one or more germ cells. These divide by mitosis and become synchronously proliferating oogonia with the start of the prophase of meiosis. In the fetal period, they become primordial follicles through deposition of a single layer of follicle cells (**F10**). Most of the roughly two million primordial follicles are lost before birth, so the ovaries of a newborn girl contain only several hundred thousand.

Descent of the gonads. The testis and ovary move caudally from their original position at the level of the first lumbar vertebra. The testis (**G–I11**) first reaches the lesser pelvis, (**transabdominal descent, GH**), and passes the inguinal canal in a second phase (**transinguinal descent, I**). Descent of the testis depends on testosterone and is guided by the **gubernaculum testis** (**G–I12**), which arises from the mesonephros. Ventral to the gubernaculum testis, the parietal peritoneum forms the funnel-shaped **processus vaginalis of the testis** (**H13**), which continues into the scrotum like the other layers of the abdominal wall. The testis migrates downward behind the gubernaculum testis. When descent is complete, the processus vaginalis is obliterated and the testis invaginates the serosal cavity in the scrotum (**I14**).

The ovary descends along the ovarian gubernaculum as far as the wall of the lesser pelvis. The suspensory ligament of the ovary derives from its cranial end, and the round ligament of the uterus from the caudal end, which passes through the inguinal canal and ends in the labium majus.

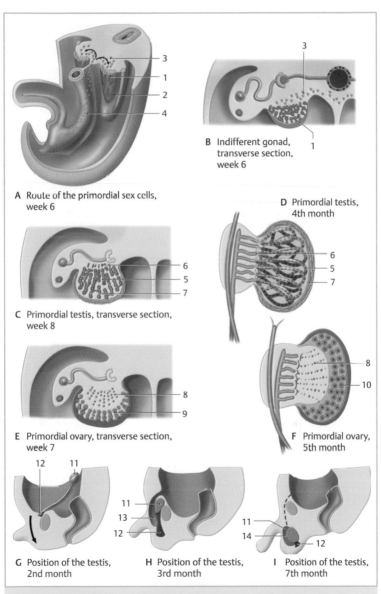

A Route of the primordial sex cells, week 6

B Indifferent gonad, transverse section, week 6

C Primordial testis, transverse section, week 8

D Primordial testis, 4th month

E Primordial ovary, transverse section, week 7

F Primordial ovary, 5th month

G Position of the testis, 2nd month

H Position of the testis, 3rd month

I Position of the testis, 7th month

Fig. 8.21 Genital system.

Development of the Genital System, cont.

The primordial genital ducts are indifferent at first; they are present in both sexes lateral to the mesonephros, as the mesonephric (Wolffian) duct (**AB1**) and paramesonephric (Müllerian) duct (**AB2**).

Male genital ducts. *Antimüllerian hormone* (**AMH**) produced by Sertoli cells causes almost complete degeneration of the Müllerian duct in the male embryo but the Wolffian duct is preserved under the influence of testosterone despite regression of the mesonephros. The Wolffian duct becomes the ductus deferens (**C1a**) and the segment next to the testis forms the epididymis (**C1b**), which receives the openings of the efferent ductules originating from mesonephric tubules (**C3**). The seminal vesicle develops from the terminal portion of the mesonephric duct, while the prostate arises from epithelial buds from the urethra and the surrounding mesenchyme.

Female genital ducts. While the Wolffian ducts degenerate in the female embryo, the Müllerian ducts (**D2**) become the important genital ducts, developing into the tubes (**D4**), uterus (**D5**), and upper part of the vagina (**D6**). The cranial parts of the Müllerian ducts become the tubes (**E–G4**), while the caudal segments on both sides fuse medially to form the uterovaginal canal (**EF7**), with a broad ligament of the uterus on both sides. A temporary septum can be identified in the uterus; this differentiates gradually into the body and cervix (**E8**). The fused caudal end of the Müllerian ducts (**E9**) reaches the urogenital sinus (**EF6, 10**), which in turn produces paired sinuvaginal horns by epithelial proliferation. These become a solid vaginal plate (**F11**), which proliferates toward the uterovaginal canal and gradually acquires a lumen (**FG12**). The vaginal epithelium therefore develops from at least two primordial tissues but the boundary between them remains unclear.

The urogenital sinus and vaginal lumen are separated by the hymen, a thin layer of tissue (**FG13**).

External genitalia. The indifferent stage of the external genitalia develops from the mesenchyme surrounding the cloaca. Urogenital (cloacal) folds (**H14**), which are slight elevations around the cloacal opening, fuse ventral to the genital tubercle (**H15**) and are accompanied laterally by genital swellings (**H16**). Following perforation of the cloacal membrane, the urorectal septum divides the cloacal opening into an anterior urogenital sinus (**J10**) and a posterior anal opening (**IJ17**); it becomes the perineum (**IJ18**).

Male external genitalia. Under the influence of testosterone, the genital tubercle grows and becomes the phallus (**I19**). The genital folds fuse to become the urethra and gradually close the urethral groove (**I20**). The scrotum (**IK21**), which develops from union of the genital (scrotal) swellings, becomes attached to the resulting penis.

Female external genitalia. When the embryo has XX chromosomes, there is little growth of the genital tubercle, which becomes the clitoris (**L22**). The genital folds form the labia minora (**L23**) and the genital swellings form the labia majora (**L24**). The urogenital sinus remains open and becomes the vestibule of the vagina, into which the urethra (**L25**) and vagina (**L26**) open.

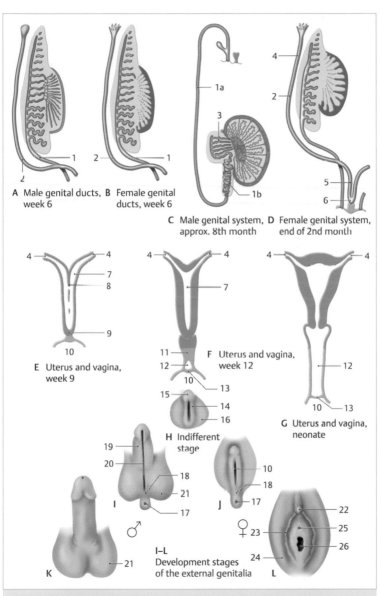

A Male genital ducts, week 6

B Female genital ducts, week 6

C Male genital system, approx. 8th month

D Female genital system, end of 2nd month

E Uterus and vagina, week 9

F Uterus and vagina, week 12

G Uterus and vagina, neonate

H Indifferent stage

I–L Development stages of the external genitalia

Fig. 8.22 Genital system, continued.

Pregnancy and Human Development

8.13 Perinatal Period

The Neonate

The average neonate weighs 3,400 g and measures 360 mm (CRL), or 50 cm (CHL). Fatty tissue makes up about 16% of its body weight, giving the neonate a plump appearance. Its head is the largest body part in terms of proportion; its trunk is oval-shaped, and its largest diameter is in the liver region. The thorax of the neonate is barrel-shaped (**A1**), the abdomen long (**A2**), and the pelvic region (**A3**) poorly developed. The proportionately shorter legs are bowed (varus position), and the feet are supinated. The amount of hair on the head varies greatly, and it usually falls out shortly after birth. At the time of birth, the human infant is relatively immature and helpless, compared to the offspring of other primates. Completion of development and maturation of organ systems is postponed until postnatal life. The morphological and functional characteristics can be summarized as follows:

Musculoskeletal system. The bones of a neonate are spongier than those of the adult and contain more bone marrow. The neurocranium is considerably larger in proportion to the viscerocranium. Between the bones of the calvaria are **fontanelles**, the largest of which is the **anterior fontanelle** (**A4**) overlying the superior sagittal sinus; pulsation from the superior sagittal sinus is transmitted to the overlying skin. This fontanelle closes within the 2nd year. Ossification is particularly advanced in the long bones (see Vol. 1). A sign of maturity is the presence of a secondary ossification center in the distal femoral epiphysis (**A5**).

Cardiovascular system. The heart (**A6**) of the neonate is relatively large. The heart rate is 120–140 beats per minute. Conversion of the fetal circulation occurs with closure of the foramen ovale shortly after birth (see p. 8).

Respiratory system. After taking its first spontaneous breath, the neonate has a respiratory rate of 40–44 breaths per minute. Its ribs are more horizontal, resulting in abdominal breathing, with the flatter diaphragm performing most of the work of breathing.

Alimentary system. In the first months of life, the organs of the digestive system are equipped for digestion of the mother's milk, that is, fluid ingestion. In the first few days of life, the neonate excretes a viscous, greenish intestinal discharge called *meconium*. The large liver (**A7**) makes up about 4% of the neonate's body weight.

Urinary system. The urinary bladder (**A8**) has not yet reached its final position in the lesser pelvis, and the ureters do not yet have a pelvic part.

Male genital system. Descent of the testes into the scrotum (**A9**) is a sign of maturity in the male neonate. The external male genitalia are relatively large.

Female genital system. The large ovaries lie in the iliac fossa and have not yet reached their final position in the pelvis. The cervix of the uterus makes up about two-thirds of the uterus. The external female genitalia appear relatively large at the time of birth. Covering of the labia minora by the labia majora is a sign of maturity in the female neonate.

Nervous system. Since the head of the neonate makes up one quarter of the entire body in terms of size, the brain is also proportionately large. The spinal cord extends to L2–L3 and myelinization of the corticospinal tract begins.

Skin. The skin of the neonate is thick and has only sparse lanugo hair and a well-developed subcutaneous layer of fat (**A10**). The fingernails extend beyond the fingertips, and there is a deep fold in the plantar surface of the foot.

Clinical note. The overall appearance of the neonate is assessed as soon as possible after delivery. Clinical evaluation includes heart rate, respiratory effort, muscle tone, reflexes, and skin color. Parameters are set according to the Apgar score.

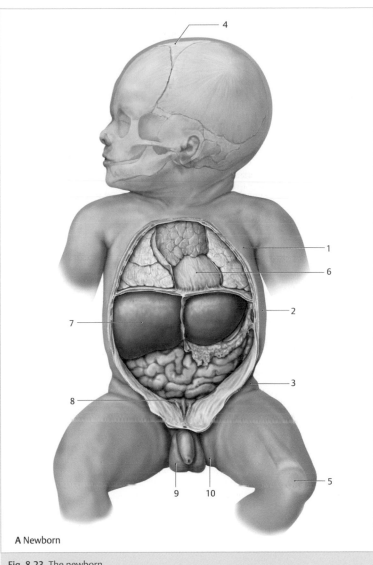

A Newborn

Fig. 8.23 The newborn.

Pregnancy and Human Development

8.14 Postnatal Period

The **neonatal period** is followed by **infancy**, which lasts until the end of the 1st year. Infancy is followed by **early childhood** (2–6 years), **late childhood/preadolescence** (7–10 years), and **adolescence** (11–20 years). **Puberty** describes the developments (sexual maturation) occurring in conjunction with hormonal changes that begin around the age of 10. It is characterized by a growth spurt and development of secondary sex characteristics and ends when adult height is reached and sexual maturity is complete.

Body weight. The average weight of the neonate at birth is 3,400 g. By the age of 5 months, its weight has doubled, and by 1 year it has tripled. By 2.5 years, the weight of the infant is four times its birth weight, by 6 years it is six times greater, by 10 years it is ten times greater. Growth and development are measured during routine check-ups, in terms of *percentiles*. The 50th percentile represents the average figure in the healthy population, for instance, for weight relative to height (A), 94% of children are between the 3rd and 97th percentile.

Height. The neonate is about 50–51-cm long. The first 2 years of life are a period of rapid growth, after which growth slows for several years before speeding up again at the beginning of adolescence (*"growth spurt"*). An important criterion is the relationship between height and weight. With proper diet, height and weight percentiles should be roughly identical (**B**).

Acceleration describes an accelerated increase in height and weight—compared with earlier decades—beginning at 7 years of age. Related to this is the earlier onset of *menarche* (first menstrual period), which occurs on average 2 years earlier than in previous generations.

Body proportions. The proportions of the body change dramatically between the neonatal period and adulthood, owing to disproportionate growth of the limbs compared to the head and trunk. In the neonate, the head comprises about one quarter of the total length of the body and in the adult this proportion is only about one eighth (**C**). The center of the neonate's body is near the navel; in the adult female, it is at the upper margin of the pubic symphysis and in the adult male, it is in the lower margin.

Body surface area. The relationship between the body's surface area and volume is greater in the neonate and child than in the adult. The surface area is about 0.25 m^2 in the neonate, 0.5 m^2 in a 2-year-old, 1 m^2 in a 9-year-old, and 1.73 m^2 in an adult. This must be taken into consideration for drug dosages and is also an important factor in prognosis and management of burn injuries.

Skeletal age. Physical growth of the child can be precisely assessed in terms of skeletal age in relation to chronological age. To determine the number, size, and appearance of ossification centers, for instance, a hand radiograph (wrist radiograph) can be useful and can also quite accurately predict adult height.

Head circumference. The growth of the cranium is monitored during the first 4 years and is measured in terms of head circumference, which in most children corresponds to the percentile curves. Changes in size or delayed closure of fontanelles or cranial sutures can be signs of *microcephaly* and *hydrocephaly*.

See **Deciduous Teeth** (p. 162) and **Development of the Teeth** (p. 164).

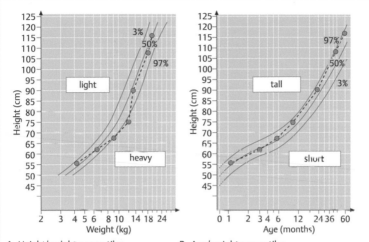

A Height/weight percentiles   **B** Age/weight percentiles

The dashed red curve illustrates typical changes in height and weight during the first 6 years of life of a healthy girl

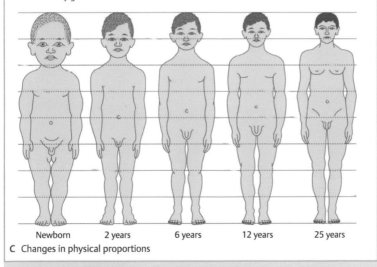

C Changes in physical proportions

Fig. 8.24 Development during the postnatal period.

9 Secretion, Glandular Epithelium, Endocrine System

9.1 Overview and Classification of Exocrine Glands

Glandular cells are epithelial cells whose principal task is to synthesize and **secrete** substances with a special biological function. Secretion is the process of intracellular production and release from the cell. A gland is an entire organ consisting of glandular cells or clusters of glandular cells. A basic distinction is made between exocrine and endocrine glands: while exocrine glands secrete their product directly or through a duct system onto an internal or external surface, endocrine glands release their secretory product, which is termed a **hormone**, into the bloodstream or surrounding tissue, by the process of **incretion**.

Classification of Exocrine Glands

Distribution. There are numerous different exocrine glands in the skin (sweat glands [**A1**], sebaceous glands [**A2**], scent glands [**A3**], mammary glands [**A4**]) and on internal body surfaces (lacrimal glands [**A5**], salivary glands [**A6**], bronchial glands [**A7**], liver [**A8**], pancreas [**A9**]).

Number and position. Isolated **unicellular intraepithelial glands** (goblet cells [**B1**]) occur in some surface epithelia, and **multicellular intraepithelial** glands in others (e.g., in the nasal mucosa and conjunctiva [**B2**]). **Multicellular extraepithelial glands** originally grow in the form of solid masses of epithelial tissue; the connection with the epithelial surface becomes the excretory duct (e.g., Brunner glands in the duodenum; sweat, scent, and sebaceous glands in the skin) (**B3**). The glandular tissue can lose its direct contact with the original surface epithelium and become a separate **extramural** gland, e.g., lacrimal gland and salivary glands of the oral cavity (p. 170). These glands arise embryologically from clusters of epithelial cells (in the respiratory tract, digestive tract, genital tract, and skin), which grow into the underlying connective tissue. They become differentiated into clusters of secretory cells and form **glandular acini**. The acini are connected to the surface by an **excretory duct** or duct system.

Form and growth habit of the secretory units. Depending on their shape, secretory units are described as **tubular** (**C1**) (e.g., colon crypts), **acinar** ("grape-like") (**C2**) (e.g., pancreas), or **alveolar** (**C3**) (e.g., scent glands). There are also mixed forms such as **tubuloacinar** (e.g., submandibular gland) or tubuloalveolar (e.g., **lactating breast**). Simple glands (e.g., merocrine sweat glands) have a separate duct that opens on an epithelial surface (**C1–C3**), while branching glands (e.g., pyloric glands) consist of several secretory units that open into a single duct (**C4–C6**); in compound glands (e.g., salivary glands), the secretory units, regardless of their form, open into a branching system of ducts (**C7–C8**). The general structure of compound extraepithelial glands can be illustrated by the salivary glands (p. 170).

The liver (p. 224), with the linked biliary tract, and the gallbladder as well as the pancreas (p. 234) are also regarded as **accessory glands** of the digestive system.

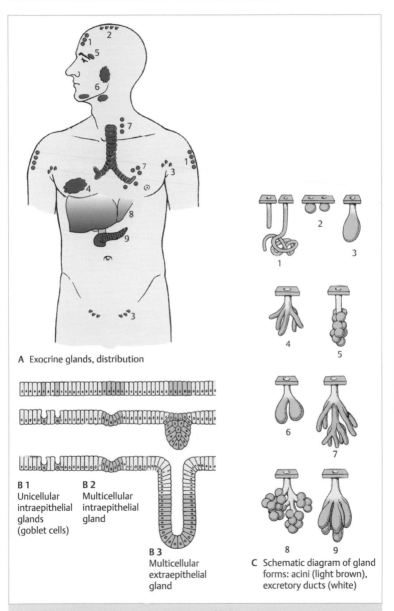

A Exocrine glands, distribution

B 1
Unicellular
intraepithelial
glands
(goblet cells)

B 2
Multicellular
intraepithelial
gland

B 3
Multicellular
extraepithelial
gland

C Schematic diagram of gland
forms: acini (light brown),
excretory ducts (white)

Secretion, Glandular Epithelium, Endocrine System

Fig. 9.1 Overview and classification of exocrine glands.

Classification of Exocrine Glands, cont.

Morphology of secretory cells and nature of the secretion. Secretory units are classified as **mucous** or **serous** on the basis of their morphology and staining pattern. This classification also reflects the chemical structure of the secretion. Serous secretory units (**A1**) are lined by tall, pyramid-shaped, polarized cells whose apices point toward the narrow lumen. Their **apical** cytoplasm usually contains **acidophilic** or **eosinophilic** secretory granules, while the **basal** parts are **basophilic**, owing to the well-developed rough endoplasmic reticulum (ER), which synthesizes export proteins. Serous glands produce a watery, protein-rich secretion (e.g., pancreas, parotid gland, lacrimal gland). Serous secretory units often have basal myoepithelial cells. The cytoplasm of mucous secretory units (**A2**) is light and foamy, and the flattened nuclei and rough ER are located in a narrow basal band of cytoplasm. The glands produce a viscous and mucinous secretion (e.g., sublingual gland, surface epithelium of parts of the stomach and duodenum). **Seromucous glands** contain both types of secretory units (e.g., submandibular gland).

Myoepithelial cells (**A3**) are present in some glands (e.g., sweat, mammary, salivary, and lacrimal glands). These are **contractile** epithelial cells that lie between the basal cell membranes of the secretory units and their excretory ducts to expel the secretion.

Secretory mechanism. Exocrine glands have a variety of secretory mechanisms. These include **merocrine** (**eccrine**) secretion by **exocytosis** (**B1**, **C6**), which involves extrusion without expulsion of the cell membrane. The secretion-filled vesicles, which are still surrounded by a Golgi membrane, gather along the inner surface of the cell membrane. The two membranes fuse at the site of contact, and the protein-rich contents of the vesicle are transported outside of the cell without the loss of the membrane. Secretions leaving the cell in this fashion no longer possess a membranous covering. This is the secretory mechanism of most exocrine and endocrine glands. In **apocrine** secretion (**B2**) or **apocytosis**, a part of the cell body and cell membrane is cast off. The membrane-covered secretion first produces a bulge on the apical surface of the cell and finally buds off. The secretory product is enveloped in a membrane after budding off, for example, milk fat globules in the lactating mammary gland. **Holocrine** secretion (**B3**) or **holocytosis** is limited to sebaceous glands. The cells form large lipid droplets and then die by programmed cell death (apoptosis), that is, the cells of the gland are completely transformed into secretory product. New glandular cells are continually replenished from a basal cell layer.

Electron microscopic dimension of secretion production. Materials (amino acids, sugar) are absorbed by diffusion or pinocytosis from the bloodstream (**C1**) and enter the cisterns of the rough **ER** (**C2**), where synthesis and posttranslational modification of secretory proteins, mucins, and lipoproteins occur. These are then carried by transport vesicles to the **Golgi apparatus** (**C3**) and are packaged by its membrane into **Golgi vesicles** (**C4**). The discharge-filled vesicles ultimately bud off (**C5**) or are released by exocytosis (**C6**).

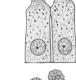

A Morphological classification of serous and mucous secretory units of salivary glands

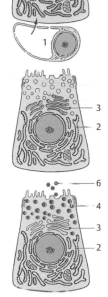

Features	Serosal secretory unit	Mucosal secretory unit
Total diameter	Smaller	Larger
Appearance	Acinus or cap	Tubule
Lumen	Very narrow	Relatively wide
Nucleus shape	Round	Flattened
Nucleus position	(almost) Basal	Basal, along the wall
Cytoplasm	Apical granules	Light, foamy
Cell borders	Less distinct	More distinct
Tight junctions	Absent	Detectable
Secretory canaliculi	Intercellular	Absent

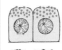

1 Exocytosis   2 Apocrine secretion   3 Holocrine secretion

B Various secretion processes, light microscopy

C Production of proteincontaining secretions and secretion process, electron microscopy

Secretion, Glandular Epithelium, Endocrine System

Fig. 9.2 Light microscopic classification of exocrine secretory units.

9.2 Endocrine System

Overview

Endocrine secretion signifies that the cells and cell aggregates of the endocrine system secrete hormones that are distributed in the body by the bloodstream (**A1**). Hormones are chemical messengers that produce specific effects in their target cells via receptors. The endocrine system is a means of communication between cells that, like the nervous system, with which it is intimately linked, coordinates and controls the body's internal workings. Most hormones are proteins, polypeptides, or steroids. The term "endocrine" distinguishes these ductless glands from exocrine glands, which release their secretion through a duct.

Hormonal signaling. Endocrine hormones (**A1**) can influence their target tissue or organ over long distances. The chemical signal is carried by the bloodstream. Autocrine or paracrine secretion (**A2**) means that hormones are released to the secreting cell itself or to nearby cells. In **neurosecretion**, the secretory cell is a neuron, which releases its transmitter into the bloodstream to act as a hormone (**A3**). This is not the same as synaptic transmission (**A4**), in which a hormone or neurotransmitter is released into the synaptic gap, analogous to paracrine secretion.

Most classic endocrine glands are derived from epithelium from which they have lost their connection. The endocrine glands include the pituitary gland (hypophysis) (**B1**), pineal gland or body (**B2**), thyroid gland (**B3**), parathyroid glands (**B4**), and adrenal glands (**B5**). The **glands** of the endocrine system occur *individually* or in *pairs* and are organized *hierarchically*. Endocrine gland activity is usually in response to specific stimuli and in many cases, it is halted by negative feedback (i.e., by an increase in hormone levels in the blood).Regulatory processes mostly involve several glands in the hierarchy of glands.

All endocrine glands have a dense capillary or sinusoid network (**C, D**).

Besides the individual endocrine glands, **endocrine cell aggregations** are found in other organs: these include the *islets of Langerhans* in the pancreas (**B6**), known collectively as the pancreatic islets, *Leydig cells* in the interstitial tissue surrounding the seminiferous tubules (**B7**) as well as *theca lutein cells, granulosa lutein cells,* and *hilar cells* of the ovary (**B8**).

The epithelium of specific organs (e.g., in the gastrointestinal tract and respiratory system) also contains individual endocrine cells, which are collectively known as the disseminated or diffuse endocrine cell system. Endocrine cells are also present in the **hypothalamus,** which contains numerous groups of neurons that produce neurohormones (p. 368).

There has been evidence recently that it is not only cells of epithelial origin that produce hormones but also mesenchymal cells (e.g., fat cells and muscle cells).

Hormones belong to different chemical groups and the ultrastructure of the corresponding endocrine cells varies greatly as a result. The hydrophilic substances include polypeptides, peptides, glycoproteins, and biogenic amines. The lipophilic substances include steroid hormones and thyroid hormones.

Clinical note: Increased or reduced hormone secretion is found in a number of diseases (e.g., diabetes mellitus, over- or underactive thyroid).

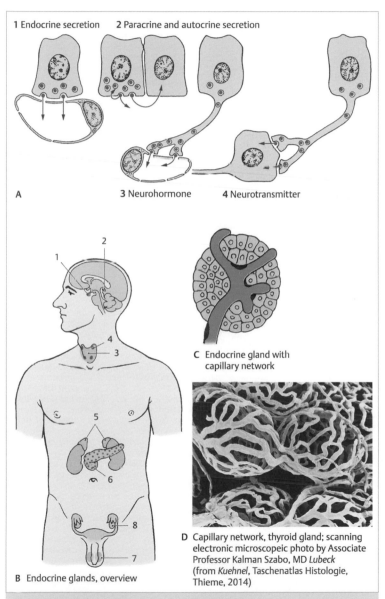

1 Endocrine secretion **2** Paracrine and autocrine secretion

A **3** Neurohormone **4** Neurotransmitter

C Endocrine gland with capillary network

B Endocrine glands, overview

D Capillary network, thyroid gland; scanning electronic microscopeic photo by Associate Professor Kalman Szabo, MD *Lubeck* (from *Kuehnel*, Taschenatlas Histologie, Thieme, 2014)

Fig. 9.3 Overview and principles of endocrine gland function.

Secretion, Glandular Epithelium, Endocrine System

9.3 Hypothalamic–Pituitary Axis

Gross Anatomy

Hypothalamus

The hypothalamus (**A1**, **B**) is formed by the **lowermost portion of the diencephalon**. Arising from its caudal portion is the tuber cinereum, from which the funnel-shaped infundibular recess extends downward and becomes continuous with the infundibulum of the pituitary gland (hypophyseal stalk) (**A2**, **B**). **Posteriorly**, it extends to the mammillary body; **rostrally**, it is contiguous with the optic chiasm (**A6**, **B**). The **anterior** surface of the hypothalamus is the only region of the diencephalon visible externally (see Vol. 3).

Function. The hypothalamus and its nuclei constitute the main control organ for autonomic function, as well as the main regulatory organ of the endocrine system, which it controls by means of its connections to the pituitary gland.

Pituitary Gland (Hypophysis)

The cylindrical pituitary gland weighs 600–900 mg, rests in the **hypophysial fossa** of the sella turcica in the sphenoid bone at the center of the skull base, and is separated from the cranial base by a sheet of dura mater, known as the *sellar diaphragm*, in the center of which is an opening for the passage of the hypophyseal stalk (**A7**, **B**). The pituitary gland may be divided into the adenohypophysis, an epithelial structure, and the neurohypophysis.

Adenohypophysis (**A3**, **B**) (anterior lobe of pituitary gland). The anterior lobe of the pituitary gland consists of the **pars distalis**, which makes up the bulk of the gland; the **pars tuberalis**, which covers the anterior parts of the infundibulum (**A2**, **B**) and parts of the tuber cinereum; and the **pars intermedia** (middle lobe) (**A4**, **B**), which forms a narrow, intermediate zone bordering on the surface of the neurohypophysis.

Neurohypophysis (**A5**, **B**) (posterior lobe of pituitary gland). This contains only unmyelinated axons, axon terminals, glial cells (*pituicytes*), and wide-lumen capillaries. It is connected to the hypothalamus by the **infundibulum** (hypophyseal stalk) (**A2**, **B**). The funnel-shaped **infundibular recess** (**B**) projects into the initial portion of the hypophyseal stalk from the third ventricle; the bulge on its posterior wall is known as the **median eminence** (**B**). The posterior lobe of the pituitary gland houses a functionally important vascular area (see p. 356).

Topography. The pituitary gland may be divided into the suprasellar and infrasellar parts. The **suprasellar** part consists of the *hypophyseal stalk* (*infundibulum* and *pars tuberalis of adenohypophysis*), which lies in close proximity to the optic chiasm anteriorly. The tuber cinereum rests on the sellar diaphragm, surrounded by the cerebral arterial circle. The **infrasellar** part consists of the *anterior and middle lobes of the adenohypophysis*, as well as the *neurohypophysis* (*posterior lobe*) (extradural position).

Blood circulation (see pp. 355 and 357 and Vol. 3). The pituitary gland is supplied by four arteries: the right and left **inferior hypophysial arteries** arise from the *cavernous part of the internal carotid artery* and join to form an arterial ring around the neurohypophysis (mantle plexus). The inferior hypophysial arteries anastomose with the **superior hypophysial arteries**, which originate from the *cerebral portion of the internal carotid artery*. The superior hypophysial arteries pass to the anterior portion of the hypothalamus, the pars tuberalis of the adenohypophysis, and the hypophyseal stalk; a trabecular artery ascends in front of the hypophyseal stalk, passes through the adenohypophysis, and feeds the capillary loops of the neurohypophysis. The *adenohypophysis is not directly supplied by these arteries* but instead receives its blood supply from a **system of portal veins:** after entering the hypophyseal stalk, the two **superior hypophysial arteries** divide into hairpin-shaped capillary loops ("special vessels") (**primary plexus**). Blood from the plexus drains into one or two **portal vessels** (hypophysial portal veins), which carry it to the adenohypophysis. There the vessels divide again to form a sinusoid capillary network (**secondary plexus**) surrounding the glandular cells. Blood drains from the secondary plexus to the superficial **veins**, which empty into the **cavernous sinus**. The capillary network of the posterior lobe anastomoses with that of the anterior lobe but is also directly connected with the blood vessels of the general circulation. There is no portal venous system between the hypothalamus and the posterior pituitary.

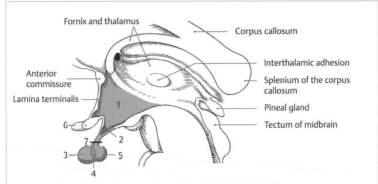

A Pituitary gland and hypothalamus (diencephalon), overview

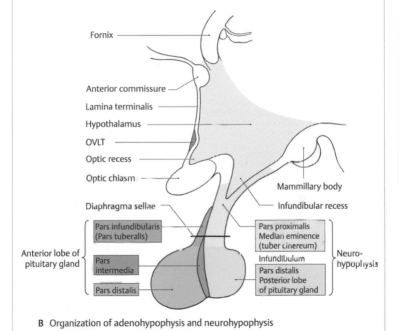

B Organization of adenohypophysis and neurohypophysis

Fig. 9.4 Macroscopic structure of the hypothalamus and pituitary gland.

Secretion, Glandular Epithelium, Endocrine System

Microscopic Anatomy of the Pituitary Gland

The pituitary gland is surrounded by a thin **connective tissue capsule** (**A1**). At the pars tuberalis (**A2**) the capsule also surrounds the *portal vessels* and *arteries* supplying the adenohypophysis. The veins underneath the capsule form a *venous plexus*.

Adenohypophysis (Anterior Lobe of Pituitary Gland)

The anterior lobe of the pituitary gland (adenohypophysis) is composed of irregular **strands and nests of epithelial cells** that are surrounded by wide-lumen **sinusoid capillaries** with fenestrated endothelium, and by **reticular fibers**. Located between the anterior and posterior lobes of the pituitary is the pars intermedia, which contains colloid-filled cysts (**A6**, **D**).

Glandular cells (**A4**, **B**). Various staining techniques may be used to examine the cells of the anterior lobe. Azan stain can be used to distinguish three groups of cells: acidophilic (α-cells; **B7**), basophilic (β-cells; **B8**), and chromophobic (γ-cells; **B9**) (poorly staining). Acidophilic and basophilic cells secrete various hormones (either polypeptides or glycoproteins). The protein hormones *somatotropin* (*STH*), known internationally as growth hormone (**GH**), and *prolactin* (*PRL*) are secreted by nonglandotropic **acidophilic** cells and stain orange with Orange G. The protein hormone *corticotropin* (*adrenocorticotropic hormone, ACTH*) and the glycoprotein hormones *thyrotropin* (*thyroid-stimulating hormone, TSH*), *follitropin* (*follicle-stimulating hormone, FSH*), *lutropin* (*luteinizing hormone, LH*), *lipotropin* (*lipotropic hormone, LPH*), and *melanotropin* (*melanocyte-stimulating hormone, MSH*) are produced by glandotropic **basophilic** cells that stain with periodic acid-Schiff stain (PAS).

Chromophobic cells are probably not directly involved in hormone production and are thus not included in the figure on p. 359. It is currently believed that these cells are either precursors of hormone-producing cells (*stem cells*) or *degranulated* (*emptied*) *cells* of any type. Chromophobic **follicular** (**stellate**) **cells** have long, thin processes that extend through the entire gland, incompletely surrounding the groups of glandular cells and dividing the anterior lobe into regions.

These cells are apparently associated with glia.

Immunohistochemical techniques can also be used to identify glandular cell types by light and electron microscopy, based on their hormonal secretions.

Cell arrangement. The various glandular cells in the anterior pituitary are neither strictly distributed by type nor evenly dispersed throughout the gland. About 50% are chromophobic, 10% basophilic, and 40% acidophilic. The acidophilic cells producing **STH** and **PRL** lie mainly in the *lateral parts of the pars distalis*, while the basophilic cells containing **ACTH**, **MSH**, and **LPH** are mostly found in the *central* and *anterior portions of the gland*. The cells of the *pars tuberalis* predominantly produce the gonadotropins **FSH** and **LH**. TSH-producing basophilic cells are frequently located in the *anterior, central part of the pars distalis* of the gland. Chromophobic cells are not specific to any particular part.

Electron microscopic appearance. The variously staining cells are characterized under electron microscopy by their **membrane-enclosed granules** (vesicles with electron-dense nuclei), the size of which depends on the hormone contained within the cell and ranges from 60 to 900 nm. Cells also differ in terms of the shape and position of the granules, as well as the appearance of ergastoplasm (endoplasmic reticulum) and Golgi complexes. Hormone transport is by exocytosis.

Neurohypophysis (Posterior Lobe of Pituitary Gland)

Over 70% of the posterior lobe of the pituitary gland, or neurohypophysis (**A5**), consists of **unmyelinated axons** with cell bodies in hypothalamic nuclei, axon endings, specialized glial cells called **pituicytes**, and a complex system of wide-lumen **capillaries**. It does not contain any nerve cells. Hormones synthesized in the hypothalamic nuclei are conveyed via axonal transport along the unmyelinated nerve fibers to the site of release from the posterior pituitary into the bloodstream (**neurosecretion**) (see Vol. 3).

A3 Infundibulum (hypophyseal stalk), **B10** γ-cell, **B11** ε-cell

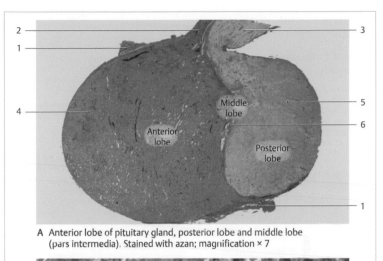

A Anterior lobe of pituitary gland, posterior lobe and middle lobe (pars intermedia). Stained with azan; magnification × 7

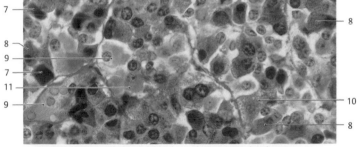

B Staining patterns of cells in adenohypophysis. Stained with azan; magnification × 400

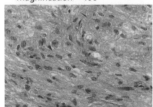

C Posterior lobe of pituitary gland. Bundle of unmyelinated nerve fibers. Stained with hematoxylin and eosin; magnification × 100

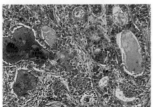

D Middle lobe with colloid cysts and basophil invasion. Stained with azan; magnification × 80

Fig. 9.5 Microscopic structure of the pituitary gland.

Secretion, Glandular Epithelium, Endocrine System

9.4 Hypothalamus–Pituitary Connections

Efferent Connections of the Hypothalamus

The primary tasks of the hypothalamus (**A**, **B**) are **control of the autonomic nervous system and the endocrine system**. The hypothalamus receives input via receptors from the periphery of the body and other areas of the brain, which it integrates to serve broader functional tasks (e.g., regulating metabolism, body temperature, eating, and reproduction). There are two types of efferent pathways from the hypothalamus: a **neural pathway** consisting of efferent nerves that descend through the brainstem to visceromotor nuclei and also influence endocrine glands via autonomic nerves (see Vol. 3); and a **hormonal pathway** that controls other endocrine glands via the hypothalamic–pituitary unit.

Hormonal Pathway

Information is carried by **neurohormones**, which can be detected, bound to carrier proteins, in the *perikarya*, *axons*, and *axon ends* of neurosecretory cells. The neurohormones travel from the perikarya producing them along the axons to the neurohypophysis, where they are released, either in the **distal neurohypophysis** (**B4**) (*main releasing site of effector hormones*) or in the **median eminence** (**B5**) (proximal neurohypophysis, *main releasing site of regulatory hormones*). Regulatory hormones are transported by the portal vessels (**B6**) to the anterior pituitary (**B7**), where they influence the synthesis and secretion of anterior-lobe hormones. Hormones are thus transported to the anterior lobe via specialized local vessels and not the systemic circulation.

Hormones of the Hypothalamus and Pituitary Gland

Only a small number of hormones secreted by the hypothalamus or pituitary gland act directly on target organs as effector hormones. Most act indirectly as regulatory hormones; regulatory hormones secreted by the hypothalamus influence the activity of the adenohypophysis, and those secreted by the adenohypophysis influence the activity of the peripheral endocrine glands. The hypothalamus and pituitary gland form a functional unit and are connected to each other by blood vessels.

Effector hormones. The hypothalamic hormones **oxytocin** and **vasopressin** (antidiuretic hormone, ADH) act directly on target tissues, bypassing the adenohypophysis. They travel along the axons of neurosecretory cells to reach the posterior pituitary where they are released into the blood (**B4**) (see Vol. 3). The neurohypophysis serves as a site for storage and release of oxytocin and vasopressin; it does not produce any hormones. The hypophysial hormones **somatotropin**, **prolactin**, and **melanotropin** also act as effector hormones, that is, largely without involvement of peripheral endocrine glands, although there are exceptions. Somatotropin, for instance, acts via stimulation of the *somatomedins* in the liver.

Regulatory hormones. As the main control center of the endocrine glands, the hypothalamus exerts indirect control over peripheral endocrine glands by secreting **releasing hormones** (whose names are formed with the suffix **"-liberin"**) and **release-inhibiting hormones** (whose names end with **"-statin"**) which stimulate or inhibit the release of anterior pituitary hormones. Each anterior pituitary hormone has a corresponding regulatory hormone. Regulatory hormones travel along the axons to the **median eminence** of the neurohypophysis (B5) and from there through the **portal vessels** (B6) to the **capillary plexus of the adenohypophysis** (B7).

The only releasing hormones currently known are those stimulating the release of ACTH, TSH, LH, and FSH. Synthesis of these hormones is influenced by negative feedback, that is, an increase in hormone in peripheral target tissues leads to a decrease in production. The release of prolactin is inhibited by dopamine (prolactostatin or prolactin release-inhibiting factor, PIF).

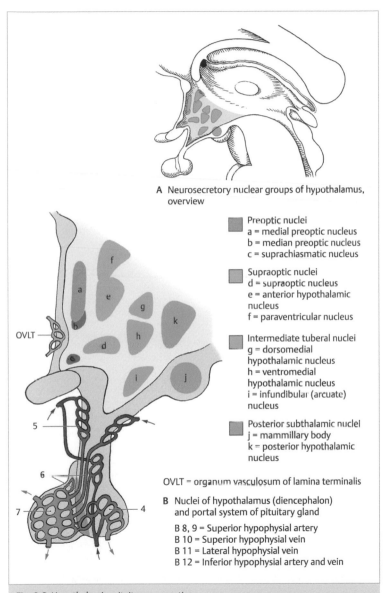

A Neurosecretory nuclear groups of hypothalamus, overview

Preoptic nuclei
a = medial preoptic nucleus
b = median preoptic nucleus
c = suprachiasmatic nucleus

Supraoptic nuclei
d = supraoptic nucleus
e = anterior hypothalamic nucleus
f = paraventricular nucleus

Intermediate tuberal nuclei
g = dorsomedial hypothalamic nucleus
h = ventromedial hypothalamic nucleus
i = infundibular (arcuate) nucleus

Posterior subthalamic nuclei
j = mammillary body
k = posterior hypothalamic nucleus

OVLT = organum vasculosum of lamina terminalis

B Nuclei of hypothalamus (diencephalon) and portal system of pituitary gland

B 8, 9 = Superior hypophysial artery
B 10 = Superior hypophysial vein
B 11 = Lateral hypophysial vein
B 12 = Inferior hypophysial artery and vein

Secretion, Glandular Epithelium, Endocrine System

Fig. 9.6 Hypothalamic–pituitary connections.

Hypothalamic–Posterior Pituitary Axis (A)

The perikarya (cell bodies) of the neurosecretory cells in the hypothalamic–posterior pituitary unit are located in the **paraventricular nucleus (A1)** and **supraoptic nucleus (A2)**, groups of large neurons in the diencephalon. The hormones *oxytocin* and *vasopressin* (antidiuretic hormone, ADH) are produced by neurosecretory cells in these nuclei and carried along their axons to the posterior lobe of the pituitary gland **(A3)**, where they are released into its capillary network. The axons carrying the neurosecretory substances form the **hypothalamicohypophysial tract (A4)**, which travels in the *internal infundibular zone*. Transport is visible as swellings of the axons, which form *Herring bodies* (see Vol. 3). Both neurohormones are bound to carrier proteins called *neurophysins*.

The **capillary network of the posterior lobe of the pituitary gland (A5)** is directly connected to the vascular system of the general circulation. Hypothalamic hormones stored in the axon terminals can thus travel directly to target tissues in the periphery of the body. As a site of storage and release, the posterior pituitary is thus a **neurohemal region for the effector hormones** vasopressin and oxytocin.

Hypothalamic–Anterior Pituitary Axis (B)

Axons from the neurons of the small-cell nuclei of the hypothalamus, the **infundibular nucleus (B1)** and the **posteromedial nucleus (B2)**, form the **tuberoinfundibular tract (B3)**, which courses in the *external infundibular zone*. The *releasing hormones* and *release-inhibiting hormones* produced in the neuron cell bodies are transported from the axon terminals, in special vessels to the **portal vessels (B4)**, and then into the **capillary network of the adenohypophysis (B5)**. Regulatory hormones stimulate the inhibition or release of anterior lobe hormones, which, in turn, mostly influence the production and release of hormones of other endocrine glands (e.g., thyroid, adrenal cortex, gonads).

The cell bodies of the regulatory hormones *luliberin (gonadotropin-releasing hormone, GnRH)*, *somatostatin (SS)*, and *thyroliberin (thyrotropin-releasing factor, TRF)* lie scattered in the **periventricular zone (B6)**. Neural cell bodies of the same hormone are grouped together, lying in separate regions that specifically produce "hypophysiotropic" hormones. *Corticoliberin (corticotropin-releasing hormone, CRH)* cell bodies lie together in the **paraventricular nucleus (A1)**; *prolactostatin (prolactin-inhibitory factor, PIF)* and *somatoliberin (growth-hormone-releasing hormone, GH-RH)* cell bodies lie scattered in the **infundibular nucleus (B1)**. The infundibular nucleus is a readily distinguishable parvocellular nucleus in the wall of the infundibulum. It receives neural afferents from other regions of the brain and regulates the release of regulatory hormones in the median eminence.

The efferent processes, consisting of unmyelinated fibers projecting from the above-named nuclei (hormone production sites) to the median eminence, form essentially separate tracts for each system within the tuberoinfundibular tract (see Vol. 3).

Median eminence (B7). The median eminence functions as a **neurohemal region for hypothalamic regulatory hormones**. It consists of *capillary loops* that radiate from outside into the pituitary gland. The capillary loops are surrounded by *perivascular connective tissue spaces*, in which the axons of the neurohormonal neurons end. Neurohormones from the nuclei of the hypothalamus are released here and are carried by the **portal vessels (B4)** to the **adenohypophysis**, where they stimulate the release or inhibition of anterior lobe hormones. Neurohormones appear in the axons and axon terminals as variably large vesicles with dense nuclei. The production and release of neurohormones can be regulated either by humoral mechanisms, that is, via blood vessels from regions containing hypothalamic nuclei, or by the central nervous system (e.g., influence of the psyche on the ovarian cycle, influence of tactile stimulation of the nipple on lactation, etc.)

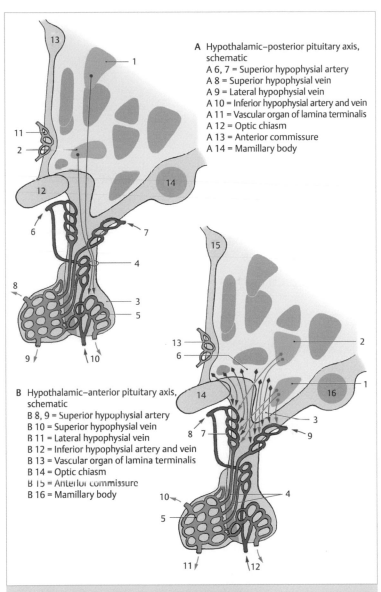

A Hypothalamic–posterior pituitary axis, schematic
A 6, 7 = Superior hypophysial artery
A 8 = Superior hypophysial vein
A 9 = Lateral hypophysial vein
A 10 = Inferior hypophysial artery and vein
A 11 = Vascular organ of lamina terminalis
A 12 = Optic chiasm
A 13 = Anterior commissure
A 14 = Mamillary body

B Hypothalamic–anterior pituitary axis, schematic
B 8, 9 = Superior hypophysial artery
B 10 = Superior hypophysial vein
B 11 = Lateral hypophysial vein
B 12 = Inferior hypophysial artery and vein
B 13 = Vascular organ of lamina terminalis
B 14 = Optic chiasm
B 15 = Anterior commissure
B 16 = Mamillary body

Fig. 9.7 Hypothalamic–pituitary connections, continued.

Secretion, Glandular Epithelium, Endocrine System

Hormones of the Hypothalamic–Posterior Pituitary Axis		
Hypothalamic hormones and synonyms	**Release site**	**Effect**
Oxytocin (OXT) (effector hormone)	Posterior pituitary	Contraction of sensory smooth muscle cells in the uterus (contractions), contraction of myoepithelial cells in the mammary gland; deficiency leads to weak contractions
Vasopressin (VP) or **antidiuretic hormone (ADH)** (effector hormone)	Posterior pituitary	Increases blood pressure and supports reabsorption of water in the kidneys; deficiency leads to diabetes insipidus
Regulatory Hormones–Releasing Hormones		
Folliberin Follicle-stimulating hormone releasing hormone (or factor) (FSH-RH* or FSH-RF)	Along the loops of the portal vessels in the external infundibular zone	Stimulates production and secretion of FSH in acidophilic cells of the adenohypophysis
Luliberin Luteinizing-hormone-releasing hormone (or factor) (LHRH or LHRF) Gonadotropin-releasing hormone (GnRH)	Along the loops of the portal vessels in the internal infundibular zone	Stimulates production and secretion of FSH and LH in acidophilic cells of the adenohypophysis
Corticoliberin Corticotropin-releasing hormone (or factor) (CRH or CRF)	Along the loops of the portal vessels in the external infundibular zone	Stimulates production and secretion of ACTH in basophilic cells of the adenohypophysis
Thyroliberin Thyrotropin-releasing hormone (or factor) (TRH or TRF)	Along the loops of the portal vessels in the external infundibular zone and median eminence	Stimulates production and secretion of TSH in basophilic cells of the adenohypophysis
Somatoliberin Somatotropin-releasing hormone (or factor) or growth hormone releasing hormone (or factor) (GH-RH or GH-RF)	Along the loops of the portal vessels in the median eminence	Stimulates release of somatotropin (STH) and growth hormone (GH) in acidophilic cells of the adenohypophysis
Prolactoliberin Prolactin-releasing hormone (or factor) (PRH or PRF)	?	Stimulates production and secretion of prolactin in acidophilic cells of the adenohypophysis
Melanoliberin Melanotropin-releasing hormone (or factor) (MRH* or MRF)	?	Substance released in the posterior lobe of the pituitary gland that presumably influences production and secretion of melanotropin in the middle lobe
Regulatory Hormones–Release-inhibiting Hormones		
Prolactostatin Prolactin-release-inhibiting hormone (or factor) (PIH or PIF) (= dopamine, DOPA)	?	Inhibits secretion of prolactin in acidophilic cells of the adenohypophysis

Fig. 9.8 Hypothalamic–pituitary system.

Regulatory Hormones – Release-inhibiting Hormones (cont.)

Somatostatin Somatotropin-release- inhibiting **h**ormone (or factor) (SRIH or SRIF)	Along the loops of the portal vessels in the external infundibular zone	Inhibits secretion of somatotropin in the adenohypophysis, inhibits TRH-induced secretion of TSH; also present in disseminated endocrine cells of the digestive tract
Melanostatin Melanotropin-release- inhibiting **h**ormone (or factor) (MIH* or MIF)	?	Presumably inhibits secretion of melanotropin in the middle lobe of the pituitary gland

*The existence of these substances is postulated on the basis of indirect findings; their chemical composition is still unknown.

Anterior Pituitary Hormones

Hormone and synonyms	Cell description (staining pattern)	Granule diameter (TEM)* (nm)	Effect
Somatotropin Growth hormone (GH) Somatotropic hormone (STH)	Somatotropic cells (acidophilic)	300–500	Stimulates growth in height; influences carbohydrate and lipid metabolism
Prolactin (PRL) Mammotropic hormone Luteotropic hormone (LTH)	Mammotropic or lactotropic cells (acidophilic)	600–900	Stimulates proliferation of mammary gland tissue and lactation
Follitropin Follicle-stimulating hormone (FSH)	Gonadotropic cells (basophilic)	350–400	Affects gonads; stimulates follicular maturation and spermatogenesis; stimulates proliferation of granulosa cells, estrogen production, and expression of lutropin receptors
Lutropin Luteinizing hormone (LH) or interstitial cell- stimulating hormone (ICSH)		170–200	Triggers ovulation, stimulates proliferation of follicular epithelial cells and synthesis of progesterone; stimulates testosterone production in the interstitial cells (Leydig cells) of the testes; general anabolic effect
Thyrotropin Thyrotropic hormone or thyroid-stimulating hormone (TSH)	Thyrotropic cells (basophilic)	200–300	Stimulates thyroid activity; increases O_2 intake and protein synthesis; influences carbohydrate and fat metabolism
Corticotropin Adrenocorticotropic hormone (ACTH)	Corticotropic cells (basophilic)	200–500	Stimulates hormone production in the adrenal cortex; influences water and electrolyte levels as well as carbohydrate production in the liver
β-/γ-Lipotropin (LPH)	Lipotropic cells (basophilic)	200–500	Not sufficiently understood in humans
α-/β-Melanotropin (MSH)	Melanotropic cells (basophilic)	200–500	Melanin production, skin pigment- ation, protection against UV rays
β-Endorphin	(basophilic)	200–400	Opioid effect

*TEM = Transmission electron microscope

Secretion, Glandular Epithelium, Endocrine System

Fig. 9.9 Hypothalamic and pituitary hormones, overview.

9.5 Pineal Gland

Gross Anatomy

The **pineal gland** (**AB1**, **C**), **or pineal body**, is about 10-mm long and weighs about 160 mg. The pine-cone-shaped (hence the name) pineal gland lies between the *habenular commissure* (**C14**) and the *posterior commissure* (**C15**), on the posterior wall of the third ventricle. The greater part of the gland projects caudally beyond the roof of the ventricle, lying in a depression between the two *superior colliculi* (**AB3**) of the tectal plate. Between the two commissures is the **pineal recess** (**BC6**), which is covered by ependyma. The remaining surface is surrounded by pia mater. The pineal gland is a **circumventricular organ** and is considered a **neurohemal organ** (see Vol. 3). It is supplied by the medial and lateral posterior choroidal arteries which arise from the right and left lateral posterior cerebral arteries. Venous drainage is via the great cerebral vein.

Development. The pineal gland is derived from the neuroepithelium of the diencephalon in the roof of the third ventricle and remains connected to other parts of the brain via the habenulae (**AB2**). During the course of phylogenesis, the pineal gland underwent a complex transformation, from originally functioning as a photosensory organ (**parietal "eye" present in reptiles**) to serving as a **neuroendocrine gland**.

A4 Thalamus, **A5** Choroid line, **B7** Anterior commissure, **B8** Lamina terminalis, **B9** Optic chiasm, **B10** Pituitary, **B11** Third ventricle, **B12** Corpus callosum, **B13** Fornix, **C7** Roof of the third ventricle.

Microscopic Anatomy

The highly vascularized pineal gland is made up of **parenchymal pinealocytes** embedded in a stroma of astrocytes processes. They are divided into lobules (**D17**) by connective tissue septa (**D16**). The pinealocyte processes, which have knoblike ends, contain synaptic ribbons that are associated with synaptic vesicles and terminate together with sympathetic nerve fibers in the pericapillary compartment.

Regression. Pineal tissue begins to deteriorate early in life and is replaced by **areas of glial cells**, which are formed by *fibrous astrocytes*. These merge to form fluid-filled cysts that may force the parenchyma into a narrow peripheral zone. Nearly all adults have brain sand, or **corpora acervulus** (**D18**), composed of layered *colloidal organic matter* that is impregnated with *calcium salts*. Winding around larger calcium concretions (**corpora arenacea**, **D18**), are reticular fibers. Larger accumulations of brain sand enable identification of the pineal gland in radiographs.

Innervation. The pineal gland is innervated by *sympathetic* (*noradrenergic*) *nerves*, whose cell bodies are located in the **superior cervical ganglion**. The nerve fibers enter the cranium via the *internal carotid nerve plexus* and pass to the pineal gland via the *periarterial nerve plexuses*. The pinealocytes are **modified photoreceptor cells**, which receive information about environmental lighting (quantity of light) from the retina. Interspersed along the neuron chain that passes from the retina to the pineal gland are *hypothalamic* (suprachiasmatic nucleus) and *sympathetic nuclei*.

Hormones. Pinealocytes synthesize and secrete indole and peptides, especially **α-melanocyte-stimulating hormone** (**α-MSH**) and **melatonin**. In amphibians, MSH induces the contraction of melanocytes and thus lightens skin pigmentation. It acts as an antagonist to melanotropin which is secreted by the adenohypophysis. Melatonin, which is produced only in darkness, is produced enzymatically from serotonin. In humans it inhibits the release of gonadotropic hormones and thus gonadal development. The thyroid is also thought to be a target organ of melatonin.

> **Clinical note:** The biological significance of melatonin is not fully understood. It is believed to influence the rhythm of biological processes and helps to counteract insomnia and jet lag. Certain forms of **pubertas praecox** (precocious puberty) are generally believed to be caused by hypofunction of the pineal gland. Pineal tumors can block the circulation of cerebrospinal fluid by compression of the cerebral aqueduct, leading to **closed hydrocephalus**.

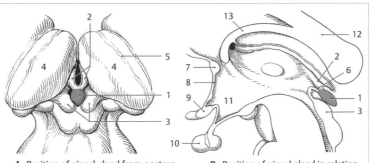

A Position of pineal gland from postero-superior, view of roof of diencephalon, midbrain and tectal plate

B Position of pineal gland in relation to third ventricle, sagittal section through diencephalon

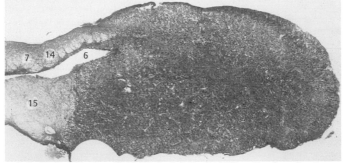

C Sagittal section through pineal gland. Stained with hematoxylin and eosin; magnification ×30

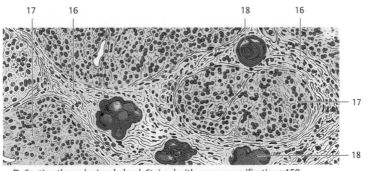

D Section through pineal gland. Stained with azan; magnification ×150

Fig. 9.10 Macroscopic and microscopic structure of the pineal gland.

Secretion, Glandular Epithelium, Endocrine System

9.6 Adrenal Glands

Gross Anatomy

Each of the paired, retroperitoneal **adrenal glands** (**suprarenal glands**) (**A1–A2**) contains two endocrine glands of differing phylogenetic origin which merged to form a compact organ and are surrounded by a common connective tissue capsule. A *mesodermal part*, that is, the outer **adrenal cortex** (**D9**), is derived from the epithelium lining the posterior coelom cavity and surrounds an *ectodermal part* (*sympathoblasts of the neural crest*), forming the **adrenal medulla** (**D10**). Each of the adrenal glands, weighing 4.2–5.0 g, is enclosed in a *perirenal fat capsule* and rests atop the superior pole of the kidney (**AB1, AC2**). On the posterior aspect of each gland, there is the **hilum**, which allows *veins* and *lymphatic vessels* to exit. *Arteries* and *nerves* enter through numerous sites in its **surface**.

Topography. When viewed from **anterior**, the **right** adrenal gland (**AB1**) is triangular in shape with a distinct *apex*. The **base** of the adrenal surface lies directly on the *superior pole of the kidney* and is curved to fit its contours. Its **lateral** portion lies against the *medial crus of the diaphragm*, overlying both the *greater splanchnic nerve* and the right parts of the *celiac ganglion*. Its **anterior** surface is covered by the *right lobe of the liver* and partly by the *inferior vena cava*.

The **left**, more crescent-shaped adrenal gland (**AC2**), does not have an apex and lies on the *upper, medial margin of the kidney*. It covers the *greater splanchnic nerve* and **anteriorly** is in close contact with the *omental bursa* and *posterior wall of the stomach*.

The adrenal glands project toward the posterior wall of the abdomen at the height of the necks of the 11th and 12th ribs. A characteristic feature of each of the adrenal glands is the close proximity of the *celiac ganglion* or *celiac nerve plexus* (**A3**), as well as the dense and branching **suprarenal nerve plexus** whose fibers arise from the *celiac nerve plexus*, *splanchnic nerve*, *phrenic nerve*, and *vagus nerve* and that pierce the organ through its surface.

Vessels, Nerves, and Lymphatic Drainage

Arteries. Each adrenal gland is supplied by a subcapsular arterial network lying on its surface that is fed by three sources: the **superior suprarenal artery** arising from the *inferior phrenic artery*; the **middle suprarenal artery** arising from the *abdominal aorta* (**A4**); and the **inferior suprarenal artery** arising from the *renal artery* (**A5**). There are numerous exceptions to the typical pattern of arteries. Those near the surface of the adrenal gland give rise to short arterioles that branch to form a **capillary network**, which ultimately passes to the cortical and medullary sinuses from which blood travels into the medullary veins. The sinusoidal **medullary veins** have strong, irregularly distributed bundles of longitudinal muscle that act to constrict the vein (*"throttle mechanism"*), temporarily blocking hormone-rich blood flow, which can be released rapidly into the circulation when needed. The adrenal glands are also supplied by **perforating arteries**, which pass directly to the adrenal medulla.

Veins. Venous blood collects in a single *central vein* located in each adrenal gland. The central veins exit through the hilum of the respective adrenal gland as the **left suprarenal vein**, which empties into the *renal vein* (**A6**), or **right suprarenal vein** emptying into the *inferior vena cava* (**A7**).

Nerve supply. The nerves supplying the adrenal glands are mainly preganglionic sympathetic fibers from the splanchnic nerves, coming from the intermediolateral nucleus of the thoracic spine (T5–T12). The innervation of the chromaffin medullary cells is cholinergic.

Lymphatic drainage. The majority of lymphatic vessels leaving the adrenal glands follow the course of the arteries. The primary lymph nodes of both adrenal glands are the **para-aortic** and **lumbar lymph nodes** (**A8**). A few lymphatic vessels accompany the thoracic splanchnic nerves; after passing through the diaphragm, they reach the **posterior mediastinal lymph nodes**.

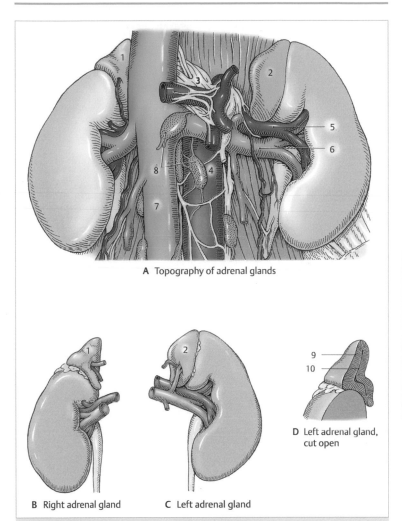

A Topography of adrenal glands

B Right adrenal gland

C Left adrenal gland

D Left adrenal gland, cut open

Fig. 9.11 Macroscopic structure of the adrenal glands.

Microscopic Anatomy of the Adrenal Cortex

The glandular epithelium of the adrenal cortex is surrounded by basal laminae and a reticular fiber network. Rich in lipids, it appears yellow to the naked eye. The adrenal cortex (**A, C**) consists of three zones:

Zona glomerulosa (**AC1**). This is composed of **small**, **round cells** with compact nuclei and dense, granulated cytoplasm. They contain *abundant smooth endoplasmic reticulum*, scattered *lysosomes*, and *lipid droplets*. The mitochondria are predominantly of the crista type. Coursing between clusters of cells are **wide capillary sinuses** that pass toward the interior of the organ to continue as the radiating sinusoid capillaries of the zona fasciculata. Their endothelium is fenestrated.

Zona fasciculata (**AC2, B**). Its cells lie in **parallel cords** and **sheets**. They are rich in *lipids, cholesterol,* and *cholesterol esters*, which are liberated during the tissue preparation, producing a foamy appearance (spongiocytes). They are also rich in vitamin *A* and *vitamin C*, and contain *tubular* or *saccular mitochondria*.

Zona reticularis (**AC3**). Its parenchymal cells are arranged in **networks** or **clusters**. The cells are relatively small and contain few lipids; their cytoplasm is acidophilic. With advancing age, increasing amounts of lipofuscin granules accumulate.

Cortical remodeling processes (**D**). In the fetal adrenal gland, the zona reticularis is highly developed. Just before birth, it begins to undergo a **physiological involution**, and continues to atrophy during early postnatal life (decrease in human chorionic gonadotropic hormone). From the age of 3 onward, the definitive cortex develops (**remodeling phase**) and the proportion of cortical to medullary tissue increases. The zona glomerulosa and zona fasciculata remain highly developed during adult life. At the onset of the menopause in women, and from the age of 60 onward in men, the zona fasciculata becomes thicker, while the volume of the zona glomerulosa and zona reticularis decreases. Cortical remodeling zones are known as transitional zones. The **outer transitional zone** corresponds to the region comprising the capsule, zona glomerulosa, and outer fasciculata region; and the **inner transitional zone** corresponds to the inner zona fasciculata region and the zona reticularis.

A4 Adrenal medulla, **A5** Connective tissue capsule

The adrenal cortex produces steroid hormones, which can be divided into three main groups based on their functions:

Mineralocorticoids. These are mainly produced in the *zona glomerulosa*. They influence **potassium and sodium levels** by increasing potassium excretion and sodium reabsorption. The most important mineralocorticoids are **aldosterone** and **deoxycorticosterone**.

> **Clinical note:** Increased secretion of mineralocorticoids leads to primary hyperaldosteronism (**Conn syndrome**). Symptoms include *high blood pressure* and *hypokalemia*. Aldosterone and cortisol deficiency cause **Addison disease**, which is marked by clinical signs of low blood pressure, hyperkalemia, hyperpigmentation, and weakness or fatigue.

Glucocorticoids. These chiefly influence **carbohydrate** and **protein metabolism** as well as the **immune system**, increasing blood glucose levels, reducing blood lymphocytes, and inhibiting phagocytosis (immunosuppressive and anti-inflammatory effect). They are mainly secreted in the *zona fasciculata* and *zona reticularis*. The most important are **cortisol**, **cortisone**, and **corticosterone**.

> **Clinical note:** Increased secretion of glucocorticoids can lead to **Cushing syndrome**, which is characterized by truncal obesity, a round face (moon face), elevated blood sugar, high blood pressure, muscular wasting in the periphery of the body, and osteoporosis. Similar signs can occur with high-dose glucocorticoid therapies.

Androgens. Produced in the *zona reticularis*, the most important are **dehydroepiandrosterone** (DHEA) and **androstenedione**. Testosterone is synthesized in small amounts.

> **Clinical note:** Excess production of adrenal androgens can cause **adrenogenital syndrome**.

Normal function of the two inner adrenal cortical zones is dependent on secretions of the pituitary gland (ACTH). Except for mineralocorticoids, it is not precisely known which cell forms or zones produce which hormones. Mineralocorticoids arise in the zona glomerulosa under the influence of the renin-angiotensin system of the kidney, independently of the hypothalamus-hypophysis system.

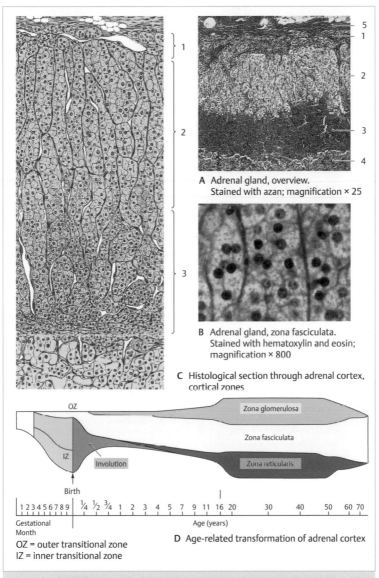

A Adrenal gland, overview.
Stained with azan; magnification × 25

B Adrenal gland, zona fasciculata.
Stained with hematoxylin and eosin;
magnification × 800

C Histological section through adrenal cortex,
cortical zones

OZ

Zona glomerulosa

Zona fasciculata

IZ

Involution

Zona reticularis

Birth

| 1 2 3 4 5 6 7 8 9 | ¼ ½ ¾ 1 | 2 3 4 5 7 9 11 16 20 | 30 | 40 | 50 | 60 70 |

Gestational
Month

Age (years)

OZ = outer transitional zone
IZ = inner transitional zone

D Age-related transformation of adrenal cortex

Secretion, Glandular Epithelium, Endocrine System

Fig. 9.12 Microscopic structure of the adrenal cortex.

Microscopic Anatomy of the Adrenal Medulla

Development. The medulla of the adrenal gland is derived from *neuroectodermal sympathoblasts* (neural crest) which, during the course of prenatal development, migrate inward through the fetal cortex and differentiate into several cell types.

Structure. The medulla is mainly composed of large epithelial cells (**A1**), which are arranged in *cords* or *clusters* with wide **sinusoidal capillaries** (**A2**) coursing between them. The cells, which are round or polygonal in shape, do not have any processes; their nuclei are loosely structured, and their weakly basophilic cytoplasm contains *fine granules* that stain brown with chromium salts, hence the terms **chromaffin or pheochrome** cells. **Catecholamines** (*epinephrine* and *norepinephrine*) are produced in the chromaffin cells and released into the venous sinuses. Medullary chromaffin cells can also be identified under light microscopy as epinephrine (E) and norepinephrine (NE) cells, based on different features of their granules.

Epinephrine (**E**) **cells**. Epinephrine-producing cells predominate (around 80%) in the human adrenal medulla. Epinephrine cells are rich in *acid phosphatase* and have a strong affinity for azocarmine, although they do not react to silver salts and do not exhibit autofluorescence.

Norepinephrine (**NE**) **cells**. Norepinephrine cells exhibit *autofluorescence* and have an *argentaffin* staining pattern. They make up about 5% of the total cell population of the medulla. Their affinity for azocarmine is low; histochemically, they exhibit a negative acid phosphatase reaction.

Electron microscopy techniques can also be used to differentiate chromaffin cells. Epinephrine cells contain electron-dense granules with an average diameter of 200 nm. Norepinephrine cells are larger, measuring about 280 nm. Given their origin, **chromaffin cells** may be considered **modified postganglionic cells of the sympathetic nervous system**. Similar to the second neuron in the sympathetic part of the (peripheral) autonomic nervous system, they are also innervated by preganglionic (sympathetic) cholinergic nerve fibers.

A number of **neuropeptides** can also be found in chromaffin cells and nerve endings using immunofluorescence and immunohistochemical techniques. These include *substance P, neuropeptide Y, vasoactive intestinal polypeptide (VIP), β-endorphin, α-melanotropin, somatostatin, oxytocin,* and *vasopressin*.

In addition to chromaffin cells, the adrenal medulla also contains nerve fibers and **multipolar sympathetic ganglion cells** (**A3**), which have long processes and are found scattered or clustered in small groups. Satellite cells lie nearby, as well as between chromaffin cells, but are difficult to distinguish from connective tissue cells.

> **Clinical note:** Chromaffin cells can degenerate and give rise to tumors called **pheochromocytomas**, generally benign adenomas that produce excess catecholamines. Clinical symptoms include high blood pressure, accompanied by severe hypertensive crises, heart palpitations, headache, sweating, and weight loss.

Paraganglia (glomus organs) (**C**) are nodular, pea-sized **epithelial structures** that contain clusters or cords of chromaffin cells secreting **catecholamines**. Paraganglia arise from the neural crest, similar to the adrenal medulla (suprarenal paraganglion), and thus are also termed *"extra-adrenal chromaffin cells"* (chromaffin bodies). Most free paraganglia, the largest of which is the (**abdominal**) **aortic paraganglion** (Zuckerkandl organs at the origin of the inferior mesenteric artery), lie irregularly dispersed in the retroperitoneal space. Other paraganglia include the **carotid glomus** (carotid paraganglion) (**C**), a chemoreceptor located in the bifurcation of the carotid artery; the **subclavian paraganglion**; the upper, middle, and lower **aorticopulmonary paraganglia**; and the **nodose paraganglion**. Paraganglia, which are permeated by fenestrated capillaries, secrete substances in response to hypoxia.

B4 Medullary cells, **B5** Muscle pad, **C6** Small groups of chromaffin cells, **C7** Capillary sinus

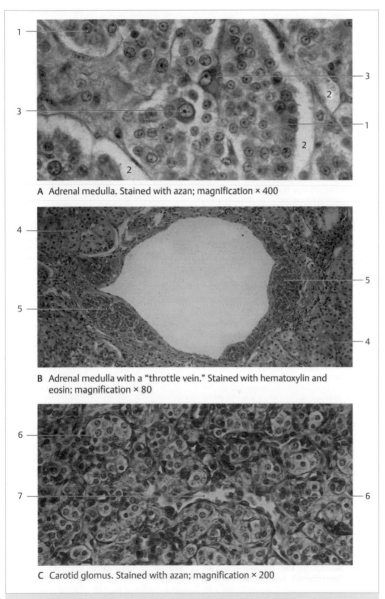

A Adrenal medulla. Stained with azan; magnification × 400

B Adrenal medulla with a "throttle vein." Stained with hematoxylin and eosin; magnification × 80

C Carotid glomus. Stained with azan; magnification × 200

Fig. 9.13 Microscopic structure of the adrenal medulla and paraganglia.

Secretion, Glandular Epithelium, Endocrine System

9.7 Thyroid Gland

Gross Anatomy

The **thyroid gland** develops from the epithelium of the floor of the mouth (foramen cecum of the tongue). It consists of two conical, lateral lobes, the **right lobe** (**A–C1**) and **left lobe** (**A–C2**), which lie on either side of the larynx, trachea, and esophagus, and are connected near their base by the **isthmus of the thyroid gland** (**AC3**).

The size and weight of the thyroid gland can vary greatly, ranging from 2–3 g in the neonate to 18–60 g in the adult. It is usually a dark brownish red in color.

Lobes of the thyroid gland. Each lobe is 4–8-cm long, 2–4-cm wide, and 1.5–2.5-cm thick in the middle. The right lobe is usually slightly wider and longer than the left. The lobes extend obliquely upward from inferior to posterosuperior and are attached to the trachea, cricoid, and thyroid cartilage by loose connective tissue (Berry ligament) and reinforcing ligaments from the capsule surrounding the organ (**C5**).

Topographical relationships. The lobes are triangular in cross section: their **anterior surfaces** are convex and their **medial surfaces**, which lie adjacent to the trachea and larynx, are correspondingly concave. Their **posterior margins** lie on either side of the sheaths of the *great vessels of the neck* (**C7**, also see figure on p. 121). The **upper poles** of the lobes extend as far as the *oblique line* of the thyroid cartilage, and the **lower poles** to the *fourth or fifth tracheal ring*. The *infrahyoid muscles* (**C8**) only partially cover the thyroid gland. The middle, or *pretracheal layer of the cervical fascia* (**C11**), extends over the thyroid gland and continues beyond it.

A22 Scalenus anterior, **A23** Thoracic duct, **A24** Thyrocervical trunk, **A25** Middle thyroid vein, **B9**, **BC10** Parathyroid gland, **C6** Fibrous capsule, **C12** Skin of neck, **C13** Platysma, **C14** Superficial layer of cervical fascia and sternocleidomastoid, **C15** Deep layer of cervical fascia, **C16** Esophagus

Isthmus and pyramidal lobe. The isthmus, which varies in size and shape and is completely absent in 20% of the cases, is 1.5–2.0-cm wide and 0.5–1.5-cm thick. A long projection extends either from its cranial border or from that of one of the lobes, usually the right lobe, and ascends toward the hyoid bone. Known as the **pyramidal lobe** (**A4**), it is a remnant of the *thyroglossal duct*, present during fetal development. It also varies in size and shape and occasionally is absent.

Fibrous capsule of the thyroid gland. The thyroid gland is surrounded by a strong fibrous capsule (**C5**, **C6**), consisting of two layers. The connective tissue **internal capsule** (**C5**) is thin and adheres closely to the parenchyma of the gland. It sends vascularized connective tissue septa into the interior of the gland, which separate larger and smaller *lobules of the thyroid gland*. The **external capsule** (**C6**) ("surgical capsule") is tougher and is considered part of the *pretracheal layer of the cervical fascia*. The **space between the loosely adherent** capsular layers is filled with loose connective tissue and contains *larger branches of vessels*, as well as the *parathyroid gland* in its posterior portion (**B9**, **BC10**). The posterior and lateral aspects of the external capsule are connected to the connective tissue of the cervical neurovascular bundle (**C7**).

Arteries. The thyroid gland is one of the most highly vascular organs in the human body. Its blood supply is provided by two pairs of arteries. **The superior thyroid artery** (**A17**), the first branch of the external carotid artery (**A21**), curves upward and gives rise to the *superior laryngeal artery* to the upper poles of the lateral lobes. It supplies the *superior, anterior*, and *lateral parts* of the thyroid gland. The **inferior thyroid artery**, a branch of the thyrocervical trunk, ascends to the level of C7, where it turns medially and inferiorly. It supplies the *inferior, posterior*, and *medial parts* of the organ. Rarely is the unpaired **thyroid ima artery** also present.

Veins. The veins draining the thyroid gland are received in the upper part of the gland by the **superior thyroid veins** (**A18**), which empty alone or with the facial vein into the *internal jugular vein* (**A19**). The **inferior thyroid veins** arise from the unpaired thyroid plexus (**A20**), situated in the pretracheal space, and open behind the sternum into the *brachiocephalic veins*.

Lymphatic vessels. The lymphatic vessels are also split up into an upper and a lower drainage basin, passing from the upper and middle parts of the gland to the **lateral cervical nodes** along the internal jugular vein. The caudal lymphatic vessels connect to the **anterior mediastinal lymph nodes**.

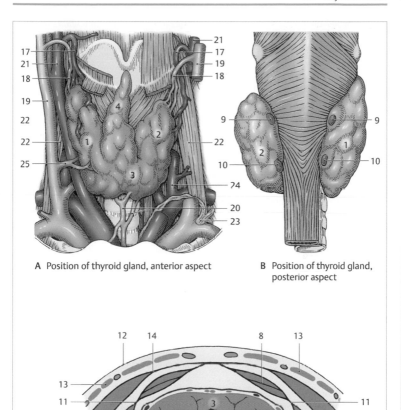

A Position of thyroid gland, anterior aspect

B Position of thyroid gland, posterior aspect

C Position of thyroid gland in relation to viscera of neck, horizontal section, diagram

Fig. 9.14 Macroscopic structure of the thyroid gland.

Secretion, Glandular Epithelium, Endocrine System

Nerves. **Sympathetic** afferents reach the thyroid gland via postganglionic fibers derived from the *superior cervical ganglion* and *cervicothoracic ganglion* of the sympathetic trunk, and enter it as periarterial networks. **Parasympathetic** supply is from the *superior laryngeal nerve* and the *inferior laryngeal nerve*.

Microscopic Anatomy

The microscopic anatomy of the thyroid gland resembles that of an exocrine gland in that it is partitioned into irregularly sized lobules consisting of **epithelial cells arranged to form approximately three million closed follicles**. Serving as a type of "final chamber," the thyroid follicles store large amounts of a hormone-containing substance called **colloid** (**AB1**).

Thyroid follicles. The walls of the variably large (50–900 μm in diameter) spherical or tubular follicles are formed by a *single layer of epithelium with tight junctions* and distinct cell boundaries. The **height of the epithelium** depends on thyroid activity. The epithelial cells are *flat* or *cuboidal*, when greater levels of secretion are stored (in the inactive gland) (**A2**); or *columnar*, or even *tall columnar*, during *secretion production* (in the active gland) (**B2**). The apical surface of the cell, which releases or resorbs secretions, bears short microvilli (**C3**). The nucleus is usually centrally located; the cytoplasm contains all known cell organelles. Lipofuscin accumulates as a person ages. The **surface of the follicle** is surrounded by *fine connective tissue fibers* (**AB4**) and a dense network *of fenestrated capillaries* (**C5, E**).

Parafollicular or C cells (**C6**). The C cells lie in the interfollicular connective tissue, as well as scattered between the polarized, follicular epithelial cells, where they lie within the basement membrane (**C7**) but are not connected with the follicle lumen. Parafollicular cells contain *abundant mitochondria*, a well-developed *Golgi apparatus*, and membrane-enclosed *granules* with a diameter of 100–180 nm. They also contain the 32-amino-acid hormone **calcitonin**, as well as serotonin and dopamine, and probably also somatostatin. C cells derive from the neural crest during embryological development and are thus of neuroectodermal origin. C cells are **APUD cells** (amine precursor uptake and decarboxylation).

Hormones. The thyroid gland produces thyroxine (T4) and triiodothyronine (T3), as well as the hormone calcitonin. The principal biosynthetic product is T4; only small amounts of T3 are synthesized.

Thyroxine and **triiodothyronine** stimulate the cellular metabolism and are essential for normal physical and mental development. **Calcitonin** lowers blood calcium levels and supports bone formation. It is the antagonist of parathormone, which is produced in the parathyroid gland, inhibiting the activity of the osteoclasts and thus bone resorption.

Clinical note: Enlargement of the thyroid gland is known as goiter or thyrocele. In patients with excess thyroid hormone production (**hyperthyroidism**, e.g., Graves disease), cells burn more fuel, resulting in weight loss, increased body temperature, a rapid heart rate, and nervous excitability. Inadequate hormone production (**hypothyroidism**, e.g., Hashimoto thyroiditis) leads to slowed metabolism, diminished growth and mental activity, and swelling of subcutaneous connective tissue, that is, *myxedema*. **Congenital hypothyroidism** can lead to *small stature* and *cretinism* (mental retardation).

Hormone production and secretion. Thyroxine and triiodothyronine are produced in a series of steps. They bind to thyroglobulin, the primary synthesis product of the follicular epithelial cells, and are stored in the lumen until they are released as needed into the bloodstream. Thus, there are two opposing sequential reactions in the thyroid: first, **thyroglobulin**, a dimeric protein, is formed in the follicular epithelial cells. **Iodide**, which is taken up from the blood by the basal part of the cells, is oxidized in the presence of H_2O_2 to form **iodine**. It binds to the **tyrosine residues** of thyroglobulin, which by now have already been secreted into the lumen of the follicle. Iodinated tyrosine residues—**tetraiodothyronine** or **triiodothyronine**—arise from various condensation processes. They are followed by the opposing process of **resorption of follicle contents** (colloid), which is stimulated by *thyrotropin* (TSH) secreted by the anterior pituitary. Vesicles are formed for transport by endocytosis. The vesicles fuse with lysosomes located in the apical cytoplasm of the follicular epithelial cells, which sever the bond between the hormone and thyroglobulin. The hormone is then released into the blood by diffusion.

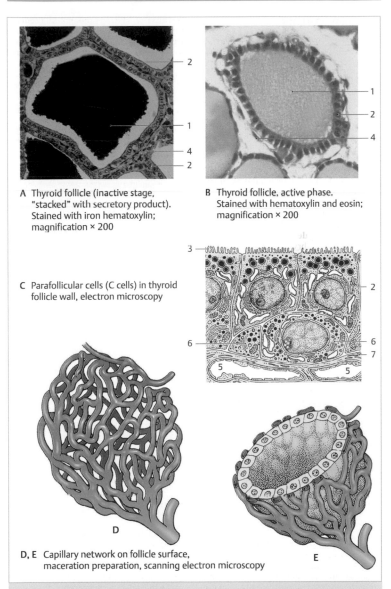

A Thyroid follicle (inactive stage, "stacked" with secretory product). Stained with iron hematoxylin; magnification × 200

B Thyroid follicle, active phase. Stained with hematoxylin and eosin; magnification × 200

C Parafollicular cells (C cells) in thyroid follicle wall, electron microscopy

D, E Capillary network on follicle surface, maceration preparation, scanning electron microscopy

Fig. 9.15 Microscopic structure of the thyroid gland.

Secretion, Glandular Epithelium, Endocrine System

Parathyroid Glands

Position. The four yellow or reddish-brown **parathyroid glands** (**B1**) are derived from the endodermal epithelium of the posterior diverticula of the third and fourth pharyngeal pouches (**A**). Each lentil-shaped gland is roughly the size of a grain of wheat (5 × 3 × 2 mm) and the glands weigh about 120–160 mg in total. They are nestled against the posterior aspect of the thyroid gland, situated between the two layers of the fibrous capsule. The paired **superior parathyroid glands** (derivatives of the fourth pharyngeal pouch) are located at the level of the *caudal margin of the cricoid cartilage*. The paired **inferior parathyroid glands** (derivatives of the third pharyngeal pouch) are located along the base of the lateral lobes at the level of the *third and fourth tracheal cartilages*. The **wide variation in position** arising during embryological development is of surgical importance.

Neurovascular supply. Each parathyroid gland is supplied by its own **parathyroid artery**, which stems from one of the thyroid arteries, usually the *inferior thyroid artery* (**B2**). The veins open into the **thyroid veins** lying on the surface of the thyroid gland, and the lymphatic vessels pass to the paratracheal nodes. The nerves to the parathyroid glands arise from the **autonomic thyroid periarterial plexuses**.

A1–A5 Pharyngeal pouches, **A6** External acoustic meatus, **A7** Cervical sinus, **A8** Inferior parathyroid gland, **A9** Superior parathyroid gland, arrows represent cell migration. **B3** Superior thyroid artery, **B4** Esophagus, **B5** Trachea, **B6** Greater horn of hyoid bone, **B7** Laimer triangle

Microanatomy. The parathyroid glands are enclosed in a **connective tissue capsule**. The **glandular epithelium** is dense in some areas and more loosely organized in others, interspersed with *connective tissue fibers* (**C1**) and *adipose cells* (**C2**) and permeated by a dense network of *fenestrated capillaries*. Two types of cells may be distinguished: chief cells and oxyphil cells. The large and distinct **water-clear chief cells** (**C3**) are especially easy to distinguish; their stained cytoplasm appears virtually empty, owing to the loss of lipids

and glycogen during preparation. The cytoplasm of the usually smaller **dark-staining chief cells**, which also contain glycogen, contains *weakly acidophilic granules* and *numerous mitochondria*. The cell bodies of the **oxyphil cells** (**C4**) are larger than those of the chief cells, and they have a marked affinity for acidic dyes (*acidophilic*), owing to their *abundant tightly packed mitochondria*. Their nuclei are small and occasionally pyknotic. With advancing age, the number of oxyphil cells increases. Their role is as yet unclear.

Hormonal effects. The polypeptide hormone **parathormone** (PTH, parathyrin), composed of 84 amino acids, is crucially important in calcium and phosphate metabolism and is believed to be produced by active chief cells. Parathormone mobilizes calcium from the bones, by stimulating osteoclasts to increase bone resorption, resulting in an **increase in the calcium concentration of the blood** (hypercalcemia). At the same time, PTH promotes phosphate excretion by the kidneys (**phosphaturia**), by inhibiting phosphate reabsorption in the distal renal tubule. Reabsorption of calcium, magnesium, and phosphate in the intestines is increased. Hormone secretion is regulated by a simple negative feedback mechanism.

Clinical note: Overactivity (**hyperparathyroidism**), for example, owing to an autonomous endocrine tumor (adenoma), causes increased excretion of phosphate in the urine and elevated blood calcium levels. Excessive secretion of parathyroid hormone can cause pathological calcium deposits in vessel walls, as well as calcium deficiency affecting the skeletal system, which is associated with a complex bone remodeling process and risk of spontaneous fracture. Parathormone deficiency (**hypoparathyroidism**) causes excessive mineralization of the bones and teeth. Low levels of calcium in the blood (hypocalcemia) can lead to generalized neuromuscular hyperexcitability, including cramps (tetany). Other hormones in addition to PTH are also involved in **bone formation** and **remodeling:** vitamin D hormone (**calcitriol**), which is produced in the kidneys, also promotes bone resorption, while **calcitonin** from thyroid C cells inhibits resorption, thus acting as a parathormone antagonist.

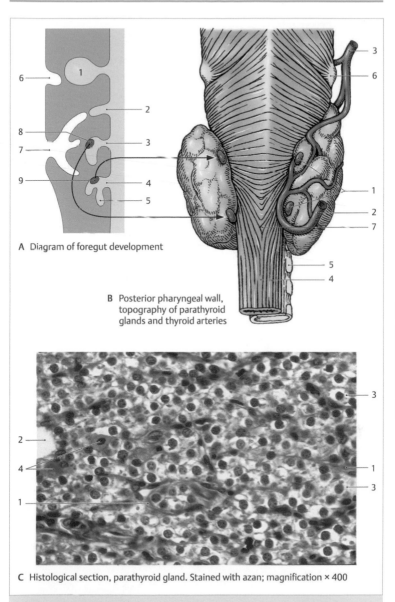

A Diagram of foregut development

B Posterior pharyngeal wall, topography of parathyroid glands and thyroid arteries

C Histological section, parathyroid gland. Stained with azan; magnification × 400

Fig. 9.16 Parathyroid glands.

Secretion, Glandular Epithelium, Endocrine System

9.8 Pancreatic Islets

Lying within or near the margin of the lobules of the exocrine pancreas (see p. 221) are the **islets of Langerhans** (**A**, **B**), collectively known as the pancreatic islets. Amid the strongly staining exocrine parenchyma, the 0.5–1.5 million islets (with a diameter of 100–200 μm and a total weight of 2–5 g) appear as pale round or ovoid areas, consisting of **columns of epithelial** cells that are vascularized by blood capillaries with fenestrated endothelium. The islets develop from endodermal epithelial buds of the ventral and dorsal primitive pancreas.

AB1 Exocrine gland acini, **A5** Vessels in the exocrine pancreas.

Microscopic Anatomy

Five different endocrine cell types can be distinguished in the islets, based on staining pattern and microscopic structure. All types produce **peptide hormones** and thus have a well-developed synthesis and transport apparatus consisting of *rough endoplasmic reticulum, Golgi apparatus.*

Alpha cells (**B3**) (about 15–20% of all islet cells). Most alpha cells lie in the periphery of the islets, abutting the capillaries. They produce the hormone **glucagon**.

> **Clinical note:** Glucagon stimulates the release of glucose from glycogen (**glycogenolysis**) in the liver. It also stimulates the formation of glucose from amino acids (**gluconeogenesis**). **In addition**, glucagon stimulates lipolysis.

Beta cells (**B4**) (nearly 70% of islet cells) produce insulin and are evenly distributed throughout the islets. They produce **insulin** and also amylin.

> **Clinical note:** Insulin increases glucose absorption in skeletal muscle and adipocytes and inhibits glycogenolysis and gluconeogenesis in the liver. When there is not enough insulin, the blood sugar level rises

(hyperglycemia). This happens in diabetes mellitus. Too much insulin leads to hypoglycemia. This can be due to an incorrect insulin dose or to drugs that increase insulin secretion and also due to B-cell tumors (known as insulinomas).

Delta cells (about 5% of all islet cells) lie mainly along the margins of the islet cords and contain homogenous secretory granules measuring about 320 nm. The granules are filled with **somatostatin**.

> **Clinical note:** Somatostatin **inhibits secretion of** many hormones, including insulin, glucagon, and growth hormone. Somatostatin analogues are therefore used in some diseases associated with increased hormone production.

PP cells (F cells) produce **pancreatic polypeptide** (PP), which is also present in the endocrine cells of the intestinal epithelium.

Other cell types. Pancreatic **D1 cells**, also called VIP cells, contain the vasoactive intestinal polypeptide (**VIP**), which dilates blood vessels and increases their permeability. Gastrin cells (**G cells**) are only found in the islets of Langerhans during embryonic and fetal development.

Blood supply and innervation. The islets of Langerhans are fed by arterioles, which arise as **afferent vessels** from the lobular arteries of the exocrine pancreas and form an **islet capillary network** (**AB2**). The capillary plexus drains via numerous **efferent vessels into the capillary system of the exocrine pancreas** (portal system). The hormone-carrying blood from the islets flows through the exocrine tissue of the pancreas and influences the acinar function before draining into the **pancreatic veins**, which empty into the **hepatic portal vein** to the liver. Sympathetic and parasympathetic nerve fibers accompany the blood vessels and can have synapses at the surface of the islet cells.

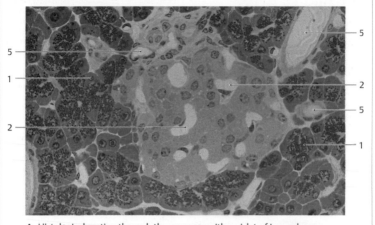

A Histological section through the pancreas with an islet of Langerhans. Stained with methylene blue and azure II; magnification × 400

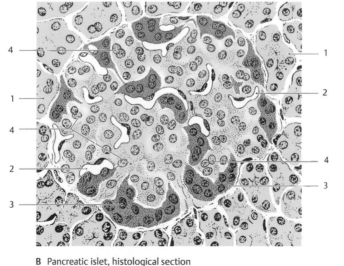

B Pancreatic islet, histological section

Fig. 9.17 Microscopic structure of the pancreatic islet.

Secretion, Glandular Epithelium, Endocrine System

9.9 Diffuse Endocrine System

Testicular Endocrine Functions

Male sex hormones (**androgens**) are produced by the interstitial **Leydig cells** (**1**) lying in the loose connective tissue (**2**) of the testes (along with unmyelinated and myelinated nerve fibers, fibrocytes, mast cells, macrophages, and lymphocytes), between the convoluted seminiferous tubules (intertubular space) directly adjacent to the capillaries (**3**). Each polygonal cell body contains a *round nucleus* with a prominent nucleolus; its *acidophilic cytoplasm* contains smooth endoplasmic reticulum, tubular mitochondria, abundant lysosomes, lipofuscin granules, and Reinke crystals (**4**), which consist of proteins and appear under light microscopy as elongated, rectangular, or rhombic elements.

Effects of Testosterone

Prenatal effects. The induction of gonadal sex and testicular differentiation during embryonic and fetal development occurs independently of testosterone. For all other organs of the male genital system, testosterone acts as a **specific growth factor**, controlling the degree of manifestation of male traits (phenotype) in genetically male fetuses, preventing obliteration of the Wolffian ducts, and promoting their development into the seminal vesicle and ductus deferens.

Postnatal effects. After birth, the Leydig cells involute; in the neonate this is expressed as a significant drop in **17-ketosteroid excretion**. At around the age of 5, ketosteroid excretion gradually begins to increase and then rises sharply during puberty, indicating that the Leydig cells are fully functional. Ketosteroid excretion reaches its maximum level by about the age of 25, after which levels begin to decline slowly.

Testosterone directly affects the seminiferous tubules, stimulating **sperm production** (spermatogenesis). Testosterone secreted into the bloodstream acts on the seminal ducts and the **development** of the **seminal vesicle** and **prostate**. Testosterone promotes the development and maintenance of **secondary sex characteristics** (muscle mass, distribution and pattern of body hair, skin pigmentation, development of the larynx, and voice changes) and stimulates the sweat and sebaceous glands (pubescent acne). It also promotes libido and virility and influences **gender-specific behaviors**. Testosterone, and its more potent metabolite, *dihydrotestosterone* (DHT) (**5**), induce the formation of androgen receptors in various target organs and the synthesis of 5α-reductase, an enzyme that converts testosterone into DHT.

Hypothalamic–Pituitary–Testicular Axis

Sperm production and testosterone secretion are controlled by gonadotropic hormones secreted by the anterior lobe of the pituitary gland, which act on the testes. Inhibition and stimulation of hormone secretion are regulated by a type of feedback mechanism: gonadotropic hormones from the anterior pituitary stimulate the testes, while rising levels of testosterone inhibit gonadotropin synthesis in the adenohypophysis. This feedback mechanism involves specific hypothalamic nuclei that secrete gonadotropin-releasing hormone (**GnRH**, gonadoliberin), which influences the production of luteinizing hormone (**LH**) and follicle-stimulating hormone (**FSH**, follitropin) in the anterior pituitary. **Luteinizing hormone** (LH, lutropin), acts on the Leydig cells to stimulate testosterone synthesis; and **follicle-stimulating hormone** promotes spermatogenesis and stimulates the production of *inhibin* (a glycoprotein) by the Sertoli cells. Sertoli cells also produce *androgen-binding protein* (ABP) (**6**).

Clinical note: Diminished secretion of inhibin due to a Sertoli cell defect causes persistently elevated serum FSH concentrations and is an indicator of severely impaired spermatogenesis—**hypergonadotropic hypogonadism**. A special form of this disease is **Klinefelter** syndrome, a congenital chromosomal aberration typical for the karyotype 47, XXY.

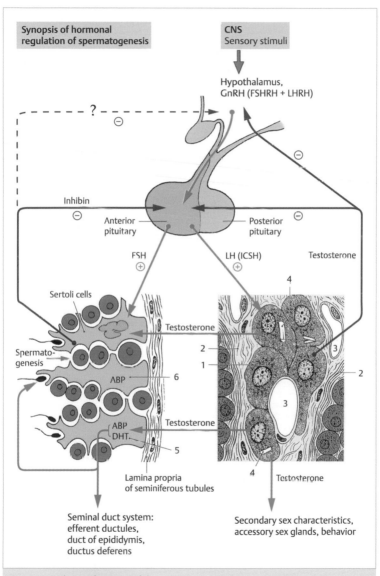

Fig. 9.18 Endocrine functions of the testis.

Ovarian Endocrine Functions

The effects that endocrine processes have on bodily functions are particularly evident with regard to the female sexual cycle. The effects of the hypothalamic–pituitary unit on the ovary are distinguished from the effects of ovarian hormones on the endometrial lining of the uterus (see p. 278), and in turn on the hypothalamus and pituitary gland.

Ovarian Cycle

Pulsatile secretion of **GnRH** (= gonadotropin-releasing hormone, gonadoliberin), a hypothalamic regulatory hormone which is transported through the hypophysial portal system to the anterior pituitary, causes it to synthesize and release the gonadotropins **FSH** (= follicle-stimulating hormone, follitropin) and **LH** (= luteinizing hormone, lutropin).

Days 1–4 of the ovarian cycle. FSH stimulates the recruitment of several **primordial follicles**.

Follicular or estrogen phase, days 5–14. During this phase, the primordial follicle matures into a primary, secondary, and then tertiary follicle. Between days 5 and 7, a dominant tertiary follicle is selected. The dominant follicle develops into a **preovulatory follicle**, which, during the late follicular phase (days 11–14), synthesizes almost all estrogen (**E**), temporarily decreasing the release of FSH in the anterior pituitary (negative feedback effect of estrogens). In addition, the dominant follicle releases inhibin, which also acts to inhibit FSH secretion. Rising estradiol levels signal the adenohypophysis to release massive amounts of LH (termed the **"LH peak,"** a positive feedback effect of estradiol), as well as FSH, which leads to complete maturation of the egg cell around day 14 of the cycle, and subsequent **ovulation**.

Luteal or gestagen phase, days 15–28. Within a matter of hours, the follicular epithelial cells differentiate (granulosa cells) forming **granulosa lutein cells**, and the cells of the theca interna (see p. 272) become estrogen-producing **thecal lutein cells** (luteinization). Transformation of the "empty" follicle into the **corpus luteum** (yellow body) can only occur under the influence of LH; if there is no LH peak, ovulation does not occur. **Progesterone (P)** and **estrogen (E)** are produced by the corpus luteum of menstruation, which exerts a negative feedback on GnRH (and in turn FSH and LH) secretion. If fertilization does not occur, the corpus luteum begins to degenerate around day 23 and progesterone levels decline, leading to ischemia of the endometrium, which is subsequently sloughed off during the **menstruation phase** (desquamation phase; days 1–5 of the new cycle).

Two additional hormones are involved in regulating the cyclical mechanism: **PRL** (= prolactin, also called mammotropic or luteotropic hormone, LTH) and **PIF** (= prolactin release-inhibiting factor, also known as prolactostatin). Prolactin stimulates growth of mammary gland tissue and induces milk synthesis and secretion.

Theca folliculi. The theca folliculi consists of the **theca interna**, which is richly vascularized, and the **theca externa**, which contains abundant connective tissue cells. The production of **androgens** (mainly androstenedione), the precursor substances for the biosynthesis of estrogen, is stimulated in the theca interna by LH.

Hilar cells. Hilar cells are epithelioid cells located in the hilum of the ovary and the adjacent mesovarium, usually lying close to vessels. They resemble the Leydig cells of the testes and produce **androgens**.

Follicular atresia. Most follicles do not mature to ovulation, but remain closed (*atretic*) and die. Primary and secondary follicles disappear without a trace, but atretic tertiary follicles leave behind theca interna cells, which form a *functional endocrine structure*, and as interstitial cells constitute a *permanent source of estrogen*.

Corpus albicans. After the corpus luteum ceases functioning, it is replaced by fibrous, glistening connective tissue scar.

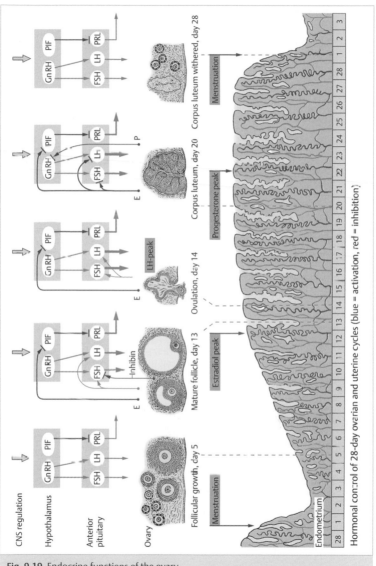

Fig. 9.19 Endocrine functions of the ovary.

Secretion, Glandular Epithelium, Endocrine System

Endocrine Functions of the Placenta

The placenta not only facilitates the selective **exchange of substances** between the mother and fetus, it also **produces numerous hormones** and **growth factors**, which regulate fetal and maternal metabolism as well as placental function. **Production** of protein hormones and growth factors mainly occurs in the placental villi, which can be divided into the multinucleated **syncytiotrophoblast** (1) and the underlying **cytotrophoblast** (2) (Langhans cells). Throughout the entire gestational period, cytotrophoblast cells are incorporated into the syncytiotrophoblast, and at birth they cover only about 20% of the inner surface of the syncytiotrophoblast.

Placental Protein Hormones

Human chorionic gonadotropin (HCG). During the first trimester, human chorionic gonadotropin, which is synthesized in the syncytiotrophoblast, is the predominant protein hormone.

Function. During pregnancy, HCG **prevents** premature degeneration (**luteolysis**) of the corpus luteum in the ovary. It also stimulates the **production of progesterone** by the corpus luteum of pregnancy, which maintains the structure and function of the endometrium that is essential for maintaining pregnancy; abnormal HCG biosynthesis results in spontaneous abortion. Additionally, HCG influences testosterone production in the Leydig cells of male fetuses and, in female gonads, estrogens and gestagens (mainly progesterone).

> **Clinical note:** HCG is excreted by the kidneys and is detectable in urine during the early stages of pregnancy. Detection of HCG, nowadays performed using immunological techniques, is the basis for most **pregnancy tests**.

Additional placental protein hormones are **chorionic thyrotropin** (HCT = human chorionic thyrotropin), **chorionic somatomammotropin** (HCS = human choriomammotropin or human placental lactogen), and **chorionic corticotropin** (HCC = human chorionic corticotropin).

Placental Steroid Hormones

Steroid hormones and their precursors are continually exchanged between the mother and fetus, through the "fetoplacental unit." This is important because the fetus and placenta are not capable on their own of producing all of the products or intermediate substances involved in steroid hormone metabolism. Toward the end of pregnancy, massive amounts of hormones are produced daily.

Progesterone. Placental **progesterone synthesis** occurs independently and increases steadily throughout pregnancy. About two-thirds of the progesterone produced in the placenta enters the mother's circulation and about one-third enters the fetal circulation.

Function. The biological function of placental progesterone is to **inhibit uterine contractions**, maintain the decidua, and to promote differentiation of the mammary gland. During the first 5–6 weeks of gestation, production of progesterone, which is stimulated by HCG, mainly occurs in the ovary. After this time, the placenta becomes the main source of progesterone.

Estrogens. The placenta also produces estrogens, which are converted from the steroid hormones *dehydroepiandrosterone sulfate* (DHEAS), which is synthesized by the fetus, and *16 a-hydroxy-DHEAS*. The predominant form of estrogen at the end of pregnancy is **estriol**. Its function is to promote growth of the uterus and mammary glands.

Other Placental Hormones and Growth Factors

Growth factors. During pregnancy, the growth processes are regulated by various hormones and growth factors. Growth of the fetus is chiefly regulated by **insulin** and insulinlike growth factors (**IGFs**, **somatomedin**). A placental growth factor is produced in the brush border of the syncytiotrophoblast, mainly during the first trimester.

Placental releasing hormones and release-inhibiting hormones. Gonadoliberin (GnRH, gonadotropin-releasing hormone), **corticoliberin** (CIF, corticotropin-release inhibitory factor), and **somatostatin** are also produced in the cytotrophoblast of the human placenta.

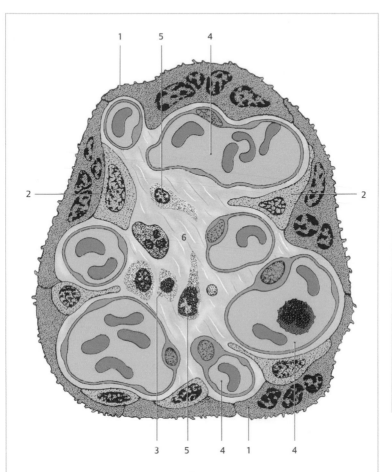

1 Syncytiotrophoblast, multinucleated, with short microvilli on the surface
2 Cytotrophoblast, Langhans cell
3 Hofbauer cell, macrophage
4 Fetal capillaries/sinusoids with erythrocytes
5 Fibroblast
6 Chorionic mesoderm

Section through terminal villus of a mature human placenta,
electron microscopy (Prof. P. Kaufmann, Aachen)

Fig. 9.20 Endocrine functions of the placenta.

Cardiac Hormones—Atrial Natriuretic Peptides

The thin-walled trabecular parts of the **atria** and the **auricles of the heart** (**A1**) contain a type of cardiomyocyte that has 0.2–0.4-µm wide membrane-covered granules with a dense core (**B4**), distinguishing it from the rest of the "working myocardium." These secretory granules store a hormone that is produced by the cardiomyocytes themselves: the 28-amino-acid **atrial natriuretic peptide** (**ANP**) (cardiodilatin/CDD, atrial peptide), and its precursor, the 131-amino-acid proANP. The presence of these hormone-producing cardiocytes, which may be referred to as **"endocrine cardiomyocytes"** (**B**), demonstrates that the heart also has endocrine functions.

Endocrine cardiomyocytes (**atrial endocrine cells**). Similar to ventricular myocytes, the atrial endocrine cell possesses one or more centrally located oval nuclei surrounded by an extensive sarcoplasm containing myofibrils with mitochondria between them. Unlike ventricular muscle cells, the atrial endocrine cells have a **well-developed secretory apparatus**, containing profiles of *rough endoplasmic reticulum* (**B2**), a *well-developed Golgi apparatus* (**B3**), which is often found below the sarcolemma, and collections of *specialized secretory granules* (**B4**), which extend nearly to the plasma membrane. These are released by exocytosis, in response to atrial stretch and stimulation of the sympathetic nervous system. Atrial endocrine cells also receive **numerous afferents** via a nerve plexus of catecholaminergic, cholinergic, and peptidergic fibers that presumably also play a role in stimulating secretion.

B5 Capillary

Function. Cardiac hormones play an important role in regulating blood pressure, blood volume, and water-electrolyte balance. **Target organs** include the *kidneys, vascular smooth muscle, adrenal cortex,* and evidently the *pituitary gland*. Atrial peptides **reduce blood volume and blood pressure:** in the kidneys, they cause dilation of arterial vessels in the renal cortex, while constricting efferent vessels. At the same time, ANP causes natriuresis, that is, an increased discharge of sodium ions (Na^+) by the kidneys. The glomerular filter widens, influencing tubular transport and altering the secretory activity of the juxtaglomerular apparatus. Atrial peptides have an important influence on cells in the zona glomerulosa of the adrenal cortex that secrete aldosterone, as well as on vasopressin release in the neurohypophysis. In both instances, activity is inhibited, which ultimately leads to a drop in blood volume and blood pressure.

Ventricular cardiomyocytes secrete a chemically related peptide with a similar effect, known as brain natriuretic peptide (BNP). Elevated plasma levels of BNP are found in patients with myocardial insufficiency.

Cardiac Ganglia

The heart contains about 550 small ganglia in the epicardial fat (*epicardial ganglia*) containing over 14,000 nerve cells, which are mainly multipolar parasympathetic neurons. The distribution of the ganglia varies. **Atrial** ganglia (**C**) are particularly numerous close to the reflection of the pericardial sac on the posterior aspect of the atria, and **ventricular** ganglia (**D**) are found mainly around the root of the aorta.

C and D Atrial and ventricular ganglia:

1 Pulmonary trunk (and valve of the pulmonary trunk)
2 Aorta (and aortic valve)
3 Superior vena cava
4 Right pulmonary veins
5 Inferior vena cava
6 Coronary sinus
7 Left pulmonary veins
8 Superior left atrial ganglia
9 Superior right atrial ganglia
10 Posteromedial left atrial ganglia
11 Posterior descending ganglia
12 Anterior descending ganglia
13 Aortic root ganglia
14 Right marginal ganglia

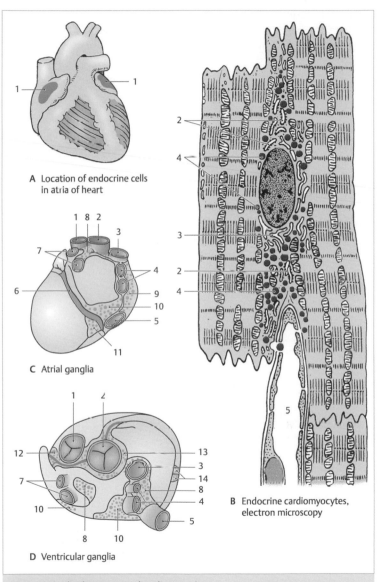

A Location of endocrine cells in atria of heart

B Endocrine cardiomyocytes, electron microscopy

C Atrial ganglia

D Ventricular ganglia

Fig. 9.21 Cardiac hormones and cardiac ganglia.

Diffuse Endocrine Cells in Various Organs

In addition to the compact endocrine glands, **dispersed endocrine cells** are also found within the epithelium of various organs throughout the body. These widely scattered cells are collectively known as the disseminated or diffuse neuroendocrine system (**DNES**). A common feature shared by the endocrine cells of the diffuse endocrine system (about 40 different types) is that they contain and secrete **biogenic monoamines** (serotonin, histamine) and various peptides, which are produced by absorption and decarboxylation of amine precursors (**APUD cell concept**). Given that many endocrine cells possess both receptor and effector functions, and thus resemble sensory and nerve cells, they are also referred to as **"paraneurons."** Diffuse polarized endocrine cells may be divided into two groups:

Open-type cells (**A1**). The narrow apical pole of these cells reaches the lumen of the hollow organ in which they are located. Open-type cells have microvilli (**A2**). The apex of the cell is thought to act as a receptor for luminal chemical stimuli.

Closed-type cells (**A3**). Closed-type cells have no connection to the free epithelial surface.

In addition, some 16 different types of disseminated endocrine cells have been distinguished, based on their secretory products and specific secretory granules.

Enteroendocrine cells. The broad-based endocrine cells of the gastrointestinal tract are oval, flask-shaped, or pyramid-shaped, and rest on the basement membrane (**AC6**). Their secretory granules are located in the basal part of the cell (**"basal granules"**) (**B8**) and are transported from there out of the cell by exocytosis (**AC4**).

A few "classic" enteroendocrine polypeptide hormones (e.g., gastrin and cholecystokinin) are also found in the endocrine pancreas (see p. 374); conversely, several hormones typical of the Langerhans islets are also found in epithelium of the gastrointestinal tract. These cells are therefore also classified as belonging to the gastroenteropancreatic (**GEP**) **system.**

Stomach. The stomach contains mostly closed-type endocrine cells, which are evenly distributed in the fundus and body of the stomach, within the epithelium of the principal glands.

Small intestine. The duodenum, especially the duodenal cap, contains abundant endocrine cells in the crypts, as well as scattered cells in the intestinal villi and duodenal glands. The jejunum and ileum contain fewer endocrine cells. **Paneth cells** (**B9**) have apical eosinophilic granules that contain antimicrobial substances such as α-defensins and lysozyme.

Large intestine. Endocrine cells of the large intestine are mainly found at the base of the crypts. **Respiratory system.** The endocrine cells of the respiratory system are scattered throughout the epithelium of the trachea and bronchi; groups of cells are found in the bronchioles. Because of their close relation to nerve fibers, these cells are also called **neuroepithelial bodies.** They are presumably *chemoreceptors* that respond to changes in O_2 and CO_2 levels in the blood.

Urogenital system. Endocrine cells are found in the epithelium of the urethra, the urethral glands, and, in wo'men, the Bartholin glands.

Regulation and Mechanism of Action

The actions of diffuse endocrine cells are regulated by signals conveyed by the bloodstream and/or the autonomic nervous system (**"innervation at a distance"**). Several of the hormones secreted by endocrine cells likewise enter the bloodstream to reach their target cells (**mechanism of endocrine action, AC5**).

A few hormones (amines or peptides) have limited local effects (**paracrine action**), that is, they stimulate or inhibit neighboring endocrine cells (**AC7**) as well as normal epithelial cells (**C10**) in the respective epithelial structure. Other possible target cells include smooth muscle cells (**C11**), nerve fibers (**C12**), and free connective tissue cells such as mast cells (**C13**). Other endocrine cells regulate *local blood flow* by directly affecting the capillaries (**AC5**) or by indirectly stimulating the release of vasoactive substances by mast cells.

Certain hormones are released by exocrine secretion at the apical pole of the cell (**AC4**). Extracellular hormones of the diffuse endocrine system can influence the secretory behavior of the endocrine cells of the same type by virtue of a feedback mechanism (**autocrine action**).

> **Clinical note:** Diffuse endocrine cells can degenerate and form tumors (neuroendocrine tumors, **NET**), for example, benign adenomas, malignant carcinomas, and carcinoids.

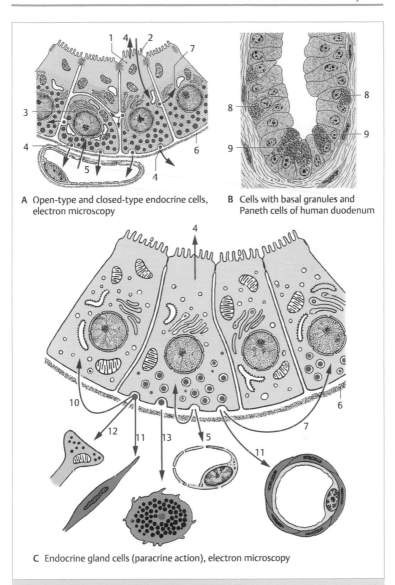

A Open-type and closed-type endocrine cells, electron microscopy

B Cells with basal granules and Paneth cells of human duodenum

C Endocrine gland cells (paracrine action), electron microscopy

Fig. 9.22 Disseminated endocrine cells in different organs.

Secretion, Glandular Epithelium, Endocrine System

Diffuse endocrine cell products and their effects

Cell type	Hormone	Site of synthesis	Stimuli activating release	Effect
A	Glucagon	Alpha cells of islets of Langerhans	Decreased blood glucose concentration (hypoglycemia), protein-rich meals, strenuous physical activity and stress	Increases blood sugar levels; antagonist to insulin in the liver; breaks down glycogen (glycogenolysis) to supply glucose from the liver, stimulates gluconeogenesis and β-oxidation of free fatty acids in the liver, lipolytic effect in adipose tissue
B	Insulin (A chain and B chain) and its precursors: proinsulin, preproinsulin (storage hormone)	Beta cells of islets of Langerhans	Increase in blood glucose concentration (hyperglycemia)	Decreases blood sugar (glucose utilization), inhibits breakdown of proteins and fats (lipogenic effect), stimulates glycogen synthesis
D	Somatostatin = somatotropin-release-inhibiting factor (SRIF)	Delta cells of islets of Langerhans; fundus, body and pylorus of stomach, small and large intestines, nerve endings	Fatty acids, glucose, peptides and bile acids in the small intestine	Reduces secretion of gastric juices and release of gastrin, reduces vagal activity, interdigestive motility, VIP and motilin release, and absorption of nutrients in the small intestine. Inhibits other endocrine cells
D1	Vasoactive intestinal polypeptide (VIP)	Neurons, nerve endings	Neurotransmitters	Causes relaxation of smooth muscle (vasodilation, sphincter control), stimulates intestinal secretion and release of various hormones, inhibits release of gastric acid and secretion of gastrin

Fig. 9.23 Synthesis products of disseminated endocrine cells and their effects.

EC	Serotonin (5-OH-tryptamine) and various peptides	Enterochromaffin cells in pylorus, small and large intestines, scattered in pancreas and bronchi, CNS	?	Causes constriction of vascular smooth muscle, intestinal walls, and bronchi; increases cholinergic secretomotor neural activity; increases intestinal motility
ECL EC-like	Histamine	Enterochromaffin cells in the fundus of the stomach, mast cells, basophils	Increased vagal nerve activity	Increases HCl and pepsinogen secretion, acts locally to increase capillary permeability; smooth muscle contraction; pruritus
ENK	Enkephalins	Stomach, predominantly antrum, small and large intestines, nerve endings	?	Inhibits effect of somatostatin
G	Gastrin	Antrum, pylorus, duodenum, proximal jejunum	Peptides in stomach; elevated pH of gastric juices, vagal efferents and high plasma catecholamine concentrations; ingestion of food	Stimulates gastric acid secretion by parietal cells and pepsinogen secretion; elevates gastric motility, especially peristaltic waves in antrum of stomach; stimulates secretion of exocrine pancreas, bile secretion, and gallbladder contraction (pancreozymin effect); diminishes water and electrolyte absorption in small intestine; trophic effect (promotes growth) on epithelial cells in stomach and duodenum
GRP	Gastrin-releasing peptide (GRP = bombesin)	Stomach and duodenum, bronchi, nerve endings	Elevated pancreatic secretion; elevated pancreozymin release	Stimulates release of gastrin and thus gastric acid secretion; presumably paracrine effects on smooth muscle of bronchial walls in the bronchi

Secretion, Glandular Epithelium, Endocrine System

Fig. 9.24 Synthesis products of disseminated endocrine cells and their effects, continued.

Secretion, Glandular Epithelium, Endocrine System

Diffuse endocrine cell product and their effects (cont.)

Cell type	Hormone	Site of synthesis	Stimuli activating release	Effect
I	Pancreozymin = cholecystokinin (CCK)	Duodenum, pancreas and brain	Fatty acids, amino acids, peptides and trypsin in duodenum; diminished pH levels in intestine	Stimulates pancreatic enzyme secretion, pepsinogen secretion, and bile duct secretion, increases gallbladder contraction reduces HCl secretion, stimulates islet cells and has trophic effect on pancreas; potentiates effect of secretions; induces feeling of satiety ("satiety hormone")
K	Glucose-dependent insulin-releasing peptide = gastric inhibitory peptide (GIP)	Jejunum	Fatty acids, amino acids and glucose in duodenum; low pH levels in duodenum	Antagonist to gastrin; promotes insulin secretion, inhibits HCl secretion and gastric motility
L	Enteroglucagon = glucagonlike peptide 1 (GLP-1)	Distal small intestine and colon	Fatty acids and glucose in ileum	Similar to A cells of pancreatic islets; increases insulin release; inhibits gastric and intestinal motility; trophic effect on epithelial cells in intestinal crypts
Mo	Motilin	Duodenum	Fatty and bile acids in duodenum; diminished somatostatin levels	Stimulates gastric emptying and motility; contraction of smooth muscle
N	Neurotensin (NT)	Duodenum	Fatty acids in small intestine	Inhibits secretion of gastric juices; meal-stimulated release causes hyperglycemia after eating; reduction of blood pressure
P	Pancreatic polypeptide (PP)	Pancreatic islets	Peptides in small intestine; vagal activity	?

Fig. 9.25 Synthesis products of disseminated endocrine cells and their effects, continued.

S	Secretin (+ serotonin)	Duodenum and jejunum	Diminished pH levels in duodenum; bile and fatty acids in duoderum	Release of HCO_3^--rich pancreatic secretion; stimulates release of pepsin as well as intestinal, pancreatic, and bile secretions; inhibits gastric emptying and has an anti-trophic effect on gastric epithelium
T	Tetragastrin (TG)	Small intestine	?	?
	Neuropeptide (NPY)	Nerve endings	Neurotransmitters	Potentiates norepinephrine
	Substance P (p = pain)	Nerve endings	Neurotransmitters	Stimulates smooth muscle contraction and stimulates secretion

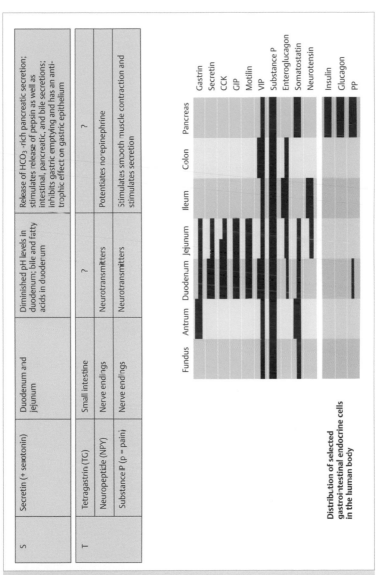

Distribution of selected gastrointestinal endocrine cells in the human body

Secretion, Glandular Epithelium, Endocrine System

Fig. 9.26 Synthesis products of disseminated endocrine cells and their effects, continued.

10 Blood and Lymphatic Systems

10.1 Blood

Components of Blood

The blood may be considered a type of fluid organ system, composed of a coagulable liquid component, blood plasma, in which formed elements, the blood cells, are suspended. Blood serum (= blood plasma without clotting factors, i.e., proteins) is obtained by allowing the blood to clot and then centrifuging it.

Blood volume. The total volume of blood in the human body is a **function of body weight**. A normal volume of blood (about 8% = one-twelfth of body weight) is necessary to maintain circulation and homeostasis. **Hematocrit** expresses the volume of red blood cells relative to total blood volume (100%), which on average is about 45%.

Function. Blood facilitates the **exchange of materials** between cells (by delivering oxygen and nutrients and removing carbon dioxide and other waste products). It also **transports** hormones, antibodies, and immune cells and allows heat transfer through the skin to the surrounding air by convection.

Erythrocytes (**A**). The red blood cell count depends on the oxygen needs of the body and oxygen supply. The human erythrocyte is 7.5 μm in diameter (see p. 395) and does not have a nucleus. Its biconcave shape makes its surface optimal for gas exchange, and its elasticity, based on its membrane skeleton, is an important feature for microcirculation. An erythrocyte consists of up to 90% iron-containing **hemoglobin**; oxygenated blood appears bright red and deoxygenated blood dark red. Immature erythrocytes (about 1%), or **reticulocytes**, contain basophilic granules and reticular structures (*reticular substance*). The **lifespan** of an erythrocyte is 100–120 days, after which it is broken down, mainly in the spleen and liver. The iron-free components of the hemoglobin give rise to bile pigments; in the liver, iron is reused for erythropoiesis in the bone marrow.

> **Clinical note:** An **increased number of reticulocytes** in the peripheral blood following blood loss is a sign of increased erythrocyte production. **Polycythemia** is a sharp increase in the number of erythrocytes; **anemia** is a decreased red blood cell count. The surface of the erythrocyte bears glycolipids and glycoproteins (glycocalyx), macromolecules that contain sugar and have antigenic properties. These determine an individual's blood group (**ABO system**).

Leukocytes (**A, B**). White (clear) blood cells (about 5000/μL blood), resemble amoebae in terms of their movements. Leukocytes serve against infection and foreign substances in the body's defense system. The number of white blood cells varies during the day, depending on factors such as digestive and physical activity. A level exceeding 10,000/μL is termed **leukocytosis** and a level below 2,000/μL is termed **leukopenia**. Types of leukocytes include *granulocytes*, *monocytes*, and *lymphocytes* (**B**).

Granulocytes (**A**). Mature granular lymphocytes have **lobulated nuclei** that are divided into individual segments by indentations, hence the term **segmented granulocyte**. Nuclear segmentation is absent in immature granulocytes, also known as **"bands" or band cells**. Depending on the stainability of their granules, they can be divided into three types of cells: **neutrophilic** granulocytes have small, azurophilic granules containing *lysosomal enzymes* and *bactericidal substances*; **eosinophilic** granulocytes have densely arranged **eosinophilic** granules, which, similar to neutrophils, are capable of *phagocytosis*, especially of antigen-antibody complexes, and are also involved in *limiting allergic reactions*. Their nuclei have *less segmentation*. **Basophilic** granulocytes contain bizarrely shaped, nonsegmented nuclei and coarse granules that appear blue-black with basic stains. Their granules contain the anticoagulant *heparin*; *histamine*, which increases vascular permeability and triggers immediate hypersensitivity; and *chemotactic factors*. A decrease in granulocytes leads to **agranulocytosis**.

Thrombocytes (**platelets**) (**A**). Blood platelets are not independent cells, but irregularly shaped *fragments of pinched-off megakaryocyte cytoplasm*. They disintegrate easily, releasing *thrombokinase*, which is active in blood clotting; they also transport the local vasoconstrictor *serotonin*.

Thrombocytopenia = platelet deficiency.

Thrombocytosis = excess platelets.

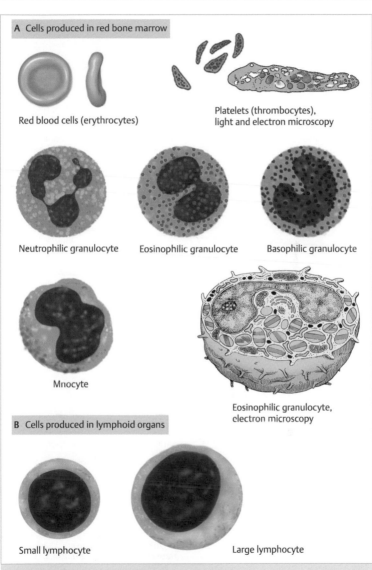

A Cells produced in red bone marrow

Red blood cells (erythrocytes)

Platelets (thrombocytes),
light and electron microscopy

Neutrophilic granulocyte   Eosinophilic granulocyte   Basophilic granulocyte

Mnocyte

Eosinophilic granulocyte,
electron microscopy

B Cells produced in lymphoid organs

Small lymphocyte

Large lymphocyte

Fig. 10.1 Components of the blood.

Blood Count (Normal Ranges) and Functions by Cell Type

Cell type	Cell count per µL of blood (normal range)	Percentage of leukocytes (average)	Lifespan/ presence in the blood	Function
Total leukocyte count	7400 (4000–9000)	100		Immune defense functions in organism
Neutrophilic granulocytes	4250 (2200–6300)	55–70	6–7 hours	Nonspecific immunity. Microphages, chemotaxis, phagocytosis, and lysis of parasites (viruses, bacteria), leukocyte diapedesis, formation of lysozyme, lactoferrin, oxygen free radicals, release of substances with leukotactic activity (leukotrienes)
• Segmented neutrophils	4150 (2000–6300)	50–70		
• Band neutrophils	285 (120–450)	3–5		
Eosinophilic granulocytes	220 (80–360)	2–4	8 hours	Defense against parasites (e.g., nematodes), synergy with mast cells and basophils, e.g., in allergic reactions
Basophilic granulocytes	45 (0–90)	0–1	5–6 hours	Release of histamine and heparin, defense against parasites and helminths
Monocytes	265 (80–540)	2–6	15–20 hours	Precursor cells of mononuclear phagocyte system (see p. 380), macrophages
Lymphocytes	2150 (1000–3300)	5–40	Months–years	B and T lymphocytes, humoral and cell-mediated immunity
Erythrocytes	♂ 4.6–5.9 mill ♀ 4.0–5.5 mill		c. 120 days	Transport of O_2 and CO_2. O_2/CO_2 exchange in the lungs
Thrombo-cytes	150 000–450 000		9–12 days	Hemostasis and coagulation

Fig. 10.2 Normal blood cell levels in the differential blood count and functions of blood cells.

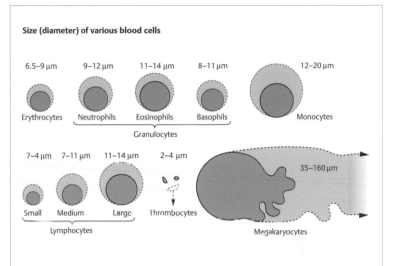

Size (diameter) of various blood cells

6.5–9 μm — Erythrocytes

9–12 μm — Neutrophils
11–14 μm — Eosinophils
8–11 μm — Basophils
(Granulocytes)

12–20 μm — Monocytes

?–4 μm — Small
7–11 μm — Medium
11–14 μm — Large
(Lymphocytes)

2–4 μm — Thrombocytes

35–160 μm — Megakaryocytes

Important Proteins in Plasma and Serum, and their Functions

Protein	Concentration (g/L)	Functions
Albumin	36–50 (55%–65%)	Maintains colloid osmotic pressure in the blood; transport of Ca^{2+}, bilirubin, fatty acids, and other lipophilic substances
α_1-Globulins	1–4 (2.5%–4%)	Transport of lipids and lipoproteins, thyroxin, and adrenal cortical hormones
α_2-Globulins	5–9 (7%–10%)	Oxidase function, plasma inhibitor
β-Globulins	6–11 (8%–12.5%)	Transport of lipoproteins and iron, complement proteins
γ-Globulins or immunoglobulins (IgA, IgD, IgE, IgG, IgM)	7–15 (11%–20%)	Majority of circulating antibodies, immune defense mechanisms
Fibrinogen	2–4.5	Coagulation (fibrin precursor)
Prothrombin	0.06–0.10	Coagulation (thrombin precursor)

Fig. 10.3 Differential blood count and plasma proteins.

Blood and Lymphatic Systems

Hematopoiesis

Prenatal Hematopoiesis

The site of embryonic and fetal production of blood cells, or **hematopoiesis**, changes several times during the course of prenatal development. Hematopoietic phases may be divided as follows (**C**):

Megaloblastic (mesoblastic) phase. About 2 weeks after fertilization, hematopoiesis begins in the **extraembryonic mesoderm of the yolk sac wall** and **embryonic body stalk**. The mesenchyme of these sites or blood islands gives rise to **hemocytoblasts** as well as **angioblasts**, precursor cells of the blood vessel endothelium. By the end of the week 3, embryonic and extraembryonic blood vessels are connected and begin to convey blood. The large red blood cells (15–18 μm in diameter), which at this point still contain nuclei, are termed *megaloblasts*. There are no granulocytes or lymphocytes. The megaloblastic period lasts until the end of the third fetal month.

Hepatolienal phase. By the start of the embryonic week 6 or 7, the **mesenchyme of the liver, spleen,** and **lymph nodes** also becomes involved in hematopoiesis. The *erythrocytes* extrude their nuclei and reach their normal size; and the number of immature erythrocytes decreases. *Megakaryocytes* and *granulocytes* appear. The hepatolienal period gradually recedes from the fifth month of pregnancy onward.

Medullary (myeloid) phase. In the fifth fetal month, hematopoiesis continues in the **bone marrow** of all bones, the final hematopoietic site ("red bone marrow"). By the end of the sixth month, most of the still immature *granulocytes* differentiate and give rise to *monocytes*. *Lymphocytes* begin forming during the fourth month, first in the liver and then in the bone marrow. Some migrate from the marrow to the thymus, which they leave as *T lymphocytes* to colonize and multiply in lymphoid organs, while others travel as *B lymphocytes* from the bone marrow directly to peripheral lymphoid organs (specific immune response, see p. 400).

Postnatal Hematopoiesis

After birth, blood cells are primarily produced in the **red bone marrow** (**A**); the lymphocytes multiply in the **lymphoid organs**, that is, the thymus, lymph nodes, and spleen. Around the age of 6, lymphopoiesis reaches adult levels.

Once growth stops, medullary hematopoiesis occurs only in the **marrow of the ends (epiphyses) of the long bones** and in the **short flat bones**. In people with chronic blood loss or marrow damage, hematopoiesis can resume in the shafts (diaphyses) of the long bones and in the connective tissue of the liver and spleen.

Bone marrow. The bone marrow fills the cavities of the long bones and the spaces in spongy bone. The total weight of the marrow is about 2,000 g. In the adult, one half is red marrow and the other half yellow marrow (fatty marrow).

Between the trabeculae and adipose cells (**B1**) of the **red marrow** is *reticular connective tissue* (fibroblastic reticular cells), in the meshwork of which lie *hematopoietic stem cells* (progenitor cells for *erythropoiesis* (**B2**) and *granulopoiesis* as well as *megakaryocytes* (**B3**) for thrombocytopoiesis). The red marrow contains wide *venous sinuses with fenestrated endothelium*, which are derived from the nourishing vessels of the bone. Mature blood cells pass through spaces in the endothelial cells into the venous sinuses; these open into veins in the marrow, which follow the same course as the arteries. Bone marrow does not contain lymphatic vessels.

B4 Eosinophilic myelocyte

Hemocytoblast. Hemocytoblasts are **pluripotent stem cells** that have the potential to give rise to any type of blood cell. They are functionally distinct, but morphologically indistinct, most closely resembling medium-sized lymphocytes. Pluripotent stem cells can remain in a resting state or divide, producing either more stem cells or differentiating into specialized cells of one of the various blood cell lines. The lymphocyte cell line is the first to branch off the common cell lineage tree (see p. 399).

Clinical note: Proliferation of connective tissue fibers in the bone marrow is known as myelofibrosis.

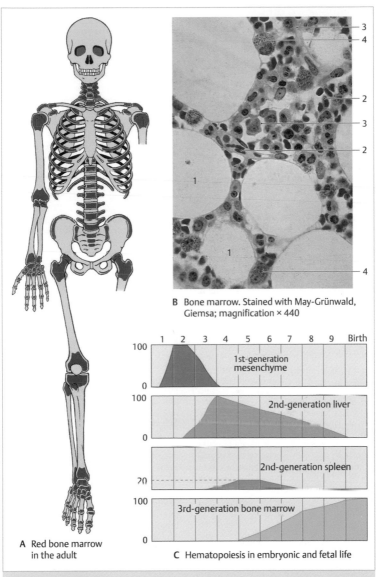

B Bone marrow. Stained with May-Grünwald, Giemsa; magnification × 440

A Red bone marrow in the adult

C Hematopoiesis in embryonic and fetal life

Fig. 10.4 Hematopoiesis.

Hematopoiesis, cont.

The cells of the blood and immune systems are produced in the red marrow (erythrocytes, granulocytes, monocytes, lymphocytes, and thrombocytes) and lymphatic organs (immune system cells). The pluripotent **hemocytoblast** (**1**) is the common stem cell of all blood cells. It divides mitotically to give rise to two cells, one of which remains a pluripotent cell, while the other becomes a committed progenitor cell (unipotent stem cell that is specific for a certain blood cell line), depending on the effect of various growth and differentiation factors. Precursor cells become blast cells and eventually mature blood cells, after progressing through a series of intermediate stages.

Erythropoiesis. About 30% of the immature blood cells in the marrow are erythropoietic cells. A single **hemocytoblast** (**1**) gives rise to a **proerythroblast** (**2**) and an **erythroblast** (**3**), both of which are morphologically identifiable. During proliferation of the polychromatic erythroblast, occurring in four stages of cell division, the cells and their nuclei shrink while the amount of hemoglobin increases (cells become acidophilic). Erythroblasts generally cluster around sinusoids in small groups, at the center of which are one or two reticular cells that provide iron for heme synthesis (*"nurse cells"*) and regulate erythropoiesis.

Erythroblast mitosis gives rise to **normoblasts** (**4**). These expel the now eccentrically located, dense nucleus, which is phagocytosed by marrow macrophages. This process gives rise to **erythrocytes** (**5**). Immature erythrocytes, **reticulocytes** (**6**), still contain remnants of basophilic ribosomes known as *reticular substance*. The most important regulatory factor in erythropoiesis is **erythropoietin**, a glycoprotein hormone produced by the kidney. *Vitamin B12*, folic acid and *growth factors* are also needed.

Iron kinetics. Senescent erythrocytes are phagocytosed and broken down in the spleen and in the liver. Iron from the **hemoglobin** is temporarily stored in the form of hemosiderin in the phagocytes of the reticular connective tissue (detectable with Prussian blue stain). **Ferritin** is liberated from hemosiderin. Two Fe^{3+} ions bind

to a protein molecule called **transferrin** and are carried by the blood to the bone marrow, where the iron is absorbed by reticular cells and taken up by surrounding erythroblasts.

Granulopoiesis. The cells in the three successive stages of the granulocytic series are: **myeloblasts** (**7**), which have virtually no granules, **promyelocytes** (**8**), and granular **myelocytes** (**9**). Myelocyte cell lines are distinguishable by granule staining as neutrophilic, eosinophilic, or basophilic, each of which gives rise to **metamyelocytes** (**10**) and **band cells** (**11**), and ultimately terminally differentiated segmented **granulocytes** (**12**). A **mature** granulocyte is one that contains a multilobed nucleus, typically with 3–4 segments produced by *threadlike indentations*. Granulocytes pass through the walls of venous sinuses in the bone marrow to enter the bloodstream. The granulocytes circulating in the blood represent a mere fraction of those contained in the bone marrow, and additional cells can be quickly mobilized if needed. New formation of granulocytes is generally stimulated by growth factors. Generalized or selective inhibition is also possible, for example, reducing eosinophils with epinephrine or glucocorticoids.

Monocytopoiesis. Monocytes (**13**) are derived from **monoblasts** (**14**) via **promonocytes**.

Thrombocytopoiesis. Megakaryocytes (**15**), giant cells of the bone marrow, arise from precursor cells called **megakaryoblasts** (**16**) and **immature megakaryocytes** (**17**). **Megakaryocytes** (**15**) have large, lobed nuclei. Their cytoplasm contains fine granules and has projections resembling pseudopodia. **Thrombocytes** (**18**) arise from fragmented megakaryocytes, which die after repeated thrombocyte production.

Lymphocytopoiesis. The immunoincompetent precursor cells leave the bone marrow and develop in the lymphoid organs into T or B lymphocytes (**19**). After primary contact with antigens, T or B **immunoblasts** (**20**) arise, the former of which in turn give rise to **immunocytes** (**21**) and the latter to **plasma cells** (**22**) or **memory T or B cells** (**23**) (see p. 402).

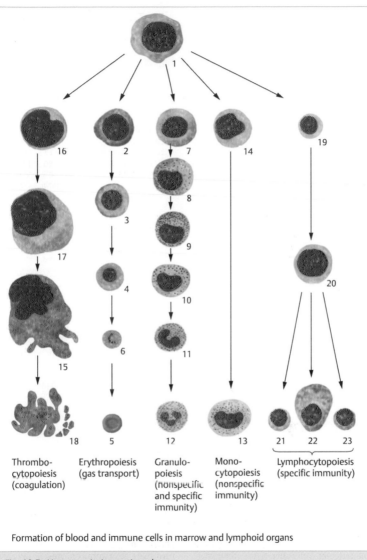

Thrombo-
cytopoiesis
(coagulation)

Erythropoiesis
(gas transport)

Granulo-
poiesis
(nonspecific
and specific
immunity)

Mono-
cytopoiesis
(nonspecific
immunity)

Lymphocytopoiesis
(specific immunity)

Formation of blood and immune cells in marrow and lymphoid organs

Fig. 10.5 Hematopoiesis, continued.

10.2 Immune System

Every day the human organism encounters a multitude of microbial pathogens (bacteria, viruses, protozoa, fungi) and toxic foreign substances that enter the body through the skin, gastrointestinal tract, and respiratory system. Considering the abundance of infectious organisms colonizing our environment and our food, the occurrence of illness is infrequent, and most infections endure only briefly, with little lasting damage. This is thanks to a highly effective **immune system**, in essence a system of complex interactions between cells and soluble proteins.

The **chief function** of the immune system is to prevent invasion by infectious microorganisms and to defend the body against bacteria and/or foreign substances that have already entered. The term **"immunity"** refers in this sense to the relationship between the ability of the body to distinguish between its own ("self") and foreign ("nonself") substances, and to produce antibodies specific to nonself substances (= *humoral immunity*) and/or specifically reactive lymphocytes (= *cell-mediated immunity*). **Antigens** are soluble substances or particulate materials that provoke an immune response. Contact with the antigen produces a type of memory in the organism, termed **immunological memory**, which elicits a rapid immune response if the same antigen is encountered again.

Specific immunity (acquired or adaptive immunity). The main agents in specific immunity are **immunocompetent T lymphocytes** (cell-mediated immune response) and soluble **antibodies** produced by **B lymphocytes** (humoral immune response). Both types of lymphocytes become **immunocompetent** as they develop from precursor cells (see p. 398). Cells belonging to the body are recognized by lymphocytes as "self" and, unlike foreign substances ("nonself"), are not attacked.

Clinical note: Immunological tolerance is the failure of cells to attack the body's own cellular components. Tolerance of foreign antigens, however, can result in death.

Conversely, hypersensitivity of the immune system, as in **autoimmune disorders**, can cause the body to attack and destroy its own structures and molecules.

Nonspecific immunity (natural or innate immunity). Innate immunity involves an essentially instantaneous response that locally destroys pathogens (foreign substances) as well as malignant cells produced by the body itself.

The most important cells in nonspecific immunity are **phagocytes:**

Neutrophilic granulocytes (see pp. 392 ff and 403 E) gather within the first hours of infection, having been attracted to the infection site by pathogens and substances produced by cellular degradation. Neutrophils ingest foreign material and destroy it, with the help of *lysosomal enzymes*. At the same time, they release *proteolytic enzymes*, which soften the inflammatory infiltrate and can lead to abscess formation. The neutrophils die in the process, giving rise to pus corpuscles.

Macrophages (see p. 403 G) develop from monocytes. They migrate as **mobile "exudate macrophages"** to infection sites, as *pleural* and *peritoneal macrophages* in serous cavities and *alveolar macrophages* in the lungs. Examples of **fixed macrophages** are the *Kupffer cells* (*stellate cells*) in the liver and *histiocytic, reticular cells* in the spleen, lymph nodes, and bone marrow. These cells are collectively known as the **mononuclear phagocytic system** (**MPS**) (formerly known as the reticuloendothelial system, RES; or reticulohistiocytic system, RHS). They also have an important function in specific immunity and, as highly active secretory cells, produce a number of humoral factors that lead to the recruitment and activation of new phagocytes. Phagocytosis and cytotoxicity are supported by humoral factors including lysosomes, acute-phase proteins, cytokines, and proteins of the complement system. Other macrophages arising from monocytes include *osteoclasts*, which resorb bone, and *microglia cells*, which are resident immune cells of the central nervous system that contribute to its protection and repair.

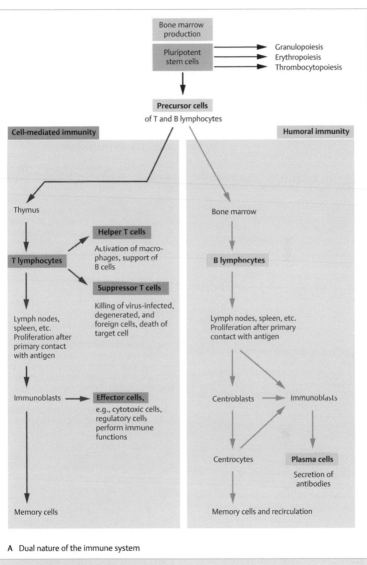

A Dual nature of the immune system

Fig. 10.6 Overview.

Blood and Lymphatic Systems

Cells of the Immune System

The lymphocytes (A) constitute the cellular part of specific (adaptive) immunity. They may be subdivided into **T cells** and **B cells**, which are characterized by a usually round nucleus that is high in chromatin (**A**).

T lymphocytes. Thymus-dependent T lymphocytes develop in the **cortex of the thymus**, into various subtypes (see below). Before leaving the thymus, T lymphocytes must undergo a selection process; only those cells that recognize self tissues and thus attack only foreign substances are released. After leaving the thymus, T lymphocytes travel in the blood to the **T-dependent regions of the lymphoid organs**, where they reenter the circulation via the lymphatic system as immunocompetent cells. Lymphocytes are characterized by certain surface molecules, and each expresses an antigen-specific **T-cell receptor**.

Subpopulations (see p. 401). T-cell sub-populations include **helper T cells**, whose primary role is *coordination of the immune response*. Helper T cells release cytokines, which influence the development, differentiation, and activation of other immune cells. B lymphocytes, for example, require the help of T cells, which specifically react to antigen in order to mount an immune response (proliferate and secrete antibodies). In a mechanism that is not yet fully understood, **suppressor T lymphocytes** can suppress the immune response of B cells, helper T cells, and **cytotoxic T cells**. Cytotoxic (killer) T lymphocytes can destroy antigenic cells such as virus-infected cells and cancer cells, by direct contact. They also play an important role in the rejection of allotransplantations. The cytotoxic peptides released by killer T cells, such as *perforin*, allow them to lyse target cells without destroying themselves.

The specificity of each of these functions is attained with the **primary response** to antigen, which activates the T lymphocyte to become the proliferative **T immunoblast** (**B**). At the same time, **memory cells** arise, which are capable of long-term recognition of the invading antigen.

B lymphocytes. These are also immunocompetent cells that mediate specific humoral immunity. They have **immunoglobulin receptors** (antibody receptors) on their membranes that bind with high specificity to their respective antigens. After contact with the "best-fitting" antigen (lock-and-key model), they proliferate and differentiate, mainly into antibody-producing plasma cells (= **direct plasma cell production**).

Plasma cells (**C, F**) are differentiated, large **basophilic** cells (15–20 µm in diameter). Their nuclei lie eccentrically and have a **spoke-wheel arrangement** (**C**) that is visible under light microscopy. They are considered the **most effective antibody producers**. Plasma cells contain an extensive rough endoplasmic reticulum (**F1**), where immunoglobulins are produced. They do not divide and have a lifespan of about 4 days. Immunoglobulins are released into connective tissues and travel through the bloodstream to the antigen, which they bind to and destroy.

Indirect plasma cell production. Specific **memory cells** are activated when a specific antigen is encountered again (**secondary response**). Memory cells possess receptors for the invading antigen, having arisen from B lymphocytes during the primary response via various intermediate stages of development (**centroblast, centrocyte**) in the germinal center of the secondary follicle (see p. 410). Memory cells are capable of reacting years later to "their" antigen and rapidly differentiate into antibody-producing plasma cells. Memory cells are thus the foundation of immunological memory.

Mast cells (**D**). These cells develop from hematopoietic precursor cells in bone marrow and contain large granules that are highly basophilic because of their content of heparin (which inhibits blood clotting) and chondroitin sulfate. Mast cells are the most important effector cells in allergic events. They are found everywhere in connective tissue and are especially abundant close to vessels and in all mucous membranes.

E Neutrophilic granulocyte with phagolysosomes (1)

G Macrophage with phagosome (1)

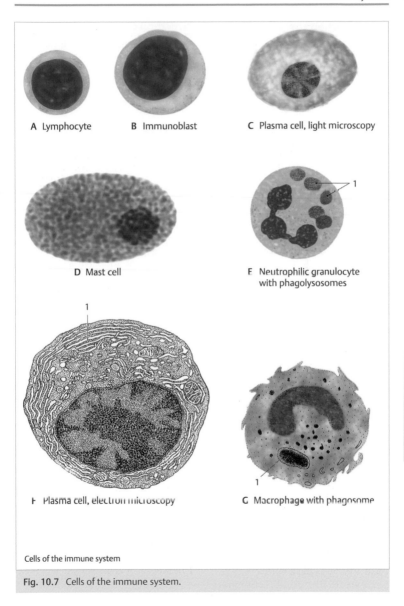

A Lymphocyte   B Immunoblast   C Plasma cell, light microscopy

D Mast cell

E Neutrophilic granulocyte
   with phagolysosomes

F Plasma cell, electron microscopy

G Macrophage with phagosome

Cells of the immune system

Fig. 10.7 Cells of the immune system.

10.3 Lymphatic Organs

Overview

The lymphatic organs are important in the specific immune response (see p. 400 ff). The **primary lymphatic organs** serve as the sites for production, development, and maturation of immune cells. **Secondary lymphatic organs** are where immune cells encounter foreign substances.

Primary Lymphatic Organs

Bone marrow. The bone marrow (see p. 396) contains lymphocyte stem cells (derived from hemocytoblasts), as well as precursor cells of the mononuclear phagocyte system (MPS).

Thymus. The role of the thymus is paramount in the development of the immune system (see p. 406).

Secondary Lymphatic Organs

Lymphoepithelial organs. These include the *pharyngeal tonsil, palatine tonsil, lingual tonsil*, and *tubal tonsil* at the opening of the auditory tube, and *lateral pharyngeal bands* in the lateral and posterior walls of the pharynx (see p. 416).

Mucosa-associated lymphoid tissue (MALT). This includes gut-associated lymphoid tissue (GALT); intraepithelial lymphocytes and lymphocytes of the lamina propria; solitary lymph nodules within the lamina propria of the small intestine; aggregated lymphoid nodules (Peyer patches) within the lamina propria and submucosa of the small intestine and vermiform appendix (see p. 418); bronchus-associated lymphoid tissue (BALT); lymphoid tissue of the urogenital system; palpebral conjunctiva; and the lacrimal drainage system.

Skin-associated Lymphoid Tissue (SALT)

Lymphoreticular organs. The lymphoreticular organs include the *lymph nodes* (see p. 410) and *spleen* (see p. 412).

Structural Components

Cellular elements. The lymphatic organs contain B and T lymphocytes; monocytes (**A**) and macrophages; polymorph nucleated granulocytes; mast cells (**B**) and plasma cells; and natural killer cells.

Reticular connective tissue. This is a special form of connective tissue that contains few fibers. Its branching **fibroblastic reticular cells** of mesenchymal origin have numerous processes and form a loosely woven three-dimensional tissue meshwork (**C**). Reticular cells form **reticular fibers** that can be impregnated with a silver salt. A special type of reticular cell is the **histiocytic reticular cell**, which is capable of phagocytosis and is viewed as a monocyte derivative. **Dendritic cells** have treelike branching processes that surround lymphocytes. Two types may be distinguished: *interdigitating dendritic cells (IDCs)* with irregularly shaped nuclei and long, fingerlike processes that can establish contact with T lymphocytes; and *follicular dendritic cells (FDCs)* which may be multi-nuclear and are present almost exclusively in germinal centers (see p. 410). Dendritic cells are *accessory cells of the immune system*.

B- and T-cell regions. The lymphatic organs and tissues have varying populations of B and T lymphocytes. B lymphocytes are the predominant cell type found in primary and secondary follicles (see p. 410), and T lymphocytes are found in various regions specific to individual organs.

Lymphatic vessels. Part of the blood from the interstices and intercellular connective tissue areas of the organs and tissues (with the exception of the central nervous system) is drained by lymphatic vessels and returned to the venous blood supply (see p. 410).

Epithelioid venules are postcapillary venules with endothelium, its form ranging from cuboidal to columnar (high endothelial venules, **HEV**). Adhesion molecules on the endothelial surface are recognizable by circulating lymphocytes and determine the level of lymphocyte return (**homing**).

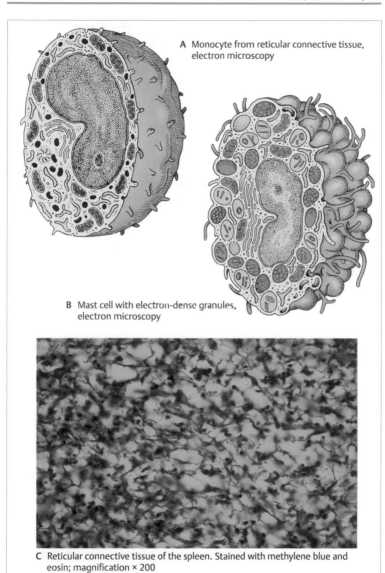

A Monocyte from reticular connective tissue, electron microscopy

B Mast cell with electron-dense granules, electron microscopy

C Reticular connective tissue of the spleen. Stained with methylene blue and eosin; magnification × 200

Blood and Lymphatic Systems

Fig. 10.8 Overview.

Thymus

The thymus is the principal lymphoid organ of the T-cell system and thus plays a **central role in regulating** the immune system function. It is considered a branchiogenic organ.

Development

The **stroma of the thymus** arises as a bilateral structure from the anterior endoderm of the third pharyngeal pouch and presumably from the ectoderm of the cervical vesicle. Its framework consists of epithelial **reticular cells**, which are distinct from the mesenchymal reticular cells forming the connective tissue that ensheathes the thymic vessels. In week 8 of embryonic development, **capillaries** begin growing in the purely epithelial thymus primordium; between weeks 9 and 12, the surface of the (epithelial) thymus primordium is indented by **mesenchymal septa** growing into it and forming *"pseudolobes."* The thymus primordium ultimately passes into the mediastinum behind the thyroid primordium and loses its connection to the pharynx. The supporting tissue framework, consisting of epithelial reticular cells, is occupied during week 8 or 9 of gestation by lymphocyte stem cells of mesenchymal origin, first by cells from the blood islands of the yolk sac, then by cells from the hematopoietic tissue of the liver and spleen, and finally, after birth, by lymphocyte precursor cells from the bone marrow. The precursor cells proliferate rapidly to produce **T lymphocytes** (thymus lymphocytes), **regulatory cells** (*helper T cells, suppressor T cells*), and **cytotoxic T cells**. All lymphoid cells of the thymus are also known as **thymocytes**.

Form and Location

The thymus is composed of **two lobes**, usually of unequal size, which may be partially fused or not at all. It lies behind the sternum in the **superior mediastinum** (**A**) in front of the great vessels, that is, the *brachiocephalic veins* and *superior vena cava*, and over the pericardium. It is bounded on either side by the lines of reflection of the costal pleural reflection onto the mediastinal pleura. The lines of reflection form the **"thymic triangle"** (red triangle pictured

in **A**), which lies at the level of the sternal attachment of the second rib, the tip of which is directed toward the apex of the "heart triangle."

In the **neonate** (**B**), each lobe is about 5 × 1.5 × 1.5 cm and weighs 11–13 g. During the first three years of life, its weight increases to about 27 g. The thymus reaches its greatest size during puberty, weighing between 20 and 30 g.

The thymus is especially well developed in the **child**. Both of its lobes extend cranially to the inferior border of the thyroid gland and caudally into the fourth intercostal space, where it may widen the radiographic shadow produced by the base of the heart. Its upper portion can project, on either or both sides, through the superior thoracic aperture behind the middle cervical fascia.

In the **adult**, the thymus is present only as a functional **thymic remnant** (**C**). It occupies considerably less space behind the manubrium of the sternum than the thymus in a young person.

Vessels, Nerves and Lymphatic Drainage

Arteries. The majority of the *thymic branches* are derived from the **internal thoracic artery** and the **pericardiophrenic arteries**;

branches also sometimes arise from the thyroid arteries.

Veins. The *thymic veins* pass to both **brachiocephalic veins**, and small veins also drain into the inferior thyroid veins.

Lymphatic vessels. Lymphatic drainage is to the **anterior mediastinal lymph nodes** along the brachiocephalic veins and aortic arch. The thymus has no afferent lymphatic vessels.

Autonomic nerves. The autonomic nerves to the thymus arise from the **vagus nerve** and **sympathetic trunk**. They accompany the cardiac nerves and their plexuses, the phrenic nerve, and the vasomotor nerves to the thymus. The vessels and nerves travel deep into the organ, within the connective tissue septa, to the corticomedullary border, where they divide and send branches into the medulla and also supply the cortex.

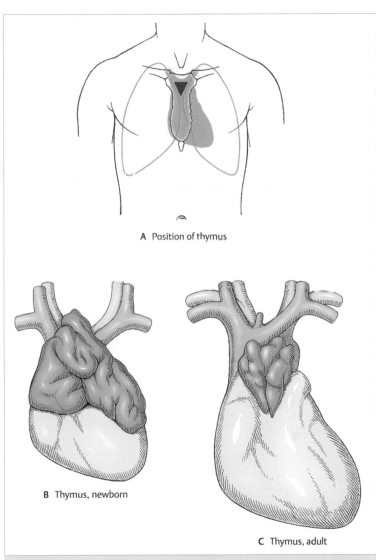

A Position of thymus

B Thymus, newborn

C Thymus, adult

Fig. 10.9 Thymus.

Microanatomy of the Thymus

The supporting framework of the thymus consists of **epithelial reticular cells** (epitheliocytes) and **lymphocytes** (lymphoepithelial organ). It is composed of branching shrublike or treelike **strands of tissue** that resemble *lobules* (**A1**, **B**) in histological sections. Each lobule has an outer **cortex** (**AB2**), with densely arranged cells and a central **medulla** (**A–C3**) containing fewer cells. The thymus is surrounded by a **connective tissue capsule** that sends short *septa* into the interior of the organ (**AB4**).

Epithelial reticular cells or thymic epithelial cells. These have large, pale nuclei and a weakly eosinophilic cytoplasm that contains cytoplasmic keratin filaments. Their long, slender **processes** are connected by *desmosomes* and form a spongelike **meshwork** containing T lymphocytes.

Cortex. The spaces within the meshwork of the epithelial cells are filled with densely packed T lymphocytes (**AB2**) and thus stain darkly. Beneath the connective tissue capsule (**B4**) is a **continuous layer of cortical epitheliocytes** with prominent *Golgi complexes* and *cisterns of rough endoplasmic reticulum*. Lymphocytes that have migrated to the thymus proliferate in the **corticomedullary zone** directly underneath, where they are surrounded by epitheliocyte projections (*"nurse cells"*).

The population of small lymphocytes arising in the thymic cortex is replenished every 3–4 days. T lymphocytes are constantly released into the blood, but in fewer numbers with advancing age. Most of the lymphocytes that migrate to the thymus die in the cortex during the selection processes that are part of the development of specific immunity.

Medulla. The dense meshwork of epithelial cells (**A–C3**) forming the medulla contains fewer lymphocytes. At the **corticomedullary junction**, **medullary reticular cells** form an aggregate of epithelioid cells. The eosinophilic **Hassall corpuscles** (**C5**) are characteristic, spherical structures (with a diameter of 30–150 μm) formed by concentric layers of *degenerated reticular cells*. They may consist of only a small number of cells or cysts that are 0.1–0.5 mm in size, with cellular debris. The significance of Hassall corpuscles, which arise in conjunction with immune processes, is uncertain.

C6 Myoid cell

Vascularization. The **thymic branches** from the pericardiophrenic artery (see pp. 52, 406) pierce the thymic capsule and travel within the *connective tissue septa* into the *thymic parenchyma* where they divide at the corticomedullary junction into arterioles and capillaries.

Cortical capillaries have a *nonfenestrated endothelium*. They are ensheathed in a *basement membrane*, *perivascular connective tissue*, and a *continuous layer of epitheliocytes*. These layers form the **blood-thymus barrier**, which limits exposure of the thymus to antigenic substances. Venous drainage follows the course of the arteries.

Age-related changes. Involution of the thymus (**D**), especially of the cortex, begins during puberty. Fat storage (**D7**) in the fibroblastic reticular cells that accompany the vessels gives rise to *thymic adipose tissue*, leaving only functional thymic rudiments (*thymic remnants*). Age-dependent involution is distinguished from **accidental involution**, which can occur after irradiation, but is more often associated with infection or poisoning.

Function. The thymus plays a critical role in the **establishment of cell-mediated immunity**. Until puberty it is the most important source of T lymphocytes. In the cortex of the thymus, proliferating lymphocytes come into contact with epithelial reticular cell processes and thus the body's own antigens. T cells are primed, that is, they are programmed to discriminate between "self" and "nonself." Since foreign antigens would interfere with priming, they are prevented by the **blood-thymus barrier** from entering the cortex. Immunocompetent T lymphocytes enter the circulation through the fenestrated endothelium of the medullary capillaries and colonize the T-dependent zones of the peripheral lymphoid organs. "Incorrectly programmed" lymphocytes are phagocytosed by macrophages. The production, differentiation, and maturation of T lymphocytes in the thymus, as well as the differentiation of peripheral lymphoid organs, are stimulated and regulated by **thymopoietin**, a polypeptide hormone produced by the epithelial reticular cells, and presumably other humoral factors (*thymosin, thymulin*) as well.

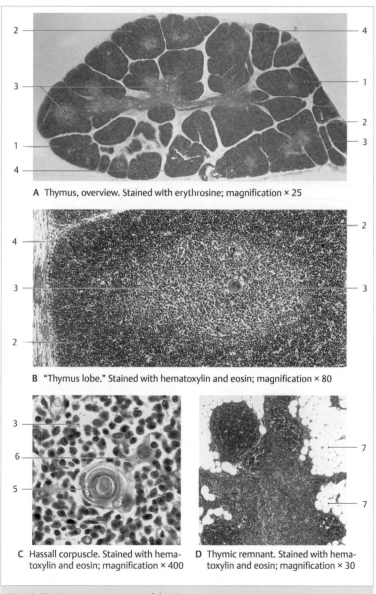

A Thymus, overview. Stained with erythrosine; magnification × 25

B "Thymus lobe." Stained with hematoxylin and eosin; magnification × 80

C Hassall corpuscle. Stained with hematoxylin and eosin; magnification × 400

D Thymic remnant. Stained with hematoxylin and eosin; magnification × 30

Fig. 10.10 Microscopic structure of the thymus.

Lymph Nodes

Lymph nodes are bean-shaped lymphoreticular organs (**A**) of variable size (ranging from a few millimeters to more than 1 cm in length) which are located in the paths of the lymphatic vessels and serve as biological filters. **Regional lymph nodes** are the first filtering station for lymph and the antigens it carries from an organ or specific region of the body. **Collecting nodes** receive lymph from several regional lymph nodes.

Structure. Each lymph node is enclosed in a **connective tissue capsule** (**ABD1**), from which **trabeculae** (**AB2**), connective tissue septa, radiate into its interior, forming a supporting framework and partitioning the node into segments. Several **afferent lymphatic vessels** (**A3**) carry lymph to the node, piercing its convex surface at various sites; **efferent lymphatic vessels** (**A4**) carry lymph away and exit at the hilum.

In the parenchyma, the **cortex**, **paracortical zone**, and **medulla** can be distinguished. The dense arrangement of cells causes the cortex to stain darkly in histological preparations (**AB5**). In the paler-staining medulla (**AB6**), the lymphocytes are less densely packed.

Functional Organization

Sinuses. Afferent lymphatic vessels drain into the subcapsular **marginal sinuses** (**AD7**), which contain few lymphocytes and are traversed by individual *reticular sinus cells*. Radiating **peritrabecular sinuses** (**A8**) empty into the centrally located, wide-lumen **medullary sinuses** (**AB9**), which communicate with efferent vessels at the hilum. The sinuses are lined by flat endothelial cells and contain lymphocytes as well as macrophages and monocytes.

Vessels. Small arteries enter and small veins leave the lymph node at the hilum. The arteries branch into arterioles in the medulla, and these continue in the cortex as a cortical **capillary network**, which is woven around the follicles like a basket and supplies them with blood. The paracortex (see below) contains specialized postcapillary venules with cuboidal endothelium (**high endothelial venules = HEV**) bearing *lymphocyte homing receptors*. These receptors are recognized by lymphocytes and facilitate their passage from the blood into the lymph node. Lymphocytes leave the

lymph nodes through the efferent vessels (**A4**).

Parenchyma. The cortex contains the **lymphoid follicles** (**C**) and corresponds to the B-cell region, while the paracortical zone is the T-cell region. The medullary cords contain mainly plasma cells and macrophages. **Primary follicles** are lymphoid follicles consisting of clusters of homogeneous lymphocytes (immunoincompetent B cells). The majority of the lymphoid follicles have a lighter-staining *germinal center* (**C10**), with activated B lymphocytes (*centroblasts* and *centrocytes*) and follicular dendritic cells (**secondary follicles, C**) in which an antigen has already been encountered.

CD11 Band of lymphocytes in the secondary follicle.

Function. Lymph nodes serve as **filters** and ensure the **immune response**. Foreign matter, pathogens, cellular debris, cancer cells, and pigments passing through the lymph nodes are trapped by endothelial cells lining the sinuses, and phagocytosed. Antigenic material is ingested and processed by macrophages, accessory cells in the immune response, which then present the antigen to lymphocytes, eliciting a T-cell or B-cell response, depending on the quality of the antigen.

> **Clinical note:** Lymph nodes can be affected by isolated disease, that is, **lymphadenopathy**. Cancer cells that are carried to the lymph nodes can proliferate there, giving rise to **lymph node metastases**.

Lymphatic vessels. The lymphatic vessels form a **drainage system** that returns fluids from the tissues to the blood circulation. The vessels originate in the interstitial space, as tiny blind canals without an endothelial lining, and carry lymph to the thin-walled **lymphatic capillaries**. These are followed by **precollecting vessels** with funnel-shaped and leaflet valves, which continue as **collecting vessels** with a typical wall structure (*tunica intima, tunica media, tunica adventitia*). Collecting vessels pass to the lymph nodes as **afferent lymphatic vessels**. **Efferent lymphatic vessels**, also termed "postnodal" lymphatic vessels, either pass to other lymph nodes (collecting nodes) or join **lymphatic trunks**. The lymphatic trunks ultimately unite to form **lymphatic ducts**, the largest of which is the *thoracic duct*, with a diameter of several millimeters.

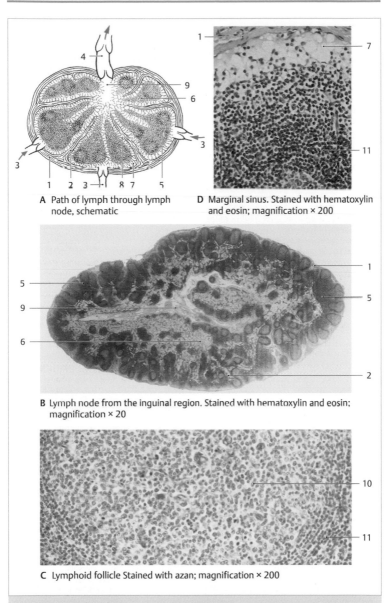

A Path of lymph through lymph node, schematic

D Marginal sinus. Stained with hematoxylin and eosin; magnification × 200

B Lymph node from the inguinal region. Stained with hematoxylin and eosin; magnification × 20

C Lymphoid follicle Stained with azan; magnification × 200

Fig. 10.11 Lymph nodes.

Spleen

The spleen is an unpaired **lymphoreticular organ**. Similar to the lymph nodes, it acts as a **filter**, but, unlike the lymph nodes, it is located in the blood circulation. It also fulfills **immune system functions**.

Development. The splenic primordium is **derived from the mesoderm**. It appears during week 5 of embryonic development, as a nonvascularized mesenchymal condensation between the layers of the posterior mesogastrium. During week 16 of embryonic development, the spleen becomes **vascularized**, and the mesenchymal cells differentiate into the typical reticular tissue framework. At the same time, **lymphatic cells migrate** to the spleen. During the first few months of development, the spleen is an important **hematopoietic organ**. **Accessory spleens** can arise from masses of mesenchymal tissue. These pea-sized or egg-sized masses of splenic tissue may be singular or numerous and are usually located adjacent to the spleen or branches of the splenic artery, but also lie along the greater curvature of the stomach, in the greater omentum, and elsewhere in the body.

Gross Anatomy

The spleen is a soft, bluish-red organ (**B**) shaped like a coffee-bean, 10–12 cm × 6–8 cm × 3–4 cm in size and weighing 150–200 g.

Surfaces and margins. The convex **diaphragmatic surface** (**B**) faces superiorly and the concave, faceted **visceral surface** (**C**) faces inferiorly. The anterior margin of the spleen, called the **superior border** (**BC2**), is narrow and marked by indentations. The broad and blunt **inferior border** (**BC3**) faces posteroinferiorly. Its posterosuperior pole, or **posterior extremity** (**BC4**), extends to a point 2 cm from the body of T10. The anteroinferior pole, or **anterior extremity** (**BC5**), extends nearly to the midaxillary line and is difficult to palpate. The spleen is primarily held in position by the **phrenicocolic ligament**, which passes from the left colic flexure to the lateral wall of the trunk, forming the floor of a *sling that supports* the organ.

Splenic hilum. The **hilum** is a long, narrow **fissure** on the visceral surface of the spleen (**C**), through which vessels and nerves enter and exit the organ. It divides the visceral surface into the *upper* and *lower regions*. The area posterior to the hilum (**D6**) touches the left kidney (**D7**), and in the area anterior

to it the *stomach* (**D8**) touches the *tail of the pancreas* (**D9**) and the *left colic flexure*.

D12 Liver

Position. The **intraperitoneal** spleen is situated posteriorly in the left hypochondriac region (**A**) below the diaphragm at the level of the 9th to 11th ribs. Its long axis is parallel to the 10th rib (**A1**).

A2 Inferior border of lung

A3 Inferior border of pleura

The **gastrosplenic ligament** (**CD10**) passes from the splenic hilum to the greater curvature of the stomach (**D8**). It conveys the *short gastric arteries* and *veins* and the *left gastro-omental artery*. The shorter **splenorenal ligament** (**CD11**) passes to the posterior wall of the trunk and diaphragm. It carries the *splenic artery* and *vein*. The **splenic recess** of the omental bursa (arrow, p. 185) extends to this point. The spleen moves with respiration.

> **Clinical note:** Traumatic rupture of the spleen causes intraperitoneal hemorrhage. Patients complain of pain in the flank, with pain radiating to the left shoulder, due to phrenic nerve irritation.

Vessels, Nerves, and Lymphatic Drainage

Arteries. The **splenic artery** (see p. 44) (**C12**), the thickest branch of the celiac trunk, passes along the superior border of the pancreas (**D9**), reaching the splenic hilum via the splenorenal ligament. It divides while in the splenorenal ligament and enters the spleen with six or more *splenic branches*. **Veins**. The **splenic vein** (**C13**) is formed at the splenic hilum by the union of several veins that drain the spleen. It is one of the three major tributaries of the hepatic portal vein (see p. 216). It courses behind the pancreas (**D9**). **Lymphatic drainage**. Lymph drains via the **splenic nodes** at the splenic hilum to the **superior pancreatic nodes**, along the superior border of the pancreas and the **celiac nodes** along the celiac trunk.

Nerves. Parasympathetic and sympathetic nerve fibers, that is, *viscerosensory, visceromotor*, and *vasomotor* nerve fibers, arise from the *celiac nerve plexus* and accompany the splenic artery as the **splenic nerve plexus**, to the spleen. The myofibroblasts of the splenic trabeculae and the trabecular arteries are supplied by adrenergic nerve fibers, which regulate the capsule contraction.

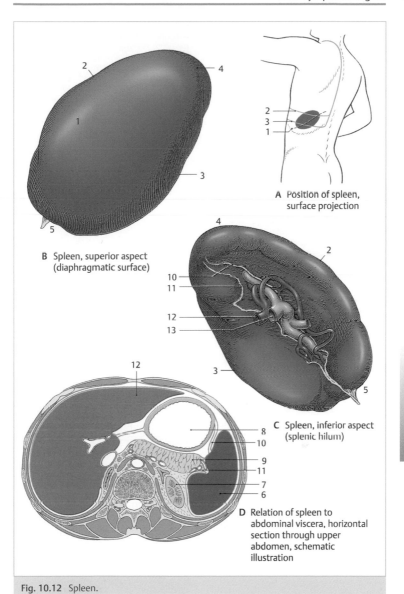

B Spleen, superior aspect (diaphragmatic surface)

A Position of spleen, surface projection

C Spleen, inferior aspect (splenic hilum)

D Relation of spleen to abdominal viscera, horizontal section through upper abdomen, schematic illustration

Fig. 10.12 Spleen.

Microscopic Anatomy of the Spleen

The spleen is surrounded by a thin **connective tissue capsule** (**AB1**), which is covered by peritoneal epithelium. The connective tissue capsule sends numerous projections called **splenic trabeculae** (**B2**) into the interior of the organ, partitioning it into segments. Most of the trabeculae are anchored to the splenic hilum. Between the capsule and the trabeculae, there is the **splenic pulp**, which is vascularized, "soft" reticular connective tissue.

Pulp. The **"red pulp"** (**A3**) is characterized by the presence of a large amount of blood and consists of **pulp cords** with **splenic sinusoids** between them. **"White pulp"** (**A4**) is made up of lymphoid nodules and periarterial lymphatic sheaths (PALS). The **marginal zone** (**B9**), containing less densely packed cells (mainly B-lymphocytes), lies around the nodules at the border between the red and white pulp.

Blood vessels. The structure of the spleen can best be understood in terms of its vascular architecture. The branches of the **splenic artery** enter the organ through the hilum and travel within the trabeculae (**B2**) as **trabecular arteries** (**B5**), accompanying the trabecular veins (**B6**). The trabecular arteries continue into the parenchyma as **pulp arteries**. Within the white pulp they are completely enclosed by *periarterial lymphatic sheaths* (PALS), containing mainly T lymphocytes, and continue as **central arteries** (**B7**) in the cords of the lymphatic tissue and, to a lesser extent, in the lymphoid nodules (**B8**). Each central artery gives rise to numerous smaller branches, which supply the meshwork of the marginal zone (**B9**) or empty directly into the venous sinuses of the red pulp. Lying along the cords of lymphatic tissue (T region) are the lymphoid nodules (B region) (**B8**). Ultimately, each central artery divides distal to the PALS, into a terminal "tree" consisting of about 50 arterioles (**penicillar arterioles**) (**B10**). These pass to the surrounding red pulp, where they divide again and continue as capillaries, a short segment of which is covered by the spindle-shaped or ovoid *Schweigger-Seidel sheath* (*ellipsoid*) (**B11**), surrounded by densely packed macrophages and contractile cells (**sheathed capillaries**). The sheathed capillaries are followed by **arterial capillaries**, the majority of which empty via the perisinusoidal **meshwork cords** of the reticular connective tissue (**B12**) into the wide **splenic sinusoids** (**B13**) of the red pulp ("*open circulation*"). A few capillaries open directly into the splenic sinusoids ("*closed circulation*"). Blood is drained from the organ via the **pulp** and **trabecular veins** (**B6**), into the **splenic vein**.

Pulp cords and splenic sinusoids. The pulp cords consist of a network of reticular cells and contain plasma cells as well as macrophages. The venous sinuses of the red pulp form a loosely woven network of wide-lumen vascular spaces that communicate with each other. The **walls of the sinuses** are composed of *spindle-shaped, longitudinally oriented endothelium* (**C14**), whose nuclei project into the lumen of the sinus. Between them are *slitlike openings* that allow blood cells (**C15**) from the surrounding pulp cord to enter the sinusoid lumen. The basement membrane of the endothelium lining the splenic sinusoids is discontinuous. They are lined by circumferential *reticulin fibers* (**C16**) and an incomplete layer of *specialized reticular cells* with *phagocytozing macrophages* (**C17**) and *reticular tissue* (**C18**).

C19 Mitosis, **C20** Macrophage

Hematopoiesis. Vast numbers of lymphocytes and plasma cells are produced in the spleen. If production of blood cells in the bone marrow is deficient, for example, due to disease, granulocyte and erythrocyte production can resume in the spleen, where it was present during fetal development.

Shedding and storage of blood cells. Senescent erythrocytes are trapped in the red pulp, engulfed by macrophages, and destroyed. **Hemoglobin**, the red pigment contained in the erythrocytes, is broken down into **bilirubin** and transported to the liver by the hepatic portal vein, to be excreted with **bile**. Hemoglobin iron is bound to a protein and transported to the bone marrow as **transferrin**, where it is again available for erythroblasts. Excess hemoglobin iron is stored in the spleen and can be detected microscopically as **hemosiderin**; in extreme circumstances, iron stores may be macroscopically visible as brown pigmentation of the organ (**hemosiderosis**).

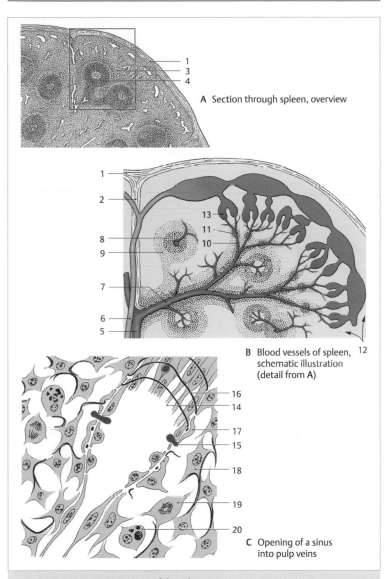

A Section through spleen, overview

B Blood vessels of spleen, schematic illustration (detail from A)

C Opening of a sinus into pulp veins

Fig. 10.13 Microscopic structure of the spleen.

The Tonsils

The **tonsils** surround the openings of the oral and nasal cavities into the pharynx and are collectively known as the **Waldeyer tonsillar ring** or **lymphoid ring**. Tonsils are secondary lymphoid organs. Given their proximity to the epithelium, they are also known as **lymphoepithelial organs**.

General structure. The tonsils contain lymphoid tissue in the form of densely packed secondary follicles lying directly beneath the mucosal epithelium, the surface of which is indented by elevations and invaginations (**crypts**). The **secondary nodules** consist of a light-staining *germinal center* and a dark-staining *lymphocyte halo*, which is thickened on the side facing the epithelium, forming a *cap of lymphocytes*. Lymphocytes and granulocytes migrate into the epithelium, especially deep in the crypts, opening the meshwork of epithelial cells like a sponge. Because of this **leukocyte diapedesis**, the epithelium and the boundary with the lymphoreticular tissue are frequently no longer detectable. **Efferent lymphatic vessels** pass from the tonsils into deeper-lying lymph nodes. The tonsils are delimited from their surroundings, by a tough capsular connective tissue covering.

Pharyngeal tonsil. The pharyngeal tonsil (**AC1**), which is shaped like a cauliflower, protrudes from behind the choanae at the level of the **roof of the pharynx**. It does not possess deep crypts, but has only **shallow infoldings** between sagittally oriented mucosal elevations. Corresponding to its location in the epipharynx, the pharyngeal tonsil is lined by pseudostratified ciliated and goblet-cell-lined columnar (respiratory) epithelium (**E12**).

> **Clinical note:** In children, the pharyngeal tonsil can become enlarged as a result of infection (adenoids or **polyps**). Obstruction of the choanae can lead to sinusitis, mouth breathing, and sleep disturbance, and, if the auditory tube is obstructed as well, chronic ear infection.

Palatine tonsil. The palatine tonsils (see p. 145) lie in the hollow formed by the palatine arches (**AB3**), known as the **tonsillar fossa**; see palatine tonsil (p. 149). They are covered by oral mucosa (stratified,

nonkeratinized squamous epithelium) and possess 10–20 cryptlike indentations known as **tonsillar pits** (**D8**). The lymphoid tissue contained in the tonsils forms **aggregated follicles** (**D7**).

The palatine tonsils are important immune system organs and the site of vigorous proliferation of B lymphocytes. They encounter pathogens that invade the body through the mouth and nose, thus ensuring early activation of the specific immune response (**"immunological early warning system"**).

> **Clinical note:** Bacterial infection can cause acute inflammation of the palatine tonsils (**tonsillitis**). Characteristic symptoms include sore throat (angina) and difficulty swallowing (dysphagia). Enlarged tonsils can be surgically removed (**tonsillectomy**).

A6 Laryngeal inlet, **C10** Sella turcica, **C11** Soft palate, **D13** Oral epithelium

Lingual tonsil. The lingual tonsil (**A4**) (see p. 149) has a bumpy surface and lies on the base of the tongue; it is flat and has numerous cryptlike infoldings of the oral mucosa, which are surrounded by secondary nodules (**lingual nodules**). The mucous-secreting posterior lingual glands open in the base of the crypts.

Tubal tonsil. The submucosal tubal tonsil (**A5**), which lies at the inner opening of the auditory tube, is viewed as a continuation of the pharyngeal tonsil. It consists of a collection of smaller secondary nodules.

> **Clinical note:** Enlargement of the tubal tonsil can obstruct the pharyngeal opening of the auditory tube, resulting in possible hearing impairment, nasal speech, and chronic ear infections.

Lateral pharyngeal bands. This term is used to refer to aggregates of lymphoid tissue in the mucosa of the lateral and posterior walls of the pharynx (**A7**). The lymphoid tissue can form small nodules on the posterior wall of the pharynx.

> **Clinical note:** Inflammatory swelling of the pharyngeal mucosa (pharyngitis, **"lateral pharyngitis"**), with symptoms of sore throat and dysphagia, also involves the **lateral pharyngeal bands**.

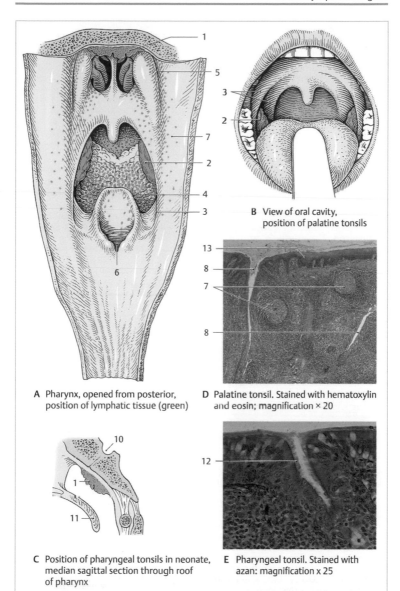

A Pharynx, opened from posterior, position of lymphatic tissue (green)

B View of oral cavity, position of palatine tonsils

D Palatine tonsil. Stained with hematoxylin and eosin; magnification × 20

C Position of pharyngeal tonsils in neonate, median sagittal section through roof of pharynx

E Pharyngeal tonsil. Stained with azan: magnification x 25

Blood and Lymphatic Systems

Fig. 10.14 Tonsils.

Mucosa-Associated Lymphoid Tissue (MALT)

Organized lymphoid tissue is also present in the lamina propria of the mucosa of the respiratory tract (**BALT**), urogenital tract, conjunctiva of the eye, skin (**SALT**), and in larger amounts in the mucosa of the gastro-intestinal tract (**GALT**).

GALT

Gut-associated lymphoid tissue (GALT), which is active in the specific immune response, comprises lymphatic tissue within the mucosal lining of the esophagus, stomach, small and large intestines, and vermiform appendix. It is made up of various components.

Solitary cells are mostly **intraperitoneal lymphocytes**. These **include suppressor cells**, (about 70%) as well as **effector cells**, which are dispersed throughout the lamina propria and include lymphocytes, plasma cells, macrophages, eosinophilic granulo-cytes, and specialized mast cells (mucosal mast cells).

Solitary lymphoid nodules. These are **nodular collections of lymphocytes** in the lamina propria of the small intestine. They can be divided into **primary nodules** whose lymphocytes form an evenly distributed mass (not yet activated by antigen exposure), and **secondary nodules**, which have a light-staining center and a dark-staining periphery of small, tightly packed lymphocytes (stimulated by antigen contact). The light-staining center serves as a germinal center for lymphocyte generation, and also acts as an "activation center" (see p. 410).

Aggregated lymphoid nodules (**Peyer patches**) (**AD1**) are **large collections of lymphoid follicles** in the lamina propria and submucosa of the vermiform appendix (**D1**) and ileum (especially opposite the mesenterial attachment). These structures projecting into the lumen measure 1–4 cm in diameter and consist of 10–50 nodules each. Villi and crypts are absent at these sites. The mucosal protrusions are referred to as "**domes**" (**AB2**), and their respective epithelial coverings as "**dome epithelium**" (**B3**). The epithelium tends to be cuboidal rather than columnar; goblet cells are absent and there are specialized enterocytes which, instead of bearing microvilli, contain microfolds in their surfaces ("microfold cells" or M cells). **M-cell areas** (**C**) with intraepithelial lymphocytes (**C8**) also have lymphocytes and macrophages (**C9**) beneath. Additional structural elements of Peyer patches are the **B lymphoblasts** (**B4**), the **corona** (mantle) (**B5**) of small B lymphocytes surrounding the nodule, and the **interfollicular region** (**B6**), which is mainly populated by T lymphocytes.

B7 Muscularis mucosae, **D2** Mucosa with crypts, **D3** Submucosa, **D4** Muscle layer

Function. As one of the mucosa-associated lymphoid tissues, GALT constitutes an **autonomous lymphoid organ complex** that encounters numerous antigens such as bacteria, parasites, viruses, and food allergens. The **contact surface area** of the intestine is about 100 m², or 60 times larger than the surface area of the skin.

B lymphocytes in the lamina propria of the mucosa mature to become antibody-secreting plasma cells, which produce all antibody classes, with 80% being immunoglobulin A (**IgA**). IgA binds to a protein produced by enterocytes and is secreted by them into the intestinal lumen. T lymphocytes are predominantly helper T cells.

At the sites of the Peyer patches, M cells in the "dome epithelium" trap antigens, which are then phagocytosed and presented to neighboring T cells. These reach the center of the lymphoid nodule, where they transmit their information to B cells, which migrate into the lymphatic circulation. The B cells reach the thoracic duct via regional lymph nodes, thus entering the general blood circulation. Most are carried by the bloodstream back to the intestinal mucosa (**lymphocyte recirculation**), where a further development into IgA-secreting plasma cells continues. Antigen contact within a Peyer patch can thus lead to a generalized immune response throughout the entire small intestine. Activated B cells migrate through the blood and lymph circulation into other secretory organs, for example, into the mammary, salivary, or lacrimal glands, where they lead to production of IgA, which is secreted with the specific secretory products of these glands.

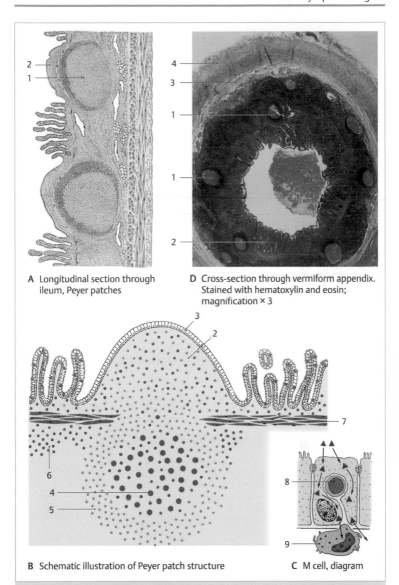

A Longitudinal section through ileum, Peyer patches

D Cross-section through vermiform appendix. Stained with hematoxylin and eosin; magnification × 3

B Schematic illustration of Peyer patch structure

C M cell, diagram

Fig. 10.15 Mucosa-associated lymphatic tissue (MALT).

Blood and Lymphatic Systems

11 The Integument

11.1 Skin

General Structure and Functions

The **skin** (**integument**) has a total surface area of 1.6–2.0 m², depending on body size. It functions as a protective covering of the body, forming the boundary between the internal and external environments. Consisting of an **epidermis** and a **dermis**, the skin makes up about 16% of the total body weight. Epidermal and dermal thicknesses vary depending on the body region, ranging between 1 and 5 mm. In cross section the epidermis is 0.04–0.3-mm thick (especially thick at sites exposed to strong mechanical forces, such as the palms of the hands and soles of the feet, measuring 0.75–1.4 mm; calloused skin is 2–5 mm). Women tend to have thinner skin than men. At the openings of the body, the skin is continuous with the mucous membranes of the mouth, nose, rectum, urethra, and vagina. "**Appendages of the skin**" are specific structures associated with the skin such as *skin, glands, hair,* and *nails.*

Functions

As an organ, the skin fulfils a variety of functions, serving to **protect** the body from mechanical, chemical, and thermal trauma, as well as a multitude of pathogens.

The immunocompetent cells of the skin are involved in immune processes, and hence it is a highly active **immune organ**.

The skin also contributes to **thermoregulation** by adjusting blood circulation as well as fluid secretion from skin glands (protection against heat loss).

It is also involved in maintaining **fluid levels**, by preventing dehydration and releasing fluids and salts in glandular secretions (regulation of fluid levels and excretion).

The skin also contains **nervous system structures** that make it a sensory organ capable of detecting pressure, touch, temperature, and pain.

It also functions in the **transformation of provitamin D** into bioactive metabolites. **Synthesis of vitamin D** takes place in the skin via photo-oxidation of 7-dehydrocholesterol, which is mediated by ultraviolet light.

The skin acts as an **organ of communication**, for example, blushing, paling, "hair-raising."

It also possesses **electrical resistance**, which changes under psychological stress (the underlying principle of lie detectors).

Skin characteristics. The skin is characterized by its **soft, elastic, distensible** quality and by **keratinization** of its epithelium. Except for the palms of the hands, soles of the feet, and scalp, the skin is loosely attached to the underlying tissue and thus **easily movable**. In areas overlying the joints it **forms** folds that permit adequate freedom of movement. The skin can become electrostatically charged, especially in conditions of dry ambient air and when synthetic fabrics are worn, resulting in a static charge of more than 1,000 volts.

> **Clinical note:** More than any other organ, the skin can be directly observed. Examination of the skin can thus **aid the diagnosis of a multitude of general disorders**. Blue discoloration (cyanosis), for instance, is considered a sign of heart disease, while a reddened patch of skin may be a sign of infection. Very white skin suggests anemia or depigmentation (absence of melanin), while yellow discoloration indicates the presence of bile pigments in the blood, for example, due to cirrhosis of the liver.

Skin Color

The normal color of healthy skin is determined by **four components**: melanin (brownish-black pigment) produced by melanocytes (**A**), carotene derived from dietary vegetables (**B**), and oxygenated (**C**) and deoxygenated (**D**) blood in the cutaneous vessels. The influence of each of these four pigments varies by body region. Pigmentation is partly related to factors such as sun exposure and nutrition, but it is usually determined genetically and by the person's sex. **Melanin pigmentation** (**A**) is strongest in the regions about the axillae, external genitalia, inner thighs, and perianal skin. **Carotene** (**B**) produces a yellowish tinge, mainly about the face, palms of the hands, and soles of the feet. The red color of **arterial blood** (**C**) determines the color of the skin of the face, palms of the hands, soles of the feet, upper half of the trunk, and buttocks. The bluish hue produced by **venous blood** (**D**) predominates in the lower half of the trunk and on the posterior aspects of the hands and feet.

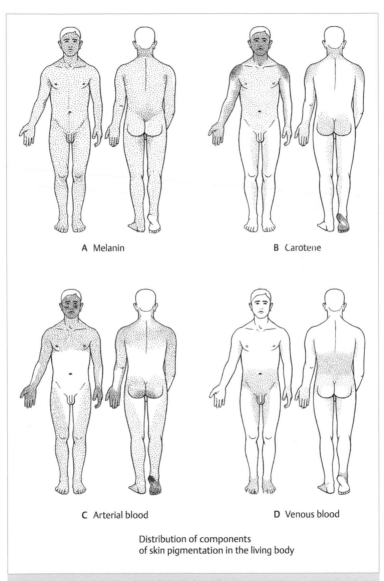

A Melanin

B Carotene

C Arterial blood

D Venous blood

Distribution of components
of skin pigmentation in the living body

Fig. 11.1 General structure of the skin and skin color.

Surface of the Skin

The outward appearance of the skin is characterized by **furrows** and **folds**, as well as **plateaus** and **ridges**. Coarse furrows are present in the form of *flexion creases* at the joints and *as facial movement lines*.

Skin tension lines. Lines of greatest and least tension are visible on the skin. The **lines of greatest tension** (**A**), or relaxed skin tension lines, arise from the action of underlying muscles, and knowledge of their location is important for surgery. Relaxed skin tension lines are usually oriented perpendicular to muscle fiber orientation and often correspond to folds (wrinkles) in aging skin.

> **Clinical note:** Properly made **skin incisions** follow the lines of greatest tension, allowing wound closure with a minimum of tension. Incisions made perpendicular to the lines of greatest tension can result in gaping wounds, delayed healing, and an unsatisfactory cosmetic outcome.
> **Excessive stretching,** such as of the abdominal skin during pregnancy or weight gain, can cause tears in the dermis (see p. 428). The resulting **striae distensae**, or stretch marks, are initially bluish red in color but later become white. They usually develop perpendicular to the direction of stretch.

Hair-bearing skin (**B**). Most of the skin covering the human body has a relief pattern of crossing furrows that form triangular, rhombic, or polygonal plateaus. On top of these **plateaus** *eccrine sweat glands* open, and at certain sites *apocrine sweat glands* as well. The **furrows** contain the *hair* and the *pores of the sebaceous glands*. The connective tissue papillae of the papillary layer (see p. 426 ff) are often poorly developed. In the surface of the hair-bearing skin, the dermal papillae are arranged with hair follicles and sweat gland excretory ducts, to form what may be described as *cockade-shaped epithelial ridges* and *rosette-shaped epithelial rows*.

Glabrous skin (**C**). The skin on the soles of the feet and the palms of the hands (especially on the finger pads) possesses fine, parallel ridges measuring about 0.5-mm wide, on top of which the sweat glands (**C1**) open. This skin is hairless and does not contain any sebaceous or apocrine sweat glands. The ridges are formed by **rows of papillae of the papillary layer** of the dermis (see p. 428), resulting in a rougher texture that enhances gripping. The genetically determined, characteristic pattern unique to each individual makes it possible to use fingerprinting (*dactylogram*) as a means of identification (*dactyloscopy*). The **four types of ridge patterns** on the finger pads are highly variable: *arch* (**DI**), *loop* (**DII**), *whorl* (**DIII**), and *double loop* (**DIV**).

Regeneration of skin. The skin has an efficient renewal system. Following an injury (wounds, loss of substance), immune cells in the dermal layer fight local infections, and capillaries and connective tissue structures are restored. The surface is re-epithelized as skin grows from around the periphery of the injury site over the regenerating connective tissue. The resulting **scar** is initially red, owing to capillary formation, but later appears white, owing to collagen fibers visible through the epithelium. Accessory skin structures (e.g., glands and hair) cease to form at the site of the scar.

Age-related skin changes. The effects of aging on the skin include *degeneration* (*atrophy*) *of the dermis, thinning of the epidermis, flattening of the dermal papillae,* and *loss of subcutaneous fatty tissue* (see p. 426 ff). These changes do not only occur with the overall aging of the body, but are also determined by long-term exogenous factors (e.g., sunlight, weather, and climate) and the level of skin pigmentation. Age-related changes are most evident in fair-skinned people and on sun-exposed parts of the body (e.g., face, neck, posterior surfaces of the hands and forearms). Changing chemical properties of the connective tissue ground substance causes fluid loss and a reduction in elastic fibers in the dermis and subcutaneous tissue. The skin becomes increasingly loose, thin, slack, susceptible to wrinkling, and fragile; if a fold of skin is pinched ("pinch test"), it is slow to return to the normal level of the surrounding skin; pigmentation becomes irregular. Ultraviolet rays (sunlamps) accelerate the loss of skin elasticity.

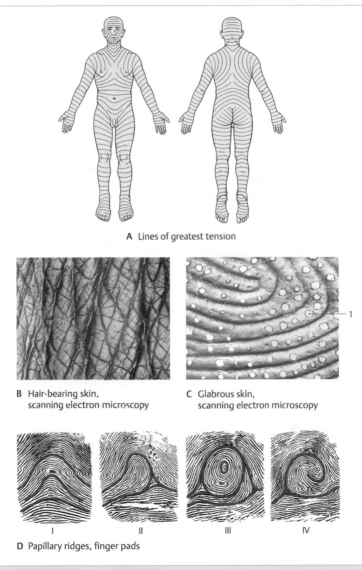

A Lines of greatest tension

B Hair-bearing skin,
scanning electron microscopy

C Glabrous skin,
scanning electron microscopy

I II III IV

D Papillary ridges, finger pads

Fig. 11.2 Skin surface.

The Integument

The Layers of the Skin

The skin is made up of the **epidermis** (**AB1**), which consists of *stratified, keratinizing, squamous epithelium*, and the **dermis** (corium) (**A–D2**), which is a *layer of connective tissue*. The **dermis** can be divided into a *papillary layer*, containing conical projections that interdigitate with the epidermis (**CD2**), and a reinforcing *reticular layer*. The epidermis and dermis are separated by a distinct boundary, but there is usually not a sharp transition between the connective tissue forming the dermis and that of the subcutaneous tissue (subcutis) (**AB3**). The **subcutaneous tissue**, which connects the skin with underlying structures (e.g., fascia or periosteum), contains *adipose tissue* and *larger vessels and nerves* (see p. 428).

Glabrous skin: A4 Merocrine sweat glands (**D4** excretory duct), **A5** Vater-Pacini lamellar corpuscles, **A6** Meissner tactile corpuscles.

Hairy skin: B7 Hair, **B8** Sebaceous gland, **B9** Arrector pili muscle, **B10** Apocrine sweat gland

Epidermis

New cells are continuously being produced by mitosis in the basal layer of the epidermis. These cells migrate to the surface of the skin within 30 days, producing keratin as they move upward. The boundaries formed between the epidermal layers as a result of this process are most distinct in the glabrous skin (**A**), and only faintly detectable in hair-bearing skin (**B**).

Regeneration layer. The germinative layer comprises the basal and spinous layers of the epidermis. The **basal layer of the epidermis** consists of a single layer of *tall prismatic cells* (**C11**) lying directly on the basement membrane. Above the basal layer is the **spinous layer** (prickle cell layer) (**CD12**), consisting of 2–5 layers of *large polygonal keratinocytes* whose spine like processes are interconnected by *desmosomes*. The cytoplasm contains a dense network of *intermediate filaments* (keratin filaments, tonofilaments) that radiate into the desmosomes. The 18–20-µm wide intercellular spaces form a cavity system.

Keratinization layer. The keratinization layer comprises the granular layer (**CD13**) and the clear layer (**CD14**). The flattened keratinocytes, which now lie parallel to the skin surface, forming the thin **granular layer** (2–3 layers of cells), contain *lamellar bodies* (*Odland bodies*) and basophilic keratohyaline granules, which indicate the beginning of keratinization. The contents of the Odland bodies (glycoproteins, lipids, and enzymes) undergo extracellular transformation, forming lipid lamellae that fill the intercellular spaces and make them impermeable. The barrier created by the lipids protects against fluid loss. Finally, a thin, translucent layer, the **clear layer** (**CD14**), arises, in which no nuclei or cell boundaries are identifiable. This layer derives its name from the presence of the highly refractive, acidophilic substance, *eleidin*, which is found in cells undergoing keratinization.

Horny layer. In the tough and virtually impermeable **horny layer** (**CD15**), consisting of cells that no longer possess nuclei or organelles, the flat *corneocytes* and *keratin* form a cohesive layer that is continually sloughed off as horny (skin) flakes that are resistant to acid, but swell in alkaline substances. Keratinization is regulated by vitamin A; deficiency leads to excessive keratinization, a disorder known as *hyperkeratosis*.

Epidermal symbionts. Nonkeratinizing epidermal cells are collectively described as epidermal symbionts. The lower cell layers contain **melanocytes** (**C16**), which are dendritic cells of neuroectodermal origin that produce the pigment *melanin*. The cell bodies of the melanocytes rest directly on the basement membrane, and their dendritic processes extend into the intercellular spaces to the middle part of the spinous layer. Melanocytes transfer their pigment directly to the basal epidermal cells. A single melanocyte supplies about 5–12 basal cells. Melanin protects the basal layer (mitosis) from harmful ultraviolet rays.

Langerhans cells (**C17**) are suprabasal cells located in the spinous layer. These dendritic cells have extensive processes and are involved in the activity of the immune system. Originating in the bone marrow, Langerhans cells present antigens to resting helper T cells, activating them and inducing a primary immune response. Also contained in the basal layer are a small number of **Merkel cells**. These touch receptors of neuroectodermal origin lie directly on the basement membrane and are connected with adjacent basal cells via desmosomes. Beneath each Merkel cell is a Merkel disk, which is derived from a myelinated axon.

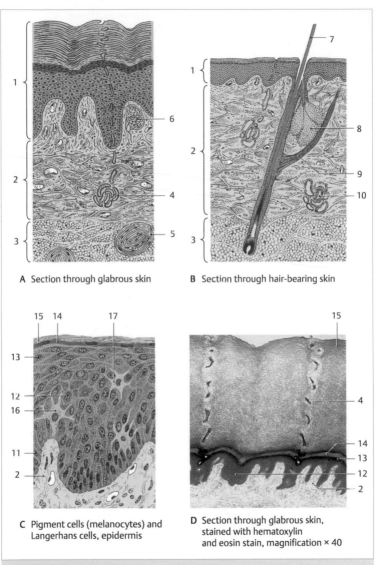

A Section through glabrous skin

B Section through hair-bearing skin

C Pigment cells (melanocytes) and Langerhans cells, epidermis

D Section through glabrous skin, stained with hematoxylin and eosin stain, magnification × 40

Fig. 11.3 Skin layers.

Dermis

The dermis (corium) (**AB2**) is much thicker than the epidermis (**AB1**). It contains accessory epidermal structures, blood and lymph vessels, connective tissue cells, free immune cells, nerves, and nerve endings and associated structures. A highly durable latticework of *interlacing bundles of collagen fibers* interspersed with *elastic fiber networks* make the dermis **tough** and **elastic**. The elasticity of the skin is mainly due to the angular motion of the meshwork of collagen fibers, with the elastic fibers acting to return the skin to its resting position. The **dermis consists of two layers:**

Papillary layer (**A4**) (papillary dermis). The papillary layer borders directly with the overlying epidermis. It contains **collagen fiber pegs**, connective tissue papillae which project upward and interdigitate with epidermal rete ridges, binding the epidermis to the underlying tissues. The height and number of dermal papillae varies by region and corresponds to the mechanical forces acting on various regions of the body; for instance, the skin of the eyelid contains fewer and smaller papillae, while that covering the knee and elbow has larger and greater numbers of papillae. The dermal papillae contain **hairpin capillary loops** (**B12**), **fine nerves**, and **sensory nerve endings**. Collagen fibers are notably thinner. In the loosely structured papillary layer of the dermis, type III collagen predominates over type I collagen.

Reticular layer (**A5**) (reticular dermis). The loosely woven delicate collagen fibers (type III collagen) of the papillary layer continue into the reticular layer as **tough collagen fiber bundles**, forming a dense fiber meshwork (type I collagen). The collagen fibers run nearly parallel to the skin surface and are accompanied by a network of **elastic fibers**. Fibroblasts, macrophages, mast cells, and small numbers of lymphocytes lie between the bundles of fibers. The interstices contain a **gel-like ground substance** that consists of proteoglycans (hyaluronic acid, chondroitin sulfate, and dermatan sulfate), proteins, and minerals. Since proteoglycans possess a high capacity for binding water, the dermis plays a vital role in regulating the *skin turgor.*

Subcutaneous Tissue

The **subcutaneous tissue** (**AB3**), or subcutis, forms the connection between the skin and the fascia covering the body (**A6**) or periosteum, and allows movement of the skin. The subcutaneous tissue contains adipose tissue in various amounts, depending on the body site. Adipose tissue serves as a *fat depot* and provides *insulation against heat loss.* Depot fat is distinguished from **structural fat**, which is partitioned by fibrous bands of connective tissue similar to a quilted cushion, for example, on the sole of the foot. **Depot fat**, such as that lying beneath the skin of the trunk (*panniculus adiposus*), is more prevalent. **Distribution of fat** is genetically determined and is also influenced by hormones. Men tend to accumulate fat around the abdomen, while women typically store fat in the hip, buttock, and breast regions. In certain places, the subcutaneous tissue is loose and devoid of fat (eyelids, auricles, lips, penis, scrotum, etc.). On the face and scalp (galea aponeurotica), the subcutaneous tissue is firmly anchored to underlying muscle and tendons (forming the basis for facial expression).

A7 Hair, **A8** Sebaceous gland, **A9** Arrector pili muscle, **A10** Merocrine sweat gland, **A11** Muscle layer

Blood vessels. The **arteries** (**B15**) form a network between the skin and subcutaneous tissue, supplying branches to the hair roots, sweat glands (**B14**), subcutaneous adipose tissue, and dermal papillae. The **subpapillary plexus** sends capillary loops (**B12**) into the individual dermal papillae. The **veins** (**B16**) form networks beneath the papillae, within the dermis as well as between the skin and subcutaneous tissue, called **cutaneous venous plexuses** (**B13**). **Arteriovenous anastomoses**, including specialized shunts known as *glomus bodies*, which are present in acral regions (e.g., fingertips, tip of the nose), can influence flow velocity. Changes in cutaneous circulation are an essential part of thermoregulation. Lymphatic vessels also form plexuses.

Nerves and sensory organs of the skin. (see p. 434).

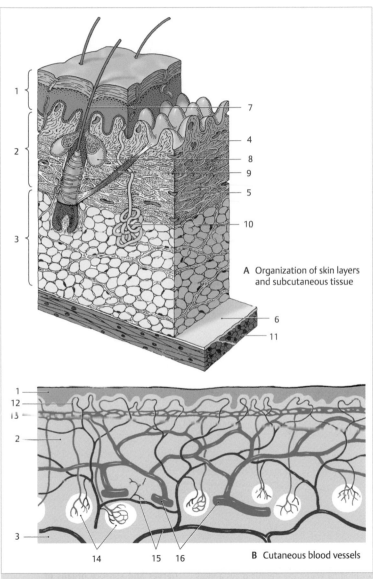

A Organization of skin layers and subcutaneous tissue

B Cutaneous blood vessels

Fig. 11.4 Dermis and subcutaneous tissue.

The Integument

11.2 Skin Appendages

Skin Glands

The skin glands (**A–E**), like the hair and nails, are also accessory structures of the skin. They derive from solid epithelial masses that project downward from the epidermis into the mesenchyme (dermis) around them and differentiate in the dermis to form various types of glands.

Sweat Glands

Eccrine sweat glands (**AB**). The 2–4 million **eccrine glands**, which are innervated by cholinergic nerves, are distributed over the entire body in a pattern that varies individually and from region to region. They are densely clustered on the forehead, palms of the hands, and soles of the feet, and scattered over the neck and thighs. Eccrine sweat glands are **narrow**, **unbranched epithelial tubes** (**AB1**) that penetrate deep into the dermis or upper portion of the subcutaneous tissue. Their terminal parts form a coil 0.3–0.5 mm in diameter (**coil glands**). The tubular **secretory units** are formed by *simple*, or occasionally pseudostratified, *cuboidal to columnar epithelium*. The cells contain lipid droplets, glycogen granules, and pigment granules. Between the glandular epithelium and the basement membrane is a discontinuous arrangement of contractile, ectodermal *myoepithelial cells* (**B2**). The secretory unit is continuous with the rather tortuous, corkscrew-shaped **excretory duct** (**A3**), which is lined by a *bilayer of cuboidal epithelium* and opens on the epidermal surface. The connective tissue surrounding the ducts contains fine fibers (**AB4**) and has a rich capillary and nerve supply.

The **acid secretion** (pH 4.5) of the eccrine glands inhibits bacterial growth (*protective acid coating*), and aids *thermoregulation* by means of perspiration and evaporation (cooling the body), and *elimination of electrolytes* Na^+, K^+, Cl^-, and HCO_3^- (the salt content of sweat is about 4%). Normally about 100–250 mL of sweat is excreted per day, but a person can lose as much as 5 L per day with heavy physical activity and high ambient temperatures.

A9 Fat vacuoles, **B10** Capillaries

Apocrine sweat glands (**C, D**). The **apocrine glands**, which are innervated by adrenergic nerves, are present on the hair-bearing skin (axillae, mons pubis, labia majora, scrotum, and perianal region), as well as on the nipple, and areola, and in the nasal vestibule. Apocrine glands are **simple coiled tubular glands**, often with widened alveolar secretory units. They are located in the subcutaneous tissue and empty into hair follicles. Their secretory ducts are lined by *simple epithelium of variable height*. Domes of cytoplasm (**C5**), which characteristically project into their lumen, are pinched off during the apocrine secretion process. Between the glandular epithelium and basement membrane are densely arranged spindle-shaped *myoepithelial cells* (**CD6**).

Apocrine sweat glands produce an **alkaline secretion** that contains *odorants*, which play a role in sexual and social behavior. Secretion begins at puberty. Apocrine sweat glands can be the site of abscesses. Modified sweat glands include the *ceruminous glands* of the external acoustic meatus, and the *ciliary glands* (Moll glands) of the eyelid.

Sebaceous Glands

The **sebaceous glands** (**E**) are holocrine glands that primarily originate from the hair germ and open into the infundibulum of the hair follicle (forming the pilosebaceous unit). Free sebaceous glands occur independently of hair follicles and are present on the vermilion border, nostrils, linea alba of the buccal mucosa, nipple, eyelid, labia minora, glans penis, and prepuce. The fully developed sebaceous glands located in the upper layer of the dermis are **individual, multilobular acinar glands** that open into a common excretory duct. Each **pear-shaped acinus** contains mitotically dividing cells and is surrounded by a peripheral layer of *proliferating matrix cells* (germinal cells) (**E7**). The matrix cells move toward the interior of the sebaceous gland, which does not contain a lumen, where they mature into polyhedral, weakly staining cells that contain increasing numbers of *lipid vacuoles* and eventually pyknotic nuclei (**E8**). The cells are ultimately completely transformed into **sebum**.

About 1–2 g of sebum are produced daily and secreted via the infundibulum onto the surface of the hair and epidermis, making them pliable and water-resistant. The fatty acids contained in sebum also give it bactericidal properties.

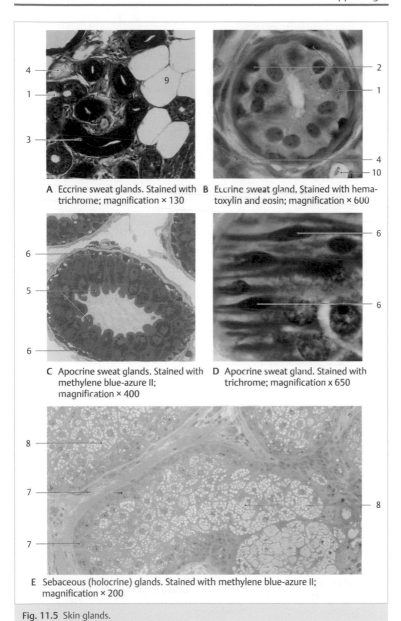

A Eccrine sweat glands. Stained with trichrome; magnification × 130

B Eccrine sweat gland. Stained with hematoxylin and eosin; magnification × 600

C Apocrine sweat glands. Stained with methylene blue-azure II; magnification × 400

D Apocrine sweat gland. Stained with trichrome; magnification x 650

E Sebaceous (holocrine) glands. Stained with methylene blue-azure II; magnification × 200

The Integument

Fig. 11.5 Skin glands.

Hair

Hairs are pliable keratinous filaments that possess a degree of tensile strength. Similar to the nails, the hair originates from the epidermis (epidermal keratinization). Hair has an important function in *touch perception* and *insulation*. Different types of hair may be distinguished: **lanugo hair** (downy or woolly hair) appears during fetal life and is present on the neonate until 6 months of age. It is short, thin, virtually colorless, and rooted in the dermis. Lanugo hair is replaced by an intermediate coat of hair (**woolly or vellus hair**), which starts to be replaced by terminal hair at puberty. **Terminal hairs** are longer, coarser, pigmented, and grouped together; they are rooted in the upper part of the subcutaneous layer. Terminal hairs develop in the axillary, pubic, and chest regions, and on the face (brows, lashes, and beard). The palms of the hands, soles of the feet, and portions of the external genitalia are devoid of hair.

Terminal hairs are positioned at an angle to the skin surface (hairline, whorls) within the cylindrical **root sheath**. Opening into the root sheath is the *sebaceous gland* (**A–D1**). Above the level of the opening of the sebaceous gland, the upper part of the hair follicle is known as the **infundibulum**; below the level of the sebaceous duct, the smooth **arrector pili muscle** (**A–D2**) has its origin. Passing beneath the epidermis, the arrector pili muscles contract in response to cold or psychological stress such as alarm or fear, causing the hair to stand upright (hair-raising, goosebumps).

Microanatomy. The hair can be divided into the root (**A3**) and the part protruding above the skin, or shaft (**A–D4**). The **hair root** rests on top of the *hair bulb* (**A5**) located above the connective tissue *hair papilla* (**A6**), a conical projection extending upward from the dermis. The *bulb, papilla,* and *surrounding connective tissue* comprise the **hair follicle**. The **hair shaft** is the fully keratinized portion of the hair. A hard *cortex* makes up most of the shaft and is composed of a shinglelike arrangement of overlapping keratinized cells, as well as keratin filaments that extend parallel to the hair axis, forming a tube surrounding the *medulla*. The shape and organization of the horny cells varies individually.

Hair development. Hair develops from a circumscribed invagination of epithelium (**A–D7**) that undergoes a process of **modified keratinization**. The hair is the keratinized tip, the epithelial root sheath (**A8**) is the epidermal funnel, and the connective tissue root sheath (**A9**) (hair follicle) its "dermal papilla." Hairs grow from cells in the hair bulb and are nourished by the papilla. If the matrix is destroyed, hair cannot regrow.

Hair color. The color of the hair is produced by **melanin deposits**. Melanin is synthesized by **matrix melanocytes**, which originate from the neural crest, and transferred to the cells of the hair bulb. Graying occurs as pigmentation decreases, melanin production ends, and the melanocytes die. There are no melanocytes in the hair bulb of white hair. The presence of air bubbles in the medulla also leads to hair whitening. In albinos, melanocytes fail to produce pigment, as a result of an enzyme deficiency.

Hair growth cycle. The lifespan of the hair depends on the type and its location on the body. Hair lives from a few weeks to several (3–5) years; eyelash and eyebrow hairs live for 100–150 days. Hair growth is cyclical. Growth (0.3–0.4 mm daily, **anagen phase**) is followed by regression (**catagen phase**) and a resting state (**telogen phase**), after which the hair falls out. About 80% of the hair follicles on the body are in the growth phase and about 15–20% in the resting phase. Some 50–100 hairs are lost each day. The matrix becomes inactive, the melanocytes temporarily cease activity, and the epithelial hair bulb (**B–D10**) detaches from the connective tissue papilla and is pushed outside of the body (**B–D**), along with the thickened, clublike lower end, hence the term *club hair* (**D11**). The remaining cells on the elongated papilla (**C12**) give rise to a new bulb (**D13**), from which a new hair will grow.

Hair growth pattern (**E**). Patterns of hair growth are influenced by hormones. **Androgens** stimulate the growth of facial and pubic hair. In men, a rhombic pattern of pubic hair growth up to the level of the navel is typical; hair also usually grows on the inner thighs, chest, and face. **Estrogens** lengthen the anagen phase, resulting in thicker hair. In women, pubic hair growth is typically in the shape of a triangle and there is less terminal hair growth on the trunk.

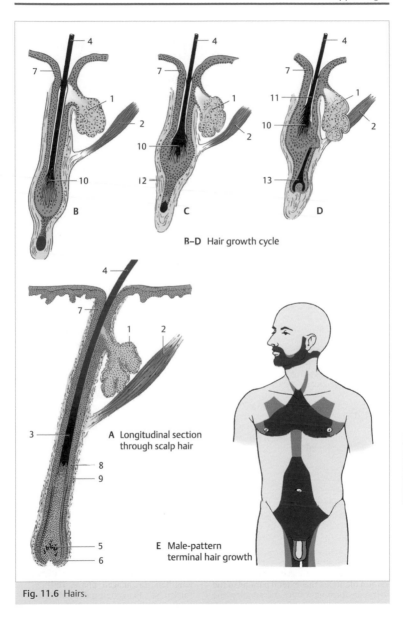

B–D Hair growth cycle

A Longitudinal section through scalp hair

E Male-pattern terminal hair growth

Fig. 11.6 Hairs.

The Integument

Nails

The **nails** also develop from the epidermis. They serve to protect the phalanges of the fingers and toes, and also aid tactile perception by providing a counter-force for tactile-pad pressure, for example, on the finger pads (**C12**). Loss of a fingernail results in decreased touch perception in the distal phalanx.

Structure. The nails are translucent, curved **keratin plates** (**BC1**) about 0.5-mm thick. They are composed of layers of polygonal, *flattened cornified cells*, which overlap like shingles and are reinforced by three layers of crossing *tonofibrils*. The nail lies on a nail bed (**BC2**) and hyponychium (**B3**) (see below). At its proximal end, it is surrounded by the **nail wall** (**BC4**), which forms the approximately 0.5-cm deep **sinus unguis** near the **nail root** (**B5**). Deep in the sinus unguis is the nail matrix (**B6**), the anterior boundary of which forms the white area known as the lunule (**A7**). Growing from the free margin of the nail wall (**BC4**) is a thin layer of epithelium called the eponychium (**C8**), which grows onto the surface of the nail and is pushed back during a manicure. The lateral border of the nail is formed by the **nail** groove (**C9**). The proximal **nail groove** is continuous distally with the **cuticle**.

Nail bed and hyponychium (**BC2**). The nail bed is produced by the **nail matrix** (**B6**), a proximal area of epithelial tissue located under the nail root (**B5**). The nail grows 0.5–1.0 mm weekly. Distal to the **lunule** (**A7**), the nail bed is continuous with the hyponychium (**AB3**) and consists of only a *germinative layer*, on which the nail is pushed distalward. There is a sharp boundary dividing the nail bed from the nail, which serves as the horny layer. The papillae consist of *narrow longitudinal ridges* that interdigitate with the respective dermal ridges. The dermis is connected with the periosteum of the distal phalanges of the fingers (**C10**) by *strong retinacula*.

The *capillary loops* in the dermal ridges give the nail its pink appearance. At its distal end, the hyponychium is continuous with the **onychodermal band** (**B11**).

> **Clinical note:** Nails can exhibit important changes in size, surface, and color that may provide important diagnostic clues. Damage to the nail matrix often results in permanent nail changes. If the matrix is completely destroyed, the nail will not regrow. Longitudinal striation often appears in the nail plate of elderly persons, sometimes with a shingled surface. The nails are abnormally brittle, cracking and splitting at their free edge (onychorrhexis).

Skin as a Sensory Organ— Organs of Somatovisceral Sensation

All skin layers are richly innervated. Part of the nerve supply is provided by **autonomic nerves**, which pass to the glands, smooth muscle cells, and vessels, but most of the nerves supplying the skin are **sensory nerves**. The sensory nerves make the skin a critically important sensory organ in humans, in terms of **touch**, **temperature**, **pain**, and **vibration** perception. The distribution in the skin of sensory qualities as well as sensory nerves varies by site on the body. **Encapsulated nerve** endings, which occur in the form of various structures (organs of somatovisceral sensation), are connected with diverse sensory qualities. Mechanoreceptors include the following: **Ruffini corpuscles** (pressure sensors) in the dermis: **Messner corpuscles** (**D1**), which detect touch and are particularly numerous in the fingertips; and **Vater-Pacini corpuscles** (**D2**) (vibration), found especially in subcutaneous tissue (**D3**). The diagram (**D**) on the facing page gives an overview of innervation of the skin. **Muscle spindles** and **Golgi tendon organs** are mechanoreceptors of the musculoskeletal system (a detailed description can be found in Vol. 3).

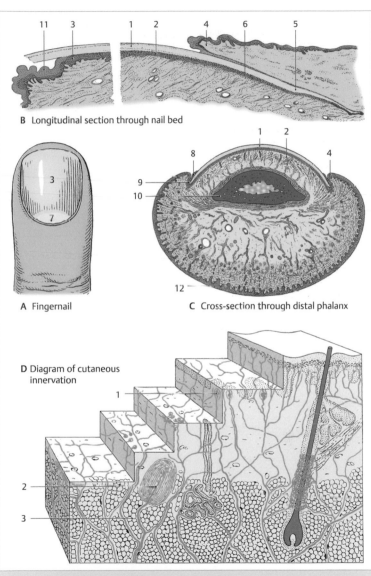

B Longitudinal section through nail bed

A Fingernail

C Cross-section through distal phalanx

D Diagram of cutaneous innervation

Fig. 11.7 Nails and sensory organs of the skin.

The Integument

11.3 Breast and Mammary Glands

The **breasts and mammary glands** are epithelial derivatives containing a connective tissue stroma; the glandular tissue derives from apocrine primordia. Breast development. In both sexes, near the end of the 1st embryonic month a bandlike condensation of epithelium called the **mammary streak** forms on either side of the trunk between the branchial arch region and tail. During week 6 of embryonic life, the mammary streak develops into the **mammary ridge** between the sites where the limbs will develop. Groups of apocrine glands begin forming within the mammary ridge. During the 3rd gestational month, the mammary ridge regresses. The remnant located over the fourth intercostal space is known as the **mammary hillocks**. The **anlage of the definitive mammary gland** is composed of about 15–20 epithelial-lined ductules with terminal end buds, which later give rise to the parenchyma of the gland.

In **neonates** of both sexes, the mammary glands develop under the influence of maternal placental hormones, forming visible and palpable eminences on the surface of the body. In the initial postnatal days, they secrete *colostral milk* (*witch's milk*). During **childhood**, breast development is gradual; its growth accelerates with the onset of puberty, and breast buds develop. Development of the female breast during **puberty** is influenced by estrogen, prolactin, and growth hormone, and exhibits great variance in terms of size, shape, and consistency. The amount of adipose tissue is another important determinant. During **pregnancy** there is strong growth of the mammary glands, and toward the end of gestation, the glands, begin to produce milk. When **lactation ceases** (**ablactation**), the mammary glands revert to the inactive state, and there is increased formation of connective tissue.

Gross Anatomy

Breast (**B**). The form of the mature female breasts may be hemispherical, or disk- or cone-shaped. The breasts lie on either side of the body on the *pectoral fascia* between the third to seventh ribs, midway between the sternum and axillae. Between the breast and the fascia is a thin layer of *interstitial connective tissue* that permits movement of the breast against the anterior wall of the thorax (**D**). Each breast is fixed in position by collagen fiber bundles known as the **suspensory ligaments of the breast** (Cooper ligaments) between the dermis and connective tissue system of the breast. The position of the breast changes only minimally with postural changes. An **axial process** or **axillary tail** frequently projects above the margin of the pectoral muscles into the axilla (**C**). The space (cleavage) between the two breasts is called the **intermammary cleft**.

Nipple. The **nipple** (**A1**) is usually located in the center of the breast, measuring 10–12 mm in diameter and pointing slightly superiorly and laterally. It is surrounded by the **areola** (**A2**). The wrinkled skin of the nipple and areola is usually darker in color than its surroundings, especially in women who have given birth. The tip of the nipple is unpigmented. In the periphery of the areola are 10–15 usually circularly arranged nodular elevations called the **areolar glands** (Montgomery tubercles) (**A3**). They contain *apocrine* and *eccrine sweat glands*, as well as (*holocrine*) *sebaceous glands*, which increase their secretion during lactation to keep the nipple moist for the nursing infant's lips.

Variants. **Flat** or **inverted nipples** can impair breastfeeding. **Accessory breasts** (polymastia) (**E**) may be present, with variably developed mammary glands. The presence of additional nipples only is known as **polythelia**.

Male breast. The anlage of the **male breast** corresponds to that in the female, but remains underdeveloped. The glandular body is about 1.5-cm wide and 0.5-cm thick and contains only isolated branching epithelial ducts. During puberty, a temporary increase in development may occur, resulting in enlargement (**gynecomastia**).

Clinical note: Abnormal breast (or nipple) mobility or asymmetry may be due to disease (cancer) or a disorder of the musculoskeletal system. The **frequency of breast cancer** by quadrant is shown in (**C**). For information on lymphatic supply of the breasts, see p. 82.

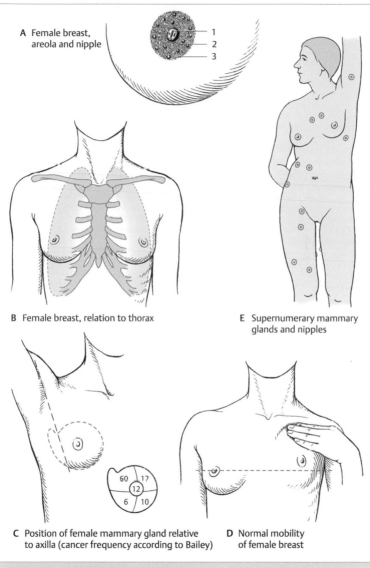

A Female breast, areola and nipple

1
2
3

B Female breast, relation to thorax

E Supernumerary mammary glands and nipples

C Position of female mammary gland relative to axilla (cancer frequency according to Bailey)

60 17
12
6   10

D Normal mobility of female breast

Fig. 11.8 Macroscopic structure of the breast.

The Integument

Microscopic Structure and Function of the Female Breast

The breast consists of the **mammary gland** (**A1**), composed of the conical *lobes of the mammary gland* and **adipose tissue** (**A2**), which is surrounded and partitioned by connective tissue. The size of the breast depends mainly on the amount of adipose tissue; in smaller breasts, the proportion of glandular tissue is greater, while in larger breasts the amount of adipose tissue predominates. The firmness of the breast is determined by the tissue characteristics of the connective tissue and the fullness of the adipose tissue chambers.

Involution of glandular tissue begins between the ages of 35 and 45. The lobes are broken down and replaced by adipose tissue, and the suspensory ligaments of the breast (**A3**) become less taut. As aging progresses, the amount of adipose tissue also decreases.

A4 Pectoral fascia, **A5** Pectoralis major, **D** Radiograph of mammary ducts (mammogram)

Nonlactating mammary gland (**B**). The architecture of the nonlactating mammary gland in the sexually mature woman is characterized by an irregular arrangement of **15–20 individual, branching tubular glands**, whose coiled terminal ends form the lobes of the mammary gland. Each lobe contains a **collecting duct** (**A–C6**) consisting of a branching epithelial tubule with a small lumen. Its branches, the **lactiferous ducts** (**AB7**), are separated by connective tissue (**BC8**). They are lined by a bilayered-to-multilayered epithelium and have budlike terminal expansions. Beneath the nipple, at the level of its base, the lactiferous ducts expand to form the 1–2-mm wide spindle-shaped **lactiferous sinuses** (**A9**), which can widen during lactation to 8 mm. The sinuses are continuous with narrow **excretory ducts**, which open on the surface of the breast. The lactiferous ducts, branching tubules, and terminal bud ends are embedded in a firm **connective tissue stroma** (**BC8**) that is somewhat less dense in the immediate vicinity of these structures, where it is also known as *mantle connective tissue* (**B10**). During the ovarian cycle, the breast increases in

size by 15–45 mL as a result of sprouting of the lactiferous ducts.

Lactating mammary gland (**C**). During week 5 or 6 of pregnancy, the lactiferous ducts begin to sprout under the influence of estrogen. At the same time, new terminal buds develop, and the connective tissue is pushed aside. Around the middle of the gestational period, the lactiferous ducts are canalized; the lateral and terminal buds differentiate under the influence of prolactin and progesterone to form alveoli (**C11**), which are lined by a single layer of cuboidal-to-columnar epithelium. As parenchymal tissue increases, the amount of connective and adipose tissue decreases. The breasts become enlarged, and their consistency changes. In the 9th gestational month, prolactin induces the production of **colostrum** (first milk), containing lipid droplets, lymphocytes, phagocytes, and cellular debris. About 3 days postpartum, the milk "comes in" (**transitional milk**). It contains lipid droplets, proteins, lactose, ions, and antibodies. Secretion of **mature breast milk** begins on about day 14 postpartum.

At the **height of lactation**, the now columnar glandular cells form **lipid droplets**, which are secreted with a membranous covering into the alveolar lumen (*apocrine secretion*). At the same time, there is a vigorous production of proteins, especially **casein**. The alveoli and lactiferous ducts are surrounded by *myoepithelial cells*, which contract under the influence of oxytocin, aiding milk ejection. Secretion of prolactin and oxytocin is maintained by tactile stimulation of the nipple (*neurohormonal reflex*). Milk stasis occurs after **cessation of suckling**; the alveoli become distended and tear, and milk production ebbs. Phagocytes remove the remaining secretory cells and the glandular tissue involutes.

Beneath the nipple and areola (see p. 436) is a system of *annular* and *radiating smooth muscle cells* (**A12**), which are anchored by strong *elastic fibers* in the skin, to the lactiferous ducts and veins. This **elastic, fibromuscular system** causes **erection of the nipple** by contracting the areola while expanding the veins and lactiferous ducts. The suckling infant uses alternating pressure from the lips and jaw to empty the sinuses, which then fill again.

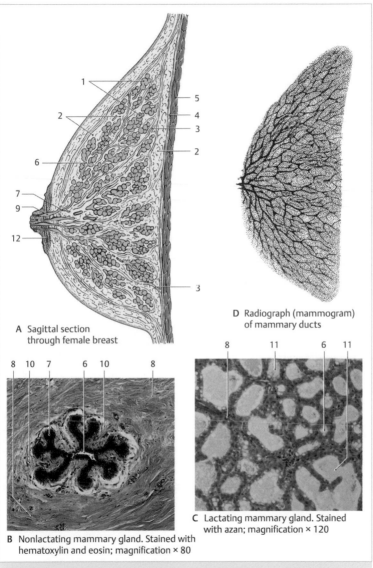

A Sagittal section through female breast

D Radiograph (mammogram) of mammary ducts

B Nonlactating mammary gland. Stained with hematoxylin and eosin; magnification × 80

C Lactating mammary gland. Stained with azan; magnification × 120

Fig. 11.9 Microscopic structure and function of the female breast and mammary gland.

References

Anatomy

Appell HJ, Stang-Voss C. Funktionelle Anatomie. 4.Aufl. Heidelberg: Springer 2008

Aumüller G. Duale Reihe Anatomie. 4. Aufl. Stuttgart, New York: Thieme 2017

Benninghoff A. Anatomie. Makroskopische Anatomie, Histologie, Embryologie, Zellbiologie. Hrsg. von Drenckhahn D. München, Jena: Urban & Fischer. Bd. 1. Zelle, Gewebe, Entwicklung, Skelett- und Muskelsystem, Atemsystem, Verdauungssystem, Harn- und Genitalsystem. 17. Aufl. 2008; Bd. 2. Herz-Kreislauf-System, Lymphatisches System, Endokrine Drüsen System, Nervensystem, Sinnesorgane, Haut. 16. Aufl. 2004

Bommas-Ebert U, Teubner P, Voß R. Kurzlehrbuch Anatomie und Embryologie. 3. Aufl. Stuttgart, New York: Thieme 2011

Buchmann P. Lehrbuch der Proktologie. 4. Aufl. Bern, Göttingen, Toronto, Seattle: Hans Huber 2002

Caspar W. Medizinische Terminologie. 2. Aufl. Stuttgart, New York: Thieme 2007

Dauber W. Pocket Atlas of Human Anatomy. 5th ed. Stuttgart, New York: Thieme 2007

Drake LR, Vogel W, Mitchell AWM. Gray's Anatomie für Studenten mit Student Consult-Zugang. Übersetzt und herausgegeben von Friedrich Paulsen. Jena, München: Elsevier-Urban & Fischer 2007

Faller A. Die Fachwörter der Anatomie, Histologie und Embryologie, Ableitung und Aussprache. 29. Aufl. München: Bergmann 1978

Faller A, Schünke M. Der Körper des Menschen. Einführung in Bau und Funktion. 17. Aufl. Stuttgart, New York: Thieme 2016

Frick H, Leonhardt H, Starck D. Allgemeine Anatomie. Spezielle Anatomie I, Extremitäten, Rumpfwand, Kopf, Hals. Taschenlehrbuch der gesamten Anatomie, Bd. I. 4. Aufl. Stuttgart, New York: Thieme 1992

Frick H, Leonhardt H, Starck D. Spezielle Anatomie II. Eingeweide, Nervensystem, Systematik der Muskeln und Leitungsbahnen. Taschenlehrbuch der gesamten Anatomie, Bd. II 4. Aufl. Stuttgart, New York: Thieme 1992

Fritsch H, Lienemann A, Brenner E, Ludwikowski B. Clinical Anatomy of the Pelvic Floor. In: Advances in Anatomy, Embryology and Cell Biology. Vol. 175. Berlin, Heidelberg, New York, Hong Kong, London, Milan, Paris, Tokyo: Springer 2004

Gertz SD. Basiswissen Neuroanatomie. Leicht verständlich, knapp, klinikbezogen. Übersetzung und Bearbeitung von Schünke M und Schünke G. 4. Aufl. Stuttgart, New York: Thieme 2003

Gilroy A. Atlas of Anatomy. 2nd ed. Stuttgart, New York: Thieme 2012

Hansen JT, Lambert DR. Netters Klinische Anatomie. Stuttgart, New York: Thieme 2006

Henne-Bruns D. Duale Reihe Chirurgie. 4. Aufl. Stuttgart, New York: Thieme 2012

Kahle W, Frotscher M, Schmitz F. Color Atlas and Textbook of Human Anatomy. Vol. 3: Nervous System and Sensory Organs. 8th ed. Stuttgart, New York: Thieme 2022

Köpf-Maier P. Wolf-Heideggers Anatomie des Menschen. Bd. 1: Allgemeine Anatomie, Rumpfwand, obere und untere Extremität. Bd. 2: Kopf und Hals, Brust, Bauch, Becken, ZNS, Auge, Ohr. 6. Aufl. Basel: Karger 2004

Lippert H. Lehrbuch Anatomie. 8. Aufl. München, Jena: Elsevier-Urban & Fischer 2011

Moses KP, Banks JC, Nava PB, Petersen D. Atlas of Clinical Gross Anatomy. Elsevier Mosby 2005

Netter FH. Atlas der Anatomie. 4. Aufl. München: Elsevier 2008

Netter FH. Atlas der Anatomie. 5. Aufl. München: Elsevier 2011

Platzer W, Shiozawa-Bayer T. Color Atlas and Textbook of Human Anatomy. Vol. 1:

Locomotor System. 8th ed. Stuttgart, New York: Thieme 2022

Rauber/Kopsch. Anatomie des Menschen. Lehrbuch und Atlas. Hrsg. von Leonhardt H, Tillmann B, Töndury G, Zilles K. Band I: Bewegungsapparat. Hrsg. und bearbeitet von Tillmann B. 3. Aufl. Stuttgart, New York: Thieme 2003; Band II. Innere Organe. Hrsg. von Leonhardt H. Stuttgart, New York: Thieme 1987; Band III: Nervensystem und Sinnesorgane. Hrsg. und bearbeitet von Krisch B, Kubik S, Lange W, Leonhardt H, Leuenberger P, Töndury G und Zilles K. Stuttgart, New York: Thieme 1987; Band IV: Topographie der Organsysteme Systematik der Leitungsbahnen. Hrsg. und bearbeitet von Leonhardt H, Tillmann B, Zilles K. Stuttgart, New York: Thieme 1988

Rohen J, Lütjen-Drecoll, E. Funktionelle Anatomie des Menschen. 11. Aufl. Stuttgart, New York: Schattauer2006

Rohen J. Topographische Anatomie des Menschen. 10. Aufl. Stuttgart, New York: Schattauer; 2000, Nachdruck 2008

Schiebler TH, Korf HW Anatomie. 10. Aufl. Berlin, Heidelberg: Steinkopff/Springer 2007

Schuenke M, Schulte E, Schumacher U. Thieme Atlas of Anatomy. General Anatomy and Musculoskeletal System. Stuttgart, New York: Thieme 2020

Schuenke M, Schulte E, Schumacher U, Ross, L, Lamperti E. Thieme Atlas of Anatomy. Head and Neuroanatomy. Stuttgart, New York: Thieme 2010

Schulze P, Donalies C. Anatomisches Wörterbuch. Lateinisch-Deutsch/Deutsch-Lateinisch. 8. Aufl. Stuttgart, New York: Thieme 2008

Schumacher GH, Aumüller G. Topographische Anatomie des Menschen. 7. Aufl. München, Jena: Elsevier - Urban & Fischer 2004

Sobotta J. Anatomie des Menschen. Der komplette Atlas in einem Band. Hrsg. von Putz R, Pabst R. München, Jena: Elsevier-Urban & Fischer 2007

Standring S. Gray's Anatomy. 41st ed. Oxford: Elsevier Ltd. 2015

Terminologia Anatomica. International Anatomical Terminology. Ed. by the Federative Committee of Anatomical Terminology (FCAT). 2nd ed. Stuttgart, New York: Thieme 2011

Thiel W. Photographischer Atlas der Praktischen Anatomie. 2. Aufl. Berlin, Heidelberg, New York, Hong Kong, London, Mailand, Paris, Tokyo: Springer 2006

Tillmann B. Atlas der Anatomie mit Muskeltrainer. 2. Aufl. Berlin, Heidelberg: Springer 2009

Tillmann B. Farbatlas der Anatomie Zahnmedizin – Humanmedizin. Kopf, Hals, Rumpf. Stuttgart, New York: Thieme 1997

Trepel M. Neuroanatomie mit Student Consult-Zugang. Struktur und Funktion. 7. Aufl. Jena, München: Elsevier – Urban & Fischer 2017

Ulfig N. Kurzlehrbuch Neuroanatomie. 1. Aufl. Stuttgart, New York: Thieme 2008

Waldeyer A. Anatomie des Menschen. Hrsg. von Anderhuber F, Pera F, Streicher J. 19. Aufl. Berlin, New York: Walter de Gruyter 2012

Whitaker RH, Borley NR. Anatomickompass. Taschenatlas der anatomischen Leitungsbahnen. 2. Aufl. Stuttgart, New York: Thieme 2003

Histology, Cell Biology, and Microscopic Anatomy

Alberts B, Johnson A, Lewis J, Raff M, Roberts K, Walter P. Hrsg. u. übers. von Schäfer U. Molekularbiologie der Zelle. 5. Aufl. Weinheim: Wiley-VCH 2011

Bucher O, Wartenberg H. Cytologie, Histologie und mikroskopische Anatomie des Menschen. 12. Aufl. Bern: Huber 1997

Junqueira LC, Carneiro J, Hrsg. Von Gratzl M: Histologie. 6. Aufl. Berlin, Heidelberg: Springer 2005

Kuehnel W. Color Atlas of Cytology, Histology, and Microscopic Anatomy. 4th ed. Stuttgart, New York: Thieme 2003

Lüllmann-Rauch R. Taschenlehrbuch Histologie. 5. Aufl. Stuttgart, New York: Thieme 2015

Michna H. The Human Macrophage System: Activity and Functional Morphology. In: Bibliotheca Anatomica. Ed. W. Lierse. Basel: Karger 1988

Rohen J, Lütjen-Drecoll E. Funktionelle Histologie. 4. Aufl. Stuttgart, New York: Schattauer 2000

Sobotta J. Atlas Histologie. Zytologie, Histologie und Mikroskopische Anatomie. Hrsg. von Welsch U. 7. Aufl. München, Jena: Urban & Fischer 2005

Sobotta J. Lehrbuch Histologie. Hrsg. von Welsch U. München, 3. Aufl. Jena: Elsevier-Urban & Fischer 2010

Ulfig N. Kurzlehrbuch Histologie. 4. Aufl. Stuttgart, New York: Thieme 2015

Embryology, Developmental Biology, and Pediatrics

Baraitser M, Winter RM. Fehlbildungssyndrome. 2. Aufl. Bern, Göttingen, Toronto, Seattle: Hans Huber 2001

Christ B, Brand-Saberi B. Molekulare Grundlagen der Embryonalentwicklung. Berlin: Lehmanns Media 2004

Christ B, Wachtler F. Medizinische Embryologie. Molekulargenetik-Morphologie-Klinik. Wiesbaden: Ullstein Medical 1998

Drews U. Color Atlas of Embryology. Stuttgart, New York: Thieme 1996

Hinrichsen KV (Hrsg.). Humanembryologie. Lehrbuch und Atlas der vorgeburtlichen Entwicklung des Menschen. Berlin, Heidelberg: Springer 1990

Moore KL, Persaud TVN, Viebahn C. Embryologie. München, Jena: Elsevier-Urban & Fischer 2007

Niessen KH. Pädiatrie. 6. Aufl. Stuttgart, New York: Thieme 2001

O'Rahilly R, Müller F, Rager G. Embryologie und Teratologie des Menschen. Bern, Göttingen, Toronto, Seattle: Huber 2002

Sadler TW. Medizinische Embryologie. 11. Aufl. Stuttgart, New York: Thieme 2008

Ulfig N, Brand-Saberi B. Kurzlehrbuch Embryologie. 3. Aufl. Stuttgart, New York: Thieme 2017

Imaging Procedures

Fleckenstein P, Tranum-Jensen J. Röntgenanatomie. Normalbefunde in Röntgen, CT, MRT, Ultraschall und Szintigraphie. München, Jena: Elsevier- Urban & Fischer 2004

Kopp H, Ludwig M. Checkliste Doppler- und Duplexsonografie. Checklisten der aktuellen Medizin. 4. Aufl. Stuttgart, New York: Thieme 2012

Koritke JG, Sick H. Atlas anatomischer Schnittbilder des Menschen. München: Urban & Schwarzenberg 1982

Moeller TB, Reif E. Normal Findings in Radiography. Stuttgart, New York: Thieme 2000

Moeller TB, Reif E. Pocket Atlas of Sectional Anatomy. 4th ed. Vol. 2. Thorax, Heart, Abdomen, and Pelvis. Stuttgart, New York: Thieme 2013

Oestmann JW. Radiologie. Vom Fall zur Diagnose. 2. Aufl. Stuttgart, New York: Thieme 2005

Weiser HF, Birth M (Hrsg.). Viszeralchirurgische Sonographie. Lehrbuch und Atlas. Berlin, Heidelberg: Springer 2000

Cardiovascular System

Anderson RH, Becker AE. Anatomie des Herzens. Ein Farbatlas. Stuttgart, New York: Thieme 1982

Balletshofer B, Claussen C, Häring HU. Herz und Gefäße. Ein handlungsorientierter Leitfaden für Medizinstudenten. Tübinger Curriculum. Stuttgart, New York: Thieme 2006

Bargmann W, Doerr W. Das Herz des Menschen. Bd. I. Stuttgart, New York: Thieme 1963

Block B. Pol-Leitsymptome. Herz-Kreislauf -System. Stuttgart, New York: Thieme 2006

Földi M, Casley-Smith JR. Lymphangiology. Stuttgart: Schattauer 1983

Kubik S. Visceral lymphatic system. In: Viamonte (jr.) M, Rüttimann A. Atlas of Lymphography. Stuttgart, New York: Thieme 1980

Loose KE, van Dongen RJAM. Atlas of Angiography. Stuttgart, New York: Thieme 1976

Staubesand J. Funktionelle Morphologie der Arterien, Venen und arteriovenösen Anastomosen. In: Angiologie. Hrsg. von Heberer G, Rau G, Schoop W, begr. von Ratschow M. 2. Aufl. Stuttgart, New York: Thieme 1974

Tomanek RJ, Runyn RB. Formation of the Heart and its Regulation. Basel: Birkhäuser 2001

Respiratory System

Becker W. Ear, Nose, and Throat Diseases. 2nd ed. Stuttgart, New York: Thieme 1994

Crystal RG, West JB, Barnes PJ, Weibel ER (eds). The Lung. Scientific Foundations. 2 Vol. 2nd ed. Philadelphia: Lippincott Williams & Wilkins 1997

Lang J. Clinical Anatomy of the Nose, Nasal Cavity and Paranasal Sinuses. Stuttgart, New York: Thieme 1994

Muarray JF. Die normale Lunge. Grundlagen für Diagnose und Therapie von Lungenkrankheiten. Stuttgart, New York: Thieme 1978

Tillmann B, Wustrow I. Kehlkopf. In Berendes J, Link R, Zöllner F. Hals-Nasen-Ohren-Heilkunde in Praxis und Klinik (S. 1–101). 2. Aufl. Bd. IV/I. Stuttgart, New York: Thieme 1982

Digestive System

Berkovitz BKB, Boyde A, Frank RM, Höhling HJ, Moxham BJ, Nalbandian J, Tonge CH. Teeth. Handbook of Microscopic Anatomy (ed. by Oksche A, Vollrath L.). Vol. V/6. Berlin, Heidelberg: Springer 1989

Block B. Pol-Leitsymptome. Gastrointestinaltrakt. Leber, Pankreas und biliäres System. Stuttgart, New York: Thieme 2006

Krentz K. Endoskopie des oberen Verdauungstraktes. Atlas und Lehrbuch. 2. Aufl. Stuttgart, New York: Thieme 1982

Liebermann-Meffert D, White H. The Greater Omentum. Berlin, Heidelberg: Springer 1983

Motta P, Muto M, Fujita T. Die Leber: Rasterelektronenmikroskopischer Atlas. Stuttgart: Schattauer 1980

Schroeder HE. The Periodontium. Handbook of Microscopic Anatomy (ed. By Oksche A, Vollrath L). Vol. V/5. Berlin, Heidelberg: Springer 1986

Schroeder HE. Orale Strukturbiologie. Entwicklungsgeschichte, Struktur und Funktion normaler Hart- und Weichgewebe der Mundhöhle und des Kiefergelenks. 5. Aufl. Stuttgart, New York: Thieme 2000

Stelzner F. Die anorectalen Fisteln. 3. Aufl. Berlin, Heidelberg: Springer 1981

Urinary System

Gosling JA, Dixon JS, Humpherson JR. Funktionelle Anatomie der Nieren und ableitenden Harnwege. Ein Farbatlas. Stuttgart, New York: Thieme 1990

Inke G. Gross Structure of the Human Kidney. Advances of Morphological Cells Tissues, p. 71. New York: Liss AR 1981

Kuhlmann U. u.a. (Hrsg.). Nephrologie. Pathophysiologie-Klinik-Nierenersatzverfahren. 6. Aufl. Stuttgart, New York: Thieme 2015

Sökeland J, Rübben H. Taschenlehrbuch Urologie. 14. Aufl. Stuttgart, New York: Thieme 2007

Male Genital System

Aumüller G. Prostate gland and seminal vesicles. In: Oksche A. Vollrath L. Handbuch der mikroskopischen Anatomie des Menschen. Bd. 7/6. Berlin, Heidelberg: Springer 1979

Holstein AF, Rossen-Runge EC. Atlas of Human Spermatogenesis. Berlin: Grosse 1981

Nieschlag E, Bartlett J. Testes. In Bettendorf G, Breckwoldt M (Hrsg.): Reproduktionsmedizin. S. 100–115. Stuttgart: Fischer 1989

Schirren C. Praktische Andrologie, 2. Aufl. Berlin: Schering 1982

Wartenberg H. Differentiation and development of the testes. In: Burger H, de Kretser D (eds.): The Testis. New York: Raven Press 1981

Female Genital System

Benirschke K, Kaufmann P, Baergen RN. Pathology of the Human Placenta. 5th ed. New York: Springer 2006

Breckwoldt M, Kaufmann M, Pfleiderer A. Gynäkologie und Geburtshilfe. 5. Aufl. Stuttgart, New York: Thieme 2007

Döring GK. Empfängnisverhütung. Ein Leitfaden für Ärzte und Studenten. 12. Aufl. Stuttgart, New York: Thieme 1990

Frangenheim H, Lindemann H-J. Die Laparoskopie in der Gynäkologie, Chirurgie und Pädiatrie. 3. Aufl. Stuttgart, New York: Thieme 1977

Horstmann E, Stegner H-E. Tube, Vagina und äußere weibliche Geschlechtsorgane. In: Handbuch der mikroskopischen Anatomie des Menschen. Erg. zu Bd.VII/1. Hrsg. von Bargmann W. Berlin, Heidelberg: Springer 1966

Kaufmann P. Plazentation und Plazenta. In: Hinrichsen KV (Hrsg.): Humanembryologie. Berlin, Heidelberg, New York: Springer 1991

Krebs D, Schneider HPG. Reproduktion, Infertilität, Sterilität. München, Wien, Baltimore: Urban & Fischer 1998

Künzel W. Schwangerschaft I. In: Bender HG, Diedrich K, Künzel W, Klinik der Frauenheilkunde und Geburtshilfe, Band 4. 4. Aufl. München, Jena: Urban & Fischer 2002

Künzel W. Schwangerschaft II. In: Bender HG, Diedrich K, Künzel W, Klinik der Frauenheilkunde und Geburtshilfe, Band 5. 4. Aufl. München, Jena: Urban & Fischer 2002

Künzel W. Geburt I. In: Bender HG, Diedrich K, Künzel W, Klinik der Frauenheilkunde und Geburtshilfe, Band 6. 4. Aufl. München, Jena: Urban & Fischer 2002

Künzel W, Wulf KH. Geburt II. In: Wulf KH, Schmidt-Matthiessen H, Klinik der Frauenheilkunde und Geburtshilfe, Band 7. 4. Aufl. München, Jena: Urban & Fischer 2002

Netter FH. NETTERs Gynäkologie. Stuttgart, New York: Thieme 2005

Weyerstahl T, Stauber M. Duale Reihe Gynäkologie und Geburtshilfe. 4. Aufl. Stuttgart, New York: Thieme 2013

Endocrine System

Allolio B, Schulte HM. Praktische Endokrinologie. 2. Aufl. München. Elsevier-Urban & Fischer 2010

Bachmann R. Die Nebenniere. In: Handbuch der mikroskopischen Anatomie des Menschen, Bd. VI/5, hrsg. von Bargmann W. Berlin, Heidelberg: Springer 1954

Bargmann W. Die Schilddrüse. In: v. Möllendorff W. Handbuch der mikroskopischen Anatomie des Menschen, Bd. VI/2. Berlin, Heidelberg: Springer 1939 (S. 2-136)

Bargmann W. Die Epithelkörperchen. In: v. Möllendorff W. Handbuch der mikroskopischen Anatomie des Menschen, Bd. VI/2. Berlin, Heidelberg: Springer 1939 (S. 137-196)

Bargmann W. Die Langerhansschen Inseln des Pankreas. In v. Möllendorff W. Handbuch der mikroskopischen Anatomie des Menschen, Bd. VI/ 2. Berlin, Heidelberg: Springer 1939 (S. 197-288)

Bargmann W. Über die neurosekretorische Verknüpfung von Hypothalamus und Neurohypophyse. Z. Zellforsch. 34: 610-634 (1949)

Bargmann W. Das Zwischenhirn-Hypophysensystem. Berlin, Heidelberg: Springer 1964

Bargmann W. Die funktionelle Morphologie des endokrinen Regulationssystems. In: Altmann HW, Büchner F, Cottier H u. Mitarb. Handbuch der allgemeinen Pathologie, Bd. VIII/1. Berlin, Heidelberg: Springer 1971 (S. 1-106)

Bargmann W., Scharrer B. Aspects of Neuroendocrinology. Berlin, Heidelberg: Springer 1970

Bloom SR, Polak JM. Gut Hormones, 2nd ed. Edinburgh: Churchill-Livingstone 1981

Böck P. The Paraganglia. In Oksche A, Vollrath L. Handbuch der mikroskopischen Anatomie des Menschen, Bd. VII/8. Berlin, Heidelberg: Springer 1973

Costa E, Trabucchi M. Regulatory Peptides, from Molecular Biology to Function. New York: Raven Press 1982

Coupland RE, Forssmann WG. Peripheral Neuroendocrine Interaction. Berlin, Heidelberg: Springer 1978

Coupland RE, Fujita T. Chromaffin, Enterochromaffin and Related Cells. Amsterdam: Elsevier 1976

Cross BA, Leng G. The Neurohypophysis: Structure, Function and Control. Progr. Brain Res. 60, 1983

Diedrich K. Endokrinologie und Reproduktionsmedizin I. In: Wulf K-H und Schmidt-Matthiesen H, Klinik der Frauenheilkunde und Geburtshilfe, Band 1. 4. Aufl. München, Jena: Urban & Fischer 2001

Diedrich K. Endokrinologie und Reproduktionsmedizin II. In: Wulff K-H und Schmidt-Matthiesen H, Klinik der Frauenheilkunde und Geburtshilfe, Band 2. 4. Aufl. München, Jena: Urban & Fischer 2003

Felig Ph, Frohman LA. Endocrinology and Metabolism, 4th ed. New York: McGraw-Hill 2001

Fujita T. Endocrine Gut and Pancreas. Amsterdam: Elsevier 1976

Fujita T. Concept of paraneurons. Arch. Histol. Jap. 40, (Suppl.): 1-12(1977)

Fuxe K, Hökfelt T, Luft R. Central Regulation of the Endocrine System. New York: Plenum Press 1979

Gardeur DG, Shoback D. Greenspan's Basic & Clinical Endocrinology, 10th ed. New York: McGraw-Hill Education 2017

Guillemin R. Control of adenohypophysial functions by peptides of the central nervous system. Harvey Lect. 71: 71-131 (1978)

Gupta D. Endokrinologie der Kindheit und Adoleszenz. Stuttgart: Thieme 1997

Hesch RD. Endokrinologie. Teil A Grundlagen. München, Wien, Baltimore: Urban & Schwarzenberg 1989

Hesch RD. Endokrinologie. Teil B Krankheitsbilder. München, Wien, Baltimore: Urban & Schwarzenberg 1989

Kalimi MY, Hubbard JR. Peptide Hormone Receptors. Berlin: de Gruyter 1987

Krieger DT, Liotta AS, Brownstein MJ, Zimmermann EA. ACTH, β-Lipotropin, and related peptides in brain, pituitary, and blood. Recent Progr. Horm. Res. 36: 277-344 (1980)

Krisch B. Immunocytochemistry of neuroendocrine systems (vasopressin, somatostatin, luliberin). Progr. Histochem. Cytochem. 13/2: 1-167 (1980)

Krisch B. Ultrastructure of regulatory neuroendocrine neurons and functionally related structures. In Ganten D, Pfaff D: Morphology of Hypothalamus and its Connections. Current Topics in Neuroendocrinology, Vol. 7. Berlin, Heidelberg: Springer 1986 (pp. 251-290)

Marischler C. BASICS Endokrinologie. München: Elsevier-Urban & Fischer 2007

Neville AM, O'Hare MJ. The Human Adrenal Cortex. Berlin, Heidelberg: Springer 1982

Oksche A, Pévet P. The Pineal Organ: Photobiology, Biochronometry, Endocrinology. Developments in Endocrinology, vol. XIV. Amsterdam: Elsevier 1981

Pearse AGE. The diffuse neuroendocrine system and the APUD concept: related "endocrine" peptides in brain, intestine, pituitary, placenta and anuran cutaneous glands. Med. Biol. 55: 115-125 (1977)

Polak JM. Regulatory Peptides. Basel: Birkhäuser 1989

Reinboth R. Vergleichende Endokrinologie. Stuttgart, New York: Thieme 1989

Scharrer E, Korf HW, Hartwig HG. Functional Morphology of Neuroendocrine Systems. Berlin, Heidelberg, New York, London, Paris, Tokyo: Springer 1987

Schulster D, Levitski A. Cellular Receptors for Hormones and Neurotransmitters. New York: Wiley 1980

Vollrath L. The pineal organ. In Oksche A, Vollrath L. Handbuch der mikroskopischen Anatomie des Menschen, Bd. VI/7. Berlin, Heidelberg: Springer 1981

Welsch U. Die Entwicklung der C-Zellen und des Follikelepithels der Säugerschilddrüse. Elektronenmikroskopische und histochemische Untersuchungen. Ergebn. Anat. Entwickl.-Gesch. 46:1-52 (1972)

Blood and Lymphatic System

Aiuti F, Wigzell H. Thymus, Thymic Hormones and Lymphocytes. London: Academic Press 1980

Begemann M. Praktische Hämatologie. Klinik, Therapie, Methodik. 11. Aufl. Stuttgart, New York: Thieme 1998

Bessis M. Living Blood Cells and their Ultrastructure. Berlin, Heidelberg: Springer 1973

Brücher H. Knochenmarkzytologie. Diagnostik und klinische Bedeutung. Stuttgart, New York: Thieme 1986

Dormann A, Luley C, Heer C. Laborwerte. 5. Aufl. München, Jena: Elsevier-Urban & Fischer 2009

Dörner K. Taschenlehrbuch Klinische Chemie und Hämatologie. 8. Aufl. Stuttgart, New York: Thieme 2013

Drößler K, Gemsa D. Wörterbuch der Immunologie. 3. Aufl. Heidelberg, Berlin: Spektrum Akademischer Verlag 2000

Eisen HN. Immunology, 3rd ed. New York: Harper & Row 1981

Frick P. Blut- und Knochenmarksmorphologie, Blutgerinnung. 19. Aufl. Stuttgart, New York: Thieme 2003

Haferlach T, Bacher U, Theml H, Diem H. Taschenatlas der Hämatologie, 6. Aufl. Stuttgart, New York: Thieme 2012

Ham AW, Axelrad AA, Cormack DH. Blood Cell Formation and the Cellular Basis of Immune Responses. Philadelphia: Lippincott 1979

Keller R. Immunologie und Immunpathologie, 4. Aufl. Stuttgart, New York: Thieme 1994

Kirchner H, Kruse A, Neustock P, Rink L. Cytokine and Interferone. Botenstoffe des Immunsystems. Heidelberg, Berlin, Oxford: Spektrum Akademischer Verlag 1993

Lennert K, Harms D. Die Milz/The Spleen. Berlin, Heidelberg: Springer 1970

Lennert K, Müller-Hermelink H-K. Lymphozyten und ihre Funktionsformen-Morphologie. Organisation und immunologische Bedeutung. Anat. Anz., Suppl. 138: 19-62(1975)

McDonald GA, Dodds TC, Cruickshank B. Atlas der Hämatologie, 3. Aufl. Stuttgart, New York: Thieme 1979

Müller-Hermelink HK. The Human Thymus, Histophysiology and Pathology. Current Topics of Pathology, Berlin, Heidelberg: Springer 1985

Müller-Hermelink HK, von Gaudecker B. Ontogenese des lympathischen Systems beim Menschen. Amat. Anz. Suppl. 74 (1980) 235-259

Noll S, Schaub-Kuhnen S. Praxis der Immunhistochemie. Hrsg. von Höfler H und Müller K-M. München, Jena: Urban & Fischer 2000

Queißer W. Das Knochenmark. Morphologie, Funktion, Diagnostik. Stuttgart, New York: Thieme 1978

Ruzicka F. Elektronenmikroskopische Hämatologie. Wien: Springer 1976

Staines N, Brostoff J, James K. Immunologisches Grundwissen. 3. Aufl. Heidelberg: Spektrum Akademischer Verlag 1999

Tischendorf F. Die Milz: In: Handbuch der mikroskopischen Anatomie des Menschen, Bd. VI/6, hrsg. von Bargmann W. Berlin, Heidelberg: Springer 1969

Skin

Breathnach AS. An atlas of the ultrastructure of human skin. London: Churchill 1971

Fitzpatrick TB, Eisen AZ, Wolff K, Freedberg IM, Austen KF. Dermatology in General Medicine, 2nd ed. New York: McGraw-Hill 1979

Halata Z. Die Sinnesorgane der Haut und der Tiefensensibilität. In: Handbuch der Zoologie, Bd. VIII Mammalia, Teilband 57. Herausgegeben von Niethammer J, Schliemann H, Starck D. Berlin, New York: Walter de Gruyter 1993

Horstmann E. Die Haut. In: Handbuch der mikroskopischen Anatomie des Menschen, Erg. zu Bd. III/1, hrsg. von Bargmann W. Berlin, Heidelberg: Springer 1957

Iggo A, Andres KH. Morphology of cutaneous receptors. Ann. Rev. Neurosci. 5: 1-31 (1982)

Kobori T, Montagna W. Biology and Disease of the Hair. Baltimore: University Park Press 1975

Odland GF. Structure of the skin. In: Goldsmith LA. Biochemistry and Physiology of the Skin. New York: Oxford University Press 1983 (pp. 3-63)

Plewig G, Landthaler M, Burgdorf WHC, Hertl M, Ruzicka T. Braun-Falco's Dermatologie, Venerologie und Allergologie. 6. Aufl. Berlin, Heidelberg: Springer 2012

Rassner G. Dermatologie. Lehrbuch und Atlas. 9. Aufl. München: Elsevier-Urban & Fischer 2009

Röcken M. Color Atlas of Dermatology. Stuttgart, New York: Thieme 2012

Index

Page numbers in *italics* refer to illustrations.
Where there is a span of page numbers, illustrations are included.

460 Index